The Research Process in Nursing

Fifth edition

Edited by

Kate Gerrish,
PhD, MSc, BNurs, RN, RM, NDN Cert
Professor of Nursing Practice Development,
University of Sheffield and Sheffield Teaching
Hospitals NHS Foundation Trust

Anne Lacey,
DPhil, MSc, BSc Hons, RGN, CertEd (FE)
Senior Research Fellow, University of Sheffield,
Director (Sheffield), Trent Research and
Development Support Unit

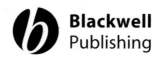

Blackwell Publishing

Editorial offices:
Blackwell Publishing Ltd, 9600 Garsington Road, Oxford OX4 2DQ, UK
   Tel: +44 (0)1865 776868
Blackwell Publishing Inc., 350 Main Street, Malden, MA 02148–5020, USA
   Tel: +1 781 388 8250
Blackwell Publishing Asia Pty Ltd, 550 Swanston Street, Carlton, Victoria 3053, Australia
   Tel: +61 (0)3 8359 1011

First published 2006 by Blackwell Publishing Ltd

ISBN-10: 1-4051-3013-X
ISBN-13: 978-1-4051-3013-4

Library of Congress Cataloging-in-Publication Data

The research process in nursing.– 5th ed. / edited by Kate Gerrish, Anne Lacey.
      p.   ;   cm.
   Includes bibliographical references and index.
   ISBN-13: 978-1-4051-3013-4 (pbk. : alk. paper)
   ISBN-10: 1-4051-3013-X (pbk. : alk. paper)
   1. Nursing–Research.   I. Gerrish, Kate, 1955– .   II. Lacey, Anne.
   [DNLM: 1. Nursing Research–methods.   2. Data Collection–methods.   3. Research Design.
WY 20.5 R4324 2006]
RT81.5.R465   2006
610.73072–dc22
            2005026464

A catalogue record for this title is available from the British Library

Set in 10 on 12.5pt Palatino
by SNP Best-set Typesetter Ltd., Hong Kong
Printed and bound in Great Britain
by TJ International Ltd, Padstow, Cornwall

The publisher's policy is to use permanent paper from mills that operate a sustainable forestry policy, and which has been manufactured from pulp processed using acid-free and elementary chlorine-free practices. Furthermore, the publisher ensures that the text paper and cover board used have met acceptable environmental accreditation standards.

For further information on Blackwell Publishing, visit our website:
www.blackwellnursing.com

Contents

Foreword

Nursing as an academic discipline has been transformed over the last few decades and this transformation has been challenging. Understanding the research process, undertaking rigorous research and implementing research findings in practice, are the fundamental building blocks of any discipline. However, 20 years ago, when the first edition of *The Research Process in Nursing* was published, research was seen as the domain of the elite few. It is now every nurses' business and the first edition of this book and the editions which followed it made a tangible contribution to this culture change. We still have a very long way to go before achieving the research capacity within the profession on the scale needed to ensure that all nursing practice is underpinned by a robust evidence base. However, developments that have taken place over the years now provide the necessary platform for sustaining nursing scholarship.

The education of students is now firmly integrated into the University sector and the proportion of nurses holding undergraduate and masters' degrees is steadily increasing. Significant numbers of nurses are now pursuing doctoral level studies and there is a growing cadre of post-doctoral nurses and established academics who are following research careers. However, the discipline will not achieve full maturity until every nurse, whatever their role, recognises the need to underpin practice with robust evidence.

This 5th edition of *The Research Process in Nursing* is timely and warmly welcomed. The new editors Kate Gerrish and Anne Lacey have brought together an outstanding group of chapter authors to produce a radically revised and contemporary resource for the profession. The content and style of the book embraces the many changes that are taking place in health care delivery with chapters on information technology, user involvement and research ethics and govermance. This excellent book offers something for everyone in education and practice. It provides a unique package of high quality material to support those undertaking research and contributing to the generation of new knowledge as well as those needing to utilise existing evidence in their professional roles.

This unique book is set fair to become another classic. It reflects the status of nursing as an established academic discipline and will provide an invaluable resource to the profession in its challenging pursuit of evidence-based nursing practice.

Professor Dame Jill Macleod Clark

Contributors

Teresa Allan MSc, BA Hons
Senior Lecturer in Health and Care Statistics, St Bartholomew School of Nursing and Midwifery, City University.

Claire Beecroft BA Hons, DPS MA
Information Officer, School of Health and Related Research (ScHARR), University of Sheffield.

Catherine Beverley MSc, BSc Hons, MCLIP
Knowledge Manager, Cumbria Social Services.

Senga Bond CBE, PhD, MSc, BA, RN
Head of the School of Population and Health Sciences, University of Newcastle upon Tyne.

Andrew Booth BA Hons, MSc, Dip Lib, MCLIP
Reader in Evidence Based Information Practice and Director of the Information Resources Section, School of Health and Related Research (ScHARR), University of Sheffield.

Steve Campbell BNurs, PhD, RGN, RSCN, RHV, NDN Cert, FRSH
Professor of Nursing Practice, School of Health, Community and Education Studies, Northumbria University and Head of Research and Development / Head of Nursing Research and Development, City Hospitals Sunderland NHS Foundation Trust.

Charlotte L Clarke PhD, MSc, PGCE, BA, RN
Professor of Nursing Practice Development Research and Associate Dean (Research) School of Health, Community and Education Studies, Northumbria University.

S José Closs BSc Hons, RGN, MPhil, PhD
Professor of Nursing Research, School of Healthcare, University of Leeds.

Jo Dumville PhD, MSc, BSc Hons
Research Fellow, Department of Health Sciences, University of York.

Mary Edmunds-Otter BA Hons
Information Librarian, Trent RDSU, Department of Health Sciences, University of Leicester.

Catherine Evans MSc, BSc Hons, RN, RHV, DN
Department of Health Research Fellow, Primary Care Nursing Research Unit, King's College London.

Jenny Freeman PhD, MSc, BSc
Lecturer in Medical Statistics, School of Health and Related Research (ScHARR), University of Sheffield.

Kate Gerrish PhD, MSc, BNurs, RN, RM, NDN Cert
Professor of Nursing Practice Development, School of Nursing and Midwifery, University of Sheffield and Sheffield Teaching Hospitals NHS Foundation Trust.

Claire Goodman PhD, MSc, BSc, RN, DN
Professor of Health Care Research, Centre for Research in Primary and Community Care, University of Hertfordshire.

Gordon Grant BSc Hons, MSc, PhD
Professor of Cognitive Disability, School of Nursing and Midwifery, University of Sheffield and Doncaster and South Humber Healthcare NHS Trust.

Helen Hancock PhD, BN, RN, Dip App Sci, Dip Crit Care, ENBcc 249
Research Fellow, Northumbria University, School of Health, Community and Education Studies and City Hospitals Sunderland NHS Foundation Trust.

Felicity Hasson Pg Dip, MSc, BA Hons
Research Fellow, Institute of Nursing Research, School of Nursing, University of Ulster.

Gill Hek MA, RGN, NDN Cert Ed FE
Reader in Nursing Research, Faculty of Health and Social Care, University of the West of England.

Immy Holloway PhD, MA, BEd
Visiting Professor, Lead, Centre for Qualitative Research Institute of Health and Community Studies, Bournemouth University.

Amanda Hunn MA Econ, BSc Hons, Cert CRGCP
OREC Manager for Yorkshire and the Humber on behalf of the Central Office for Research Ethics Committees (COREC).

Mark Johnson PhD, BSc, PG Cert HE
Professor of Pain and Analgesia, Faculty of Health, Leeds Metropolitan University.

Martin Johnson RN, MSc, PhD
Professor in Nursing and Director of the University of Salford Centre for Nursing, Midwifery and Collaborative Research.

Sinead Keeney BA Hons, MRes
Research Fellow, Institute of Nursing Research, School of Nursing, University of Ulster.

Anne Lacey DPhil, MSc, BSc Hons, RGN, CertEd (FE)
Senior Research Fellow, School of Health and Related Research (ScHARR), University of Sheffield and Director of the Sheffield site of Trent Research and Development Support Unit (RDSU).

Judith Lathlean DPhil, MA, BSc Econ
Director of Research and Professor of Health Research, School of Nursing and Midwifery, University of Southampton.

Hilary Lloyd MSc, BA Hons, RN, Cert Ed
Principal Lecturer in Nursing Practice Development and Research, School of Health, Community and Education Studies, Northumbria University and Deputy Head of Nursing Research and Development, City Hospitals Sunderland, NHS Foundation Trust.

Tony Long PhD, MA, BSc (Hons), SRN, RSCN, RNT
Senior Lecturer in Child Health, University of Salford Centre for Nursing Midwifery and Collaborative Research, and Associate Head of School for Research in the School of Nursing.

Hugh P McKenna PhD, RMN, RGN, DipN (Lond), BSc Hons, Adv Dip Ed, RNT, FFNRCSI, FEANS, FRCN
Professor and Dean of the Faculty of Life and Health Sciences, University of Ulster.

Ann McMahon MSc, BSc, RMN, RGN
Research and Development Adviser, Royal College of Nursing.

Julienne Meyer PhD, MSc, BSc, Cert Ed FE, RN, RNT
Professor of Nursing, St Bartholomew School of Nursing and Midwifery, City University.

Tricia Murphy-Black PhD, MSc, RM, RN
formerly, Professor of Midwifery, Department of Nursing and Midwifery, University of Stirling.

Andrea Nelson PhD, BSc Hons, RGN
Reader, School of Healthcare, University of Leeds.

Susan Procter PhD, BSc Hons, RGN, Cert Ed
Professor of Primary Health Care Research, Public Health and Primary Care Unit, St Bartholomew School of Nursing and Midwifery, City University.

Paul Ramcharan BA Hons, PhD
Reader in Cognitive Disability, School of Nursing and Midwifery, University of Sheffield.

Jan Reed BA, RN, PhD
Professor of Health Care of Older People, School of Health, Community and Education Studies, Northumbria University.

Angie Rees BA Hons, DPS, MA
Information Officer, School of Health and Related Research (ScHARR), University
of Sheffield.

Colin Robson PhD, BSc Hons, BSc Hons, PGCE
Emeritus Professor, School of Human and Health Sciences, University of
Huddersfield.

Angela Mary Tod MSc, MMedSci, BA Hons, RGN
Lecturer and Research Fellow, School of Nursing and Midwifery, University of
Sheffield and Sheffield Teaching Hospitals NHS Foundation Trust.

Les Todres PhD, MSoc Sc Clin Psych, BSoc Sc Hons, C Psychol
Professor of Qualitative Research and Psychotherapy, Institute of Health and
Community Studies, Bournemouth University.

Annie Topping PhD, PGCE, BSc, RGN
Head of Nursing, School of Health Studies, University of Bradford.

David Torgerson PhD, MSc
Director of the York Trials Unit, University of York.

Stephen Walters PhD, MSc, BSc, PGCE, CSTAT
Senior Lecturer in Medical Statistics, School of Health and Related Research
(ScHARR), University of Sheffield.

Hazel Watson PhD, MN, RGN, RMN, RNT
Professor of Nursing, School of Nursing, Midwifery and Community Health,
Glasgow Caledonian University.

Rosemary Whyte PhD, BA Hons, RGN, RCNT, RNT
Research Fellow, School of Nursing, Midwifery and Community Health, Glasgow
Caledonian University.

Acknowledgement

The editors wish to thank the chapter authors of this book for their valuable contributions, and their willingness to accept our editorial guidance. Thanks are also due to Sandra Szasz and Michaela Barton for their clerical assistance in producing the manuscript.

Introduction to the 5th edition

The Research Process in Nursing has had a long and honourable life as a standard and well-used research text, going through four editions and many reprints between 1984 and 2000. It has been widely used in pre- and post-registration professional courses, as well as in academic undergraduate and postgraduate level study throughout the UK.

Since 1984, however, research in nursing, as in health care in general, has grown enormously in volume, maturity, and applicability, and successive editions of *The Research Process in Nursing* have been updated to reflect this. An ever-increasing range of research methods, the increasing use of information technology in research, the growth of the evidence-based practice movement, and significant changes in health care organisation have meant that the pace of change has begun to outstrip the revision process. With the retirement of Desmond FS Cormack as Editor, the time seemed right to relaunch the book with new editors, and a completely revised format.

The 5th edition of *The Research Process in Nursing* is almost completely rewritten by new authors. We, the new editors, have been privileged to be able to commission chapter authorship from leaders of nursing research and other disciplines across the countries of the UK. We have also taken the opportunity to restructure the book, take a fresh look at old issues, and tackle some topics not previously included. We are indebted to our team of authors for their wide-ranging and authoritative contributions to the research methodology literature. We have continued to target the book at novice researchers, be they pre-registration students or those embarking on a postgraduate research degree, but the book should also be of value to many who are further on in their research careers. We have encouraged authors to write in an accessible style, but not to shrink away from complex debates and technical issues. We recognise that the academic level required of nurses undertaking their first research course has risen since 1984, and the style of writing in this new edition reflects this.

The book has been re-structured into six sections.

Section 1, *Setting the Scene*, deals with the background issues of nursing research policy, the nature of the research process, ethics and funding. A new chapter is included in this section about involving users in the research process. Readers new to the context in which nursing research is taking place will find themselves orientated to the subject and, we hope, enthused to engage with an activity that has the potential to change and improve the provision of health care.

Section 2, *Preparing the Ground*, includes chapters that take the reader through the essential steps that are necessary before a research project can begin. Some of

the most significant changes in recent years have been in the regulatory frameworks governing research in the UK, and these are highlighted in this section.
Major changes have also taken place in the explosive growth of health-related literature and other research evidence, and this section contains newly written
material from information specialists drawing on recent advances in electronic
resources.

Section 3, *Choosing the Right Approach*, is the longest section and in many ways
the heart of the book. After an introduction to the philosophical debates underlying the different research approaches available to nurses, and a chapter on sampling, nine common research approaches used in nursing research are each
explored in detail. It is perhaps a commentary on the way that nursing research
has developed that six of these nine chapters concern approaches that are essentially qualitative. In the first edition of this text in 1984, the balance was rather
different.

Section 4, *Collecting Data*, and Section 5, *Making Sense of Data*, are both practical
sections dealing with the skills required in data collection and analysis. Here the
emphasis is upon research tools, such as interviewing and statistical analysis,
common to many different research approaches. There is much that cannot be
included here, of course, but we have selected those methods most common in
nursing research and taken a generic approach to analysis.

Section 6, *Putting Research into Practice* concludes the book by taking the reader
through the process of disseminating research findings, and getting them implemented into policy and practice. As well as addressing active researchers, these
chapters will be of use to nurses who, though not wanting to engage themselves
in research, want to incorporate it into their professional lives through evidence-
based practice. The book ends with a glance into the future, and some salutary
reminders that the nursing profession must move forward if it is not to go backwards in becoming a research-based profession.

Although the book is designed in a logical fashion, as outlined above, each
chapter is also intended to be complete in itself. Many readers will dip in and
out of different sections as necessary. For this reason, we have included cross-
references wherever possible to other chapters that might be helpful, and have
provided key point summaries at the beginning of each chapter. We have also
compiled a glossary of research terms, to help the reader with new language with
which they may be unfamiliar.

Throughout the book we have adopted certain generic terms, to assist readability and reduce repetition. Foremost among these is the term 'nursing'. By this
we mean to include all the professions of nursing, midwifery, health visiting and
related specialisms. We hope that members of these professions will forgive our
shorthand, but we have tried to ensure that examples given are taken from a wide
range of health care settings. We have also used the terms 'evidence' and 'evidence-based practice' to denote the plethora of resources and implementation
activities that have become so important in health care today.

This book is intended to be used primarily by nurses, midwives and health
visitors, but it has much wider application to any health and social care practitio-

ner who wishes to learn about research. Members of the allied health professions, particularly, face many of the same debates and dilemmas as nurses in developing research capacity. The contributors to the book are not all nurses, but include statisticians, social scientists, information specialists and psychologists. We trust that as such this new edition of a well-established book will make a valuable contribution to research capacity building in nursing and health care.

Kate Gerrish and Anne Lacey
Editors to the 5th edition,
2006

Section 1
Setting the Scene

Nursing research does not exist in a vacuum, but is an applied discipline set in the context of a dynamic health care system. This section begins in Chapter 1 by considering the nature and purpose of research in nursing, and how it relates to other activities such as audit and service development. The crucial importance of implementation of research findings in evidence-based practice is highlighted, and will be picked up again later in the book in Section 6.

For the novice researcher, Section 1 then leads on to four introductory chapters, taking a broad brush approach to topics that underpin much of the rest of the book. Chapter 2 takes the reader through the essential steps in the research process, each of which will be dealt with in much more depth in later sections, but with the aim of giving an overview of the entire undertaking that is research.

Research in nursing, as in health care generally, is complicated by the fact that it is involved with vulnerable human beings, and ethical principles need to be observed from the outset of any research project. Chapter 3 therefore tackles this moral obligation on the researcher, drawing out the practical implications for researchers and setting the context for more specific ethical regulations dealt with in Section 2.

Nursing researchers cannot operate satisfactorily without personal, practical and financial support, and Chapter 4 reviews the sources from which such support may be obtained. This chapter links to discussions about nursing research policy for capacity building that begun in Chapter 1, and will be explored more fully in Section 6.

The final chapter in Section 1 is completely new to this edition of the book, focusing on user involvement in research. Government policy has raised the profile of this subject, and it is one in which nursing research is well placed to take a lead. The chapter challenges the reader to consider more than token involvement of users in the whole research process, in a range of models including participatory and emancipatory approaches.

1 Research and Development in Nursing

Kate Gerrish and Ann McMahon

Key points

- Research is concerned with generating new knowledge through a process of systematic scientific enquiry, the research process.
- Research in nursing can provide new insights into nursing practice, develop and improve methods of caring and test the effectiveness of care.
- Whereas comparatively few nurses may undertake research, all nurses should develop research awareness and utilise research findings in their practice.
- Evidence-based practice involves the integration of the best available research evidence with expert clinical opinion while taking into account of the preferences of patients.
- Current nursing research policy is concerned with increasing research capacity, developing career pathways in research for nurses, creating effective partnerships through research collaboration and exerting greater influence on the research and development (R&D) agenda.

Introduction

Significant changes in health care have taken place in the 22 years since the first edition of this book was published, and these changes are set to continue. Technological developments have led to improved health outcomes and at the same time have raised public expectations of health care services. Increased life expectancy and lower birth rates mean that the United Kingdom (UK) population is ageing. An older population is more likely to experience complex health needs, especially in regard to chronic disease, and this places additional demands on an already pressurised health service. At the same time the escalating cost of health care is leading to a shift from expensive resource-intensive hospital care to more services being provided in the primary and community care sectors. In response to these changes, government health policy is increasingly focused on improving the clinical and cost effectiveness of health care while at the same time reducing the burden of ill-health through active public health and health promotion strategies.

It is essential that nurses respond proactively to these developments in order to provide high-quality care in response to the needs of the individuals and communities with whom they work. To do this, they need up-to-date knowledge to inform their practice. Such knowledge is generated through research.

This chapter introduces the concept of nursing research and considers how research contributes to the development of nursing knowledge. In recognising that nursing is a practice-based profession the relevance of research to nursing policy and practice is examined within the context of evidence-based practice and the responsibilities of nurses in respect of research awareness, research utilisation and research activity. However, nursing research does not occur in a vacuum and a review of nursing policy and research policy in the UK provides the context for an analysis of the current position of nursing research.

The nature of nursing research and development

The definition of research provided by Hockey (1984) in the first edition of this book is still pertinent today:

> ' . . . an attempt to increase the sum of what is known, usually referred to as a 'body of knowledge' by the discovery of new facts or relationships through a process of systematic scientific enquiry, the research process' (Hockey 1984:4)

Other definitions of research emphasise the importance of the knowledge generated through research being applicable beyond the research setting in which it was undertaken, i.e. that it can be generalised to other similar populations or settings. The Department of Health, for example, defines research as:

> 'the attempt to derive generalisable new knowledge by addressing clearly-defined questions with systematic and rigorous methods' (Department of Health 2001: 4, section 1.7)

Research is designed to investigate explicit questions. In the case of nursing research these questions relate to those aspects of professional activity that are predominantly and appropriately the concern and responsibility of nurses (Hockey 1996). This may include nursing education, the management of nursing services and all aspects of nursing practice. Most nursing research investigates contemporary issues; however, some studies may take an historical perspective in order to examine the development of nursing by studying documentary sources and other artefacts.

The questions that nursing research may address vary in terms of their focus. Over 20 years ago, Crow (1982) identified four approaches that research could take; these remain pertinent today:

- research that will provide new insights into nursing practice
- research that will deepen an understanding of the concepts central to nursing care

- research that is concerned with the development of new and improved methods of caring
- research that is designed to test the effectiveness of care

Nursing research does not necessarily need to be undertaken by nurses. Indeed, sociologists have undertaken some seminal studies into nursing practice and nurse education. For example, in the 1970s Robert Dingwall, a sociologist, undertook an influential study of health visitor training (Dingwall 1977). Likewise, nurses who engage in research may not confine their area of enquiry to nursing research. The growing emphasis on multidisciplinary, multi-agency working means that nurse researchers may choose to examine questions that extend beyond the scope of nursing into other areas of health and social care.

Whereas the generation of new knowledge is valuable in its own right, the application and utilisation of knowledge gained through research is essential to a practice-based profession such as nursing. This latter activity is known as 'development'. Thus research and development, 'R&D', go hand in hand.

Research and development can be divided into three types of activity.

Basic research is original, experimental or theoretical work, primarily for the purpose of obtaining new knowledge rather than focusing on the specific use of the findings. For example, biomedical laboratory-based research falls within this category.

Applied research is also original investigation with a view to obtaining new knowledge, but it is undertaken primarily for practical purposes. Much nursing research falls within this category and is undertaken with the intention of generating knowledge which can be used to inform nursing practice and can involve both clinical and non-clinical methods.

Development activity involves the systematic use of knowledge obtained through research and/or practical experience for the purpose of producing new or improved products, processes, systems or services.

Development activity that focuses on the utilisation of knowledge generated through research can take different forms. The most common activities include clinical audit and practice development (Box 1.1). Like research, these activities often employ systematic methods to address questions arising from practice. Research, however, is undertaken with the explicit purpose of generating new knowledge, which has applicability beyond the immediate setting. By contrast, clinical audit and practice development are primarily concerned with generating information that can inform local decision-making. Yet the boundaries between action research (*see* Chapter 18) and practice development are often blurred (Gerrish & Mawson 2005).

Developing nursing knowledge

Nursing research is concerned with developing new knowledge about the discipline and practice of nursing. Nursing knowledge, like any other knowledge, is

Box 1.1   Definitions of research, clinical audit and practice development.

Research involves the attempt to extend the available knowledge by means of a systematically and scientifically defensible process of inquiry. (Clamp *et al.* 2004)

Clinical audit is a professional-led initiative which seeks to improve the quality and outcome of patient care through practitioners examining their practices and results and modifying practice where indicated. (NHSE 1996:16)

Practice development encompasses a broad range of innovations that are initiated to improve practice and the services in which that practice takes place. It involves a continuous process of improvement towards increased effectiveness in patient-centred care. This is brought about by helping health care teams to develop their knowledge and skills and to transform the culture and context of care (Garbett & McCormack 2002).

never absolute. As the external world changes, nursing develops and adapts in response. In parallel, nursing knowledge develops and changes. This year's 'best available evidence' has the potential of being superseded by new insights and discoveries. Therefore nursing knowledge is temporal and will always be partial and hence imperfect. This does not mean, however, that nurses should not continually strive to develop new knowledge to inform nursing and health care policy and practice.

Whereas the focus of this book is on the generation of knowledge through research, it is important to recognise that nursing knowledge may take different forms. In addition to empirical knowledge derived through research, nurses utilise other forms of knowledge, such as practical knowledge derived from experience and aesthetic or intuitive knowledge derived from nursing practice (Thompson 2000). It is beyond the scope of this book to examine in detail the various forms of nursing knowledge; however, Chapter 31 introduces the reader to some of these within the context of promoting evidence-based practice.

The definitions of research given earlier in this chapter emphasise the role of systematic scientific enquiry – the research process – in generating new knowledge. The research process comprises a series of logical steps, which have to be undertaken to develop knowledge. Different disciplines may interpret the research process in different ways, depending on the specific paradigms (ways of interpreting the world) and theories that underpin the discipline. A biological scientist's approach to generating new knowledge will be different from that of a sociologist. However, the basic principles of the systematic research process will be followed by all disciplines. Nursing, as a discipline in its own right, is relatively young in comparison to more established professional groups such as medicine and is in the process of generating theories that are unique to describing, explaining or predicting the outcomes of nursing actions. Nursing theories are generated through the process of undertaking research and may also be tested and refined through further research.

However, nursing also draws upon a unique mix of several disciplines, such as physiology, psychology and sociology, and any of these disciplines may be appropriate for research in nursing. For example, the management of pain can be studied from a psychological or physiological perspective; whichever approach is chosen will be influenced by the theories relevant to the particular discipline.

The research process in nursing is no different from other disciplines and the same rules of scientific method apply. Chapter 2 sets out a systematic approach to research – the scientific method in action – and subsequent chapters consider the various components of the research process in detail. At this stage, it is worth noting that in some texts, the 'scientific method' is taken to reflect a particular view of the world which values the notion that we can be totally objective in our research endeavours. Here, the term is not restricted in this way and we use the term 'scientific method' to mean a rigorous approach to a systematic form of enquiry. Chapter 11 introduces the reader to the different ways in which the scientific method can be interpreted depending on the assumptions that the researcher holds about the nature of the social world and reality.

Research awareness, utilisation and activity

Over 30 years ago, the report of the Committee on Nursing (Committee on Nursing 1972) stressed the need for nursing to become research-based to the extent that research should become part of the mental equipment of every practising nurse. Although considerable progress has been made in the intervening period, this objective still remains a challenge. In order for nursing to establish its research base, nurses need to develop an awareness of research in relation to practice, they need to be able to utilise research findings and some nurses need to undertake research activity.

Research awareness implies recognition of the importance of research to the profession and to patient care. It requires nurses to develop a critical and questioning approach to their work and in so doing identify problems or questions that can be answered through research. Nurses who are research-aware will demonstrate the ability to find out about the latest research in their area together with an openness to change their practice when new knowledge becomes available. Research awareness also implies a willingness to share the task of keeping abreast of new developments by disseminating information to others and supporting and co-operating with researchers in an informed way. Arguably, all nurses should develop research awareness as part of pre-registration nurse education programmes.

Research utilisation is concerned with incorporating research findings into practice so that care is based on research evidence. Not all research, even that which is published in reputable journals, is necessarily of high quality. Before findings can be applied a research study needs to be evaluated critically in order to judge the quality of the research. All nurses should be able to appraise a research report although specialist advice may need to be sought in regard to judging the appropriateness of complex research designs or unusual statistical tests. Chapter 8 provides guidance on how to appraise research reports.

Research studies do not always provide conclusive findings that can be used to guide practice. Different studies examining the same phenomenon may produce contradictory results. Wherever possible a systematic review of a number of studies examining a particular phenomenon should be undertaken in order to provide more robust guidance for practice than the findings of a single study would allow. Chapter 21 outlines the procedures for undertaking a systematic review. It is a time-consuming process and requires a good understanding of research designs and methods together with knowledge of techniques for analysis, including statistical tests. Whereas some nurses may develop the skills to undertake a systematic review as part of a postgraduate course, many systematic reviews are undertaken by people who are experts in the technique. For example, the Centre for Reviews and Dissemination at the University of York has been set up specifically for the purpose of undertaking systematic reviews on a range of health-related topics.

The findings from a systematic review then need to be incorporated into clinical guidelines or care protocols, which can be applied to practice. Whereas some guidelines may be developed at a national level, nurses may need to adapt national guidelines for application at a local level or develop their own guidelines where no national ones are available (*see* Chapters 31 and 32 for more information).

All nurses should be research-aware and utilise research findings in their practice; however, not all nurses need to undertake research. To carry out serious research, nurses need to be equipped with appropriate knowledge and skills. Pre-registration and undergraduate post-registration nursing programmes tend to focus on developing research awareness and research utilisation. It is generally not until nurses embark on a master's programme, or a specialist research course, that they will learn how to undertake a small-scale research study, under the supervision of a more experienced researcher. This represents the first step in acquiring the skills to become a competent researcher. Comparatively few nurses progress to develop a career in nursing research in which they undertake large-scale studies funded by external agencies. It generally requires study at doctoral level followed by an apprenticeship, working within a research team with supervision and support from experienced researchers, before being able to lead a large-scale study.

Although relatively few nurses progress to lead large research studies, many more nurses participate in research led by nurse researchers, doctors and other health professionals. Nurses working in clinical practice may be asked to undertake data collection for other researchers and their clinical nursing experience can be valuable to the research enterprise. Even if they are not leading a study, nurses who assist other researchers should have a sound understanding of the research process in order to collect valid and reliable data and to adhere to the research governance and ethical requirements outlined in Chapter 10.

Research and nursing practice

Current policy initiatives seek to promote a culture of evidence-based practice. There are generally considered to be three components to evidence-based practice, namely the best available evidence derived from research, clinical expertise and patient preferences (Sackett *et al.* 1996). In recognising that knowledge derived from research is never absolute, nurses should draw upon their own expertise and that of other more experienced nurses when deciding on an appropriate intervention. Equally, clinical expertise should not be seen as a substitute for research evidence but rather as contributing to the decision about the most appropriate intervention for a particular patient. The third component of evidence-based practice involves taking account of patient perspectives. Nurses have a responsibility to share their knowledge of the best available evidence with patients in order to assist them make informed choices about the care they receive. This is particularly important where there are alternative courses of action that can be selected. These issues are examined in more detail in Chapters 31 and 32.

Nursing's progress towards becoming evidence-based needs to be viewed within the context of wider influences on health care. The UK (England, Northern Ireland, Scotland and Wales) governments are each seeking to modernise the National Health Service through major policy reforms. Central among these initiatives has been the introduction of the concept of clinical governance, a process whereby health care organisations are accountable for continually improving the quality of their services and safeguarding high standards of care by creating an environment that promotes excellence (Currie *et al.* 2003). It is, however, difficult to achieve the aspiration of 'excellence' in health care because of financial constraints and pressure on resources (Maynard 1999). Nevertheless, the objective of seeking to develop the quality of health care together with recognition of the importance of health care organisations and the individuals who work in them being accountable for the quality of services is laudable.

In order to enhance the quality of nursing care it is important to ensure that care is clinically effective. Often referred to as 'doing the right thing right', clinical effectiveness involves providing the most appropriate intervention in the correct manner at the most expedient time in order to achieve the best outcomes for the patient. Nurses need to draw upon knowledge generated through research in order to decide which intervention is most appropriate and how and when to deliver it. Research may also highlight reasons for non-compliance. A particular dressing may have been shown through research to be effective in promoting wound healing but if it is unacceptable to the patient, problems with compliance may arise.

As mentioned earlier, the findings from a single study may not provide sufficient evidence to direct practice and wherever possible nurses should rely on knowledge generated through systematic reviews of research evidence drawn from several research studies. There are a number of national initiatives to assist nurses and other health professionals to provide clinically effective care. These include the development of clinical guidelines based on the best research evidence by, for example, the National Institute for Health and Clinical Excellence (NICE) and the Scottish Intercollegiate Guideline Network (SIGN).

Increasing demands on the finite resources within the NHS have resulted in the need to ensure that health care interventions are not only clinically effective but also cost effective. There is little point pursuing a costly intervention if a cheaper one is seen to be equally as effective. The field of health economics is concerned with examining the financial and wider resource implications of providing a specific intervention or service. Economic evaluations can be undertaken to evaluate different treatments or alternative ways of providing services from an economic perspective and providing information that can be used to inform judgements about the clinical and cost effectiveness of a particular intervention or service (Chambers & Boath 2001). NICE and SIGN guidelines take account of both clinical and cost effectiveness when making recommendations for best practice.

UK health and social care research policy

The development of nursing research is heavily influenced within each of the four countries of the UK by national health and social policy and R&D policy in particular. There is a common policy concern to promote the generation and utilisation of research evidence in order to contribute towards securing the health of the population and improve the quality and cost-effectiveness of health care services. Box 1.2 details the departments that manage NHS R&D across the UK.

Shaped by their specific health and social care priorities, each of the R&D Offices are responsible to their respective government health departments for the development of R&D policy and priorities, and for the commissioning of research to inform policy and practice.

Box 1.2   UK government health department and R&D offices.

UK country	Government health department	Government health department responsible for R&D
England	Department of Health (DH)	Research and Development (R&D)
Northern Ireland	Department of Health, Personal Social Services and Public Safety (DHPSSPS)	Health and Personal Social Services Research and Development (HPSS R&D)
Scotland	Scottish Executive Health Department (SEHD)	Chief Scientist Office (CSO)
Wales	Welsh Assembly Government	Wales Office of Research and Development for Health and Social Care (WORD)

There are a number of strategic initiatives that are addressed to different degrees within each of the four countries. These include:

- infrastructure – research support units and networks, resources to meet NHS costs of externally-funded non-commercial research, research governance arrangements
- identifying research priority areas
- commissioning and managing research to inform policy development and health services
- research capacity building initiatives including research training support schemes – from bursaries through to fellowships
- core-funded units to undertake research
- promotion of evidence-based practice

In addition to each country having its own strategic arrangements for managing R&D policy, the UK Clinical Research Collaboration (UKCRC) was established in 2004 with the intention to create a clinical research environment of international standing. The collaboration brings together the major stakeholders that influence clinical research in the UK and particularly in the NHS. Membership includes representation from the main funding bodies, academic medicine, the NHS, regulatory bodies and representatives from industry and patients. The five work streams the UKCRC is currently pursuing are listed in Box 1.3. The UKCRC is focusing its endeavours where is sees it can bring added value through collaboration. However, at the time of writing, nursing does not have a voice within the UKCRC so it is not clear whether nursing research will benefit from this initiative.

Box 1.3   UK Clinical Research Collaboration (UKCRC) work streams.

- building up the infrastructure in the NHS
- building up incentives for research in the NHS
- building up the research workforce
- streamlining the regulatory and governance processes
- co-ordinating clinical research funding

UK nursing research policy

Just as each country in the UK has developed its own priorities and strategic direction for R&D, nursing has also examined R&D policy within each of these contexts. Box 1.4 summarises the policy drivers and the current nursing R&D policy and strategy across the UK.

The strategy for nursing in England identified the need to develop a strategy to influence the research and development agenda, to strengthen the capacity to undertake nursing research, and to use research to support nursing practice (Department of Health 1999). Strictly speaking this statement of intent has never

Box 1.4 Policy drivers and the current UK R&D nursing policy.

UK country	Nursing policy context	Nursing R&D policy
England	Department of Health (1999) *Making a Difference: strengthening the nursing, midwifery and health visiting contribution to health and healthcare*. London, Department of Health 1996 and 2001 Higher Education Funding Council's Research Assessment Exercise (RAE)	Department of Health (2000) *Towards a Strategy for Nursing Research And Development. Proposals for action*. London, Department of Health. Higher Education Funding Council for England (2001) *Promoting Research in Nursing and the Allied Health Professions*. Research report 01/64
Northern Ireland	McKenna H & Mason C (1998) *Using and Doing Research: a position paper to inform strategy, policy and practice for nursing research in Northern Ireland*. Belfast, DHSS	McCance T, Fitzsimons D (2005) *Using and Doing Research: guiding the future*. Belfast, Northern Ireland Practice and Education Council for Nursing and Midwifery
Scotland	Scottish Executive (2001) *Caring for Scotland: the strategy for nursing and midwifery in Scotland*. Edinburgh, NHS Scotland 2001 Higher Education Funding Council's Research Assessment Exercise (RAE)	Scottish Executive Health Department (2002) *Choices and Challenges: the strategy for research and development in nursing and midwifery in Scotland*. Edinburgh, SEHD
Wales	National Assembly for Wales (1999) *Realising the Potential: a strategic framework for nursing, midwifery and health visiting in Wales into the 21st century*. Cardiff. National Assembly for Wales	Welsh Assembly Government (2004) *Realising the potential. Briefing Paper 6: achieving the potential through research and development*, Cardiff, Welsh Assembly Government.

been realised although 12 months after publication, recommendations detailing what a nursing R&D strategy needed to contain were published (Department of Health 2000) and these recommendations are under review at the time of writing this chapter. In addition, concern over the position of the discipline of nursing in the 1996 quadrennial assessment of research activity (Research Assessment Exercise, RAE) in UK universities led the Higher Education Funding Council for England and the Department of Health to commission research to examine why this might be so and to recommend how this could be addressed (Higher Education Funding Council for England 2001).

In Northern Ireland, a study commissioned in 1998 (McKenna & Mason 1998) examined:

- how the nursing professions could influence the overall R&D agenda
- how the nursing professions could contribute to the wider R&D programme
- priorities for research within the nursing professions

- the R&D needs of the nursing professions
- how access, dissemination and uptake of research might be improved.

This report provided a baseline assessment and the current state of play has recently been evaluated and new priorities to further the R&D agenda within nursing in Northern Ireland identified (McCance & Fitzsimons 2005).

The 2001 strategy for nursing in Scotland sought to develop the highest possible standards in education, research, innovation, accountability and professional practice (Scottish Executive 2001). The strategy acknowledged achievements to date and recognised that a future strategy for nursing research was a prerequisite to achieving the objective of creating research-aware, research-literate and research-active nurses. Further fuelled by the poor performance of nursing departments in Scottish universities in the RAE and following extensive consultation, a strategy for nursing research entitled *Choices and Challenges*, (Scottish Executive Health Department 2002) was launched in December 2002.

The 1999 Welsh strategy for nursing clearly articulated the need for the nursing professions to continue to develop a

'sound research base . . . to demonstrate conclusively the effectiveness of nursing intervention in improving health' (National Assembly for Wales 1999: section 97).

The strategy called for the development of more integrated career pathways to enable clinically-based nurses to be more research active and academically-based nurses to be more clinically engaged. A strategic framework for improving the quality and quantity of R&D carried out by the nursing professions in Wales was published five years later (Welsh Assembly Government 2004) and is currently being implemented.

Nursing research policy imperatives

There are many similarities in the research policy priorities for nursing across the UK. The necessity to develop research capacity within the nursing professions is universally recognised as a key priority. It is also acknowledged that those who develop their research capacity must be afforded the opportunity to do so within the context of a clearly-defined career pathway.

Across the board it is recognised that although the UK funding base for bio-medical research may be relatively healthy, the balance is clearly tipping in favour of basic research in areas such as genetics and immunology as opposed to clinical research, which includes nursing (Policy Research in Science and Medicine (PRISM) 1998). Nursing is therefore not only starting from a relatively low baseline (Higher Education Funding Council for England 2001) but is competing against more established disciplines such as clinical medicine for a diminishing resource. It is therefore recognised that within this context it is imperative that nursing research must become much more strategic and focused, that nursing must have a greater professional influence in R&D and nursing must develop effective partnerships to build the evidence base to inform policy and practice. Each of these policy priorities will be discussed in greater detail in Chapter 33.

Conclusion

Research is necessary to develop the knowledge base to inform nursing policy and practice. Whereas only a minority of nurses will develop a career in nursing research, all nurses should become research-aware. This means developing a critical and questioning approach in order to identify areas where practice could be improved on the basis of research findings or areas where research evidence is lacking and new knowledge needs to be generated through research. Nurses also need to utilise research findings in their day-to-day practice. However, in order to provide evidence-based care nurses should be able to evaluate the quality of published research reports. This requires a sound understanding of the research process, together with knowledge of different research designs and the methods that can be used to collect and analyse data. The following chapters of this book examine the research process, designs and methods in detail in order to equip nurses with the knowledge-base to critically appraise research reports and to engage in the process of undertaking research under the supervision of a more experienced researcher.

References

Chambers R, Boath E (2001) *Clinical Effectiveness and Clinical Governance Made Easy*, 2nd edition. Abingdon, Radcliffe Medical Press

Clamp C, Gough S, Land L (2004) *Resources for Nursing Research: an annotated bibliography*, 4th edition. London, Sage

Committee on Nursing (1972) *Report of the Committee on Nursing*. London, HMSO

Crow R (1982) How nursing and the community can benefit from nursing research. *International Journal of Nursing Studies* 19:1 37–45

Currie L, Morrell CJ, Scrivener R (2003) *Clinical Governance: a RCN resource guide*. London, Royal College of Nursing

Department of Health (1999) *Making a Difference: strengthening the nursing, midwifery and health visiting contribution to health and health care*. London, Department of Health

Department of Health (2000) *Towards a Strategy for Nursing Research and Development: proposals for action*. London, Department of Health

Department of Health (2001) *Research Governance Framework for Health and Social Care*. London, Department of Health

Dingwall R (1977) *The Social Organisation of Health Visitor Training*. London, Croom Helm

Garbett R, McCormack B (2002) A concept analysis of practice development. *NT Research* 7:2 87–100

Gerrish K, Mawson S (2005) Research, audit, practice development and service evaluation: implications for research and clinical governance. *Practice Development in Health Care* 4:1 33–39

Higher Education Funding Council for England (2001) *Promoting Research in Nursing and the Allied Health Professions:* research report 01/64. Higher Education Funding Council for England *www.hefce.ac.uk/Pubs/hefce/2001/01_64.htm*

Hockey L (1984) The nature and purpose of research. In Cormack DFS (ed) *The Research Process in Nursing*, 1st edition. London, Blackwell Science pp1–10

Hockey L (1996) The nature and purpose of research. In Cormack DFS (ed) *The Research Process in Nursing*, 3rd edition. London, Blackwell Science pp3–13

Maynard A (1999) Clinical governance: the unavoidable economic challenges. *NT Research* 4: 188–191

McCance T, Fitzsimons D (2005) *Using and Doing Research: guiding the future.* Belfast, Northern Ireland Practice and Education Council for Nursing and Midwifery

McKenna H, Mason C (1998) *Using and Doing Research: a position paper to inform strategy, policy and practice for nursing research in Northern Ireland.* Belfast, DHSS

National Assembly for Wales (1999) *Realising the Potential: a strategic framework for nursing, midwifery and health visiting in Wales into the 21st century.* Cardiff, National Assembly for Wales

National Health Service Executive (1996) *Promoting Clinical Effectiveness: a framework for action.* London, NHSE

Policy Research in Science and Medicine (PRISM) (1998) *Mapping the Landscape: national biomedical research outputs 1988–1995.* London, The Wellcome Trust

Sackett DL, Rosenberg WM, Muir Gray JA, Haynes RB, Richardson WS (1996) Evidence-Based Medicine: what it is and what it isn't. *British Medical Journal* 312: 71–72

Scottish Executive Health Department (2001) *Caring for Scotland: the strategy for nursing and midwifery in Scotland.* Edinburgh, NHS Scotland

Scottish Executive Health Department (2002) *Choices and Challenges: the strategy for research and development in nursing and midwifery in Scotland.* Edinburgh, Scottish Executive Health Department

Thompson DR (2000) An exploration of knowledge development in nursing: a personal perspective. *NT Research* 5:5 391–394

Welsh Assembly Government (2004) *Realising the Potential. Briefing Paper 6: achieving the potential through research and development.* Cardiff, Welsh Assembly Government

Websites

www.man.ac.uk/rcn/ – RCN Research and Development Co-ordinating Centre website provides links to current internet addresses to find out more about the health and nursing R&D strategies within each country, together with information on capacity building opportunities

ukcrc.org/ – UK Clinical Research Collaboration (UKCRC) provides further details of the recently established collaboration to enhance the UK position as a world leader in clinical research

www.nice.org.uk/ – National Institute for Health and Clinical Excellence (NICE) publishes recommendations on treatments and care using the best available evidence of clinical and cost effectiveness

www.york.ac.uk/inst/crd/ – Centre for Reviews and Dissemination (CRD) undertakes and publishes reviews of research about the effects of interventions used in health and social care

www.sign.ac.uk/ – Scottish Intercollegiate Guidelines Network (SIGN) publishes national clinical guidelines containing recommendations for effective practice based on current evidence

2 The Research Process

Anne Lacey

Key points

- The research process is a series of steps that need to be undertaken to carry out any piece of research.
- The precise stages of the research process, and the order in which they are undertaken, will vary depending on the nature of research, but will always follow a systematic pattern from initial ideas through to dissemination and implementation.
- Rigour in research is essential if the work is to be trustworthy and free from bias.

Introduction

The process of undertaking research is essentially the same, whether the subject matter of the research is pure science, medicine, history, or nursing. The following rather expansive definition from Graziano and Raulin (2004) sums up the breadth of scope of the research process:

> 'Research is a systematic search for information, a process of inquiry. It can be carried out in libraries, laboratories, schoolrooms, hospitals, factories, in the pages of the Bible, on street corners, or in the wild watching a herd of elephants' (Graziano & Raulin 2004: 31)

In all cases the researcher must ascertain the extent of existing knowledge, define his or her own area of enquiry, collect data and analyse it, and draw conclusions. For the pure scientist, however, the research might take place in the context of a laboratory, where experimentation is relatively straightforward as the researcher is in control of the environment and can eliminate potential confounding factors that might invalidate the research. Unless using animals or human tissue, there are few ethical considerations to take into account.

For the student of nursing research, or any research in a social context, the process is complicated by practical and ethical constraints of working in the 'real world' (Robson 2002). There is no single universally accepted way of carrying out research in the social world, but a plethora of different designs and methodologies ranging from phenomenology to randomised controlled trials, from epidemiology to action research. The range of approaches derives from different paradigms, or ways of seeing the world. However, all are valid ways of conducting research, provided the methodology used is appropriate for the research question, and is applied in a rigorous, systematic fashion.

Sarantakos (1994) put it as follows:

'Social research is a complex and pluralistic process, diverse in purpose and methods, and based on a varied theoretical and ideological structure.' (Sarantakos 1994: 30)

In this chapter the research process that is common to all nursing research will be explored, and subsequent chapters in Section 2 will look at each of the stages of research in more detail. In Section 3 of this book, different methodologies or research designs are discussed in turn, and in detail.

Although the research process will be presented as a linear, sequential process, the stages are often revisited several times during the process. In qualitative research, in particular, it is likely that the 'stages' of the research process are modified to take account of the emergent nature of the enterprise. Qualitative researchers sometimes find it difficult or even inappropriate to formulate a precise research question until they have begun to collect, and possibly even analyse, data.

However, it is helpful in the first instance to think through the entire research process in a systematic way. Many authors (Hek 1994, Kirk 1996, Parahoo 1997, Meadows 2003) have described the research process, and each comes up with a different number of stages, but essentially they contain the same elements. Box 2.1 illustrates this process as it will be described, and indicates the principal chapters in this book that deal with each stage. In this chapter a brief overview of the various stages will be given, to enable readers to see the whole before looking in more detail at each stage.

Box 2.1   The research process.

Stages in the research process	Chapters in this book
Developing the research question	6
Searching and evaluating the literature	7, 8
Choice of methodology, research design	11, 13–21
Preparing a research proposal	9
Gaining access to the data	10
Sampling	12
Data collection	22–26
Data analysis	27–29
Dissemination of the results	30
Implementation of research	31, 32

Developing the research question

Most research questions begin with a 'hunch' or initial idea that is not precisely defined. The idea might arise from clinical practice, from professional discussion among colleagues, from an issue in the media, or from reading an article or book. Alternatively the question may be derived from a 'call for proposals' from a funding body that asks for researchers to develop a proposal on a specific topic. Box 2.2 provides an example of such a call, in this case from the Department of Health Service Delivery and Organisation (SDO) Programme. The call is specific about the research question to be investigated, indicates the methods to be used, and offers £300 000 funding for the study.

Increasingly, the research community is being encouraged to include users in the process of developing research questions, so that the research agenda includes the issues of importance to those on the receiving end of health care as well as the concerns of health professionals. Chapter 5 discusses this important issue further.

A hypothetical, and somewhat frivolous research question will be used throughout this chapter to illustrate the process. Suppose a nurse has a 'hunch' that children newly diagnosed with diabetes exhibit less fear of injections if they are given a 'diabetic' teddy bear at their first contact with the diabetic nurse. She has

---

Box 2.2 Example of Service Delivery and Organisation (SDO) call for proposals.

Empirical study of the causes of poor staff morale on mental health in-patient units (August 2005)

The SDO now wishes to commission an empirical study about the factors influencing poor (or good) staff morale. This study should include morale of staff working on mental health inpatient units for children and young people, in addition to those which look after adults.

Applicants should consider the following factors, which may affect staff morale:

- characteristics of the service users, such as case mix
- characteristics of the staff group, such as the mix of professions, levels of training and staff/patient ratios
- organisational issues, such as team working, culture, climate, styles of leadership, formal and informal organisational structures
- the physical characteristics of the inpatient units

Please note that this study is *not* about interventions to improve staff morale, but about the factors that affect it.

Methods

A large, multi-site study is needed to provide sufficient high quality data. Both qualitative and quantitative research methods are likely to be necessary. Applicants should demonstrate that they have a research team in place with the appropriate research skills.

Information obtained from *www.sdo.lshtm.ac.uk/calls.htm* on 3 August 2005

observed that children are able to act out their anxieties with a new toy, and she has a hunch that such a positive experience enables them to learn new skills more easily. This idea has been supported by paediatric nurses and by parents to whom she has talked.

The initial research question might be something like:

Do children who are given a 'diabetic' teddy bear show less fear than those receiving normal care?

Several refinements could be made to this question right away. What age children are we talking about? Presumably a 12-year-old adolescent boy may not be that impressed with a teddy bear. What type of diabetes are we thinking of? Type 1 or Type 2? What sort of teddy bear? An all-singing, all-dancing one, or a basic model?

So let us assume our researcher decides on an age range of 5–10 years, and restricts the study to children with insulin dependency. After much visiting of toyshops, she decides on a Winnie the Pooh lookalike.

At this stage, the research question will look more like:

Does the provision of a teddy bear at first contact with a diabetic nurse affect anxiety in children aged 5–10 years, with insulin-dependent diabetes?

Searching and evaluating the literature

The next stage is to find out what evidence already exists in the chosen research area. It is a waste of time and money to conduct research where the answer to the question is already known. What is already known about a subject can be found from a variety of sources. Books may be a starting point, but quickly get out of date if the subject matter is topical. Academic journals are a better place to start, and access to online databases such as CINAHL (Cumulative Index of Nursing and Allied Health Literature, see Chapter 7 for more details) make this task speedy and relatively simple. If anything, the problem is that there will be too much, and Chapter 7 discusses how to refine the search. Beyond written sources, evidence may be found on the internet and various online resources. As well as locating the evidence, it must be appraised and evaluated. Not all that is written is of good quality, and evidence from one country or in one population may not necessarily generalise to other cultures or situations. Chapters 7 and 8 of this book discuss this stage in considerable detail.

Sometimes the research process may consist entirely of a review of the literature. A well-designed systematic review is an accepted research approach in its own right, systematically searching out and evaluating all the research that has been published on a particular topic. In an increasingly complex and fragmented world of information it is important to develop an evidence base that is well-validated, and on which practice can be based. Chapter 21 deals with this specialised form of research.

But to return to our example, let us suppose that a thorough search of the evidence turns up a few studies from the USA and Australia about the role of toys in relieving anxiety in children, but none from a UK source and none in diabetes. Furthermore, the studies that there are reach conflicting conclusions, use different types of toys, and use different research methods. However, there is consensus that any effect diminishes after the age of eight, and one of the studies has validated a data collection tool to measure anxiety in children. The research question might then be rewritten with a more restricted age range, and specifying the outcome measure more precisely.

Choice of methodology, research design

The majority of this book (Section 3) is devoted to a description of different research designs. In many ways, the choice of research design is the most important stage of the research process, for it affects all the others. Some questions are more appropriate for an experimental approach; others are entirely suited to an in-depth ethnographic study. Researchers often make explicit a *conceptual framework* within which they are working, which will determine the overall research approach. The kind of data collected, the types of analysis that are possible, and the way in which the results can be applied to practice will all depend upon the research design.

Some research designs are *quantitative*. This means they ultimately collect numerical data and are amenable to statistical analysis. Such research designs often have a hypothesis, or statement that can be tested, such as whether or not a certain drug reduces the size of a tumour in cancer patients. Box 2.3 (Salvesen

---

Box 2.3   Example of a quantitative experimental study.

Salvesen KA, Morkved S (2004) Randomised controlled trial of pelvic floor muscle training during pregnancy. *British Medical Journal* 329: 378–380

This study used a quantitative experimental approach to assess the effectiveness of using a structured training programme of pelvic floor exercises in reducing time spent in the second stage of labour during childbirth. Researchers in Norway recruited 301 first-time mothers during pregnancy, and randomly allocated them to either a training group (who were given an exercise programme delivered by a physiotherapist) or a control group (who had normal care). Time spent in second stage of labour was measured for the two groups. Results showed that women in the training group had a lower rate of prolonged second stage labour (25% compared to 33%) than women in the control group.

& Morkved 2004) describes a quantitative study to assess the effectiveness of training women in pelvic floor exercises during pregnancy. Other quantitative designs are observational, such as a survey using a questionnaire. Although the questions are in written form, structured answers such as ticked boxes enable the data to be coded and translated into numerical form.

Box 2.4 (Mason *et al.* 2005) gives an example of a questionnaire survey developed to measure competence in emergency nurse practitioners. Surveys may also use medical records or laboratory tests as their data source, to estimate the numbers of patients in a community who have measles, for example. Epidemiological studies of the incidence and distribution of diseases use quantitative methods.

Other research designs are *qualitative*. These designs use narrative, words, documents or graphical material as their data source, and analyse material to identify themes, relationships, concepts and, in some cases, to develop theory. Such research approaches explore an experience, culture or situation in depth, taking account of context and complexity. Qualitative designs may be used where comparatively little is known about a subject, so no hypothesis can be formulated. The purpose is exploratory rather than explanatory, although qualitative studies may certainly contribute much to our understanding of phenomena. An example of a qualitative study that aimed to generate theory and contribute to nurses' understanding of their patients and relatives is given in Box 2.5 (Johansson *et al.* 2002).

Both approaches are valid ways of advancing nursing knowledge. A quantitative study may be very good at finding out the extent of compliance with diabetic therapy, for instance, by measuring levels of the blood glucose in a sample of diabetic patients. A qualitative study, on the other hand, may tell us why it is that certain diabetic patients do not take their insulin as prescribed, by observing and talking to them, and gaining understanding of the context in which the insulin is (or is not) taken.

More than this, qualitative and quantitative methodologies are based on different philosophical assumptions and derive from different historical traditions.

Box 2.4   Example of a quantitative questionnaire survey.

Mason S, Fletcher A, McCormick S, Perrin J, Rigby A (2005) Developing assessment of emergency nurse practitioner competence: a pilot study. *Journal of Advanced Nursing* 50: 425–432

This British research team developed and tested a tool for assessment of competence in emergency nurse practitioners. The tool was developed following a questionnaire consultation with experts in emergency care, and was then piloted in a before and after study. Following an educational intervention, 17 nurses showed significant improvements since their baseline scores, and evaluated their experience of using the tool highly. The researchers concluded that the tool provided a framework for competence assessment over time, and between practitioners and departments.

> **Box 2.5** Example of a qualitative study.
>
> Johansson I, Hildingh C, Fridlund B (2002) Coping strategies when an adult next-of-kin/close friend is in critical care: a grounded theory analysis. *Intensive and Critical Care Nursing* 18:2 96–108
>
> This Swedish study used a qualitative approach called grounded theory to generate new theory about how relatives and close friends cope with the experience of their loved one being critically ill. The researchers interviewed 18 relatives/friends of intensive care unit (ICU) patients, and identified four coping strategies that they used to deal with their feelings. The use of strategies was influenced by understanding of the situation, social background, and previous experience of critical care. The researchers suggest that nurses can use the results to better understand the coping strategies employed by relatives/friends in critical care.

Chapter 11 discusses these issues in much more detail, and the reader is encouraged to get to grips with this academic debate. Nursing needs to embrace all research methodologies in order to engage with the breadth of questions that need to be asked. Ours is a discipline drawing on many different traditions of academic enquiry.

The research design (or *methodology*) is distinct from the *methods* used for data collection. A single data collection method, e.g. interview or observation may be used for many different research designs.

To return to our frivolous example, let us suppose that the researcher has decided that the best way of answering the question is to compare two groups of children newly diagnosed with diabetes. One group would be given a teddy bear at their first visit, and one group not. If the two groups were selected randomly, this study would be an experimental design. Each group will receive identical treatment in other respects, and the average anxiety for each group will be measured using the standardised scale. A qualitative design might be suitable for answering a related question about children's fears and anxieties about illness, how these can be mediated by play, and the role of soft toys in children's notions of comfort. Data would be more likely to be collected in this case by observation and interview.

Preparing a research proposal

Whether a large-scale, multi-centre study costing many thousands of pounds is planned, or a small, unfunded study for an educational degree, a formal research proposal is likely to be needed.

Such a proposal is a written statement of *what* the researcher intends to do, *why*, *how*, *when* and, often, *how much it will cost*. It is used to gain approval for the research, secure funding if that is required, and then to guide the research process during its execution. It will often be modified in the light of pilot studies or practical difficulties, but it is important that the detailed intentions are clear at the outset. It has been said that if you don't know where you are going you are unlikely to get there!

Chapter 9 sets out the content of a research proposal in detail, but the precise form of the proposal will vary according to the nature of the research and the purpose of the written proposal. A proposal written in response to a funding call from the Department of Health or the Medical Research Council is likely to be a substantial document of many pages, written by a team of experienced researchers. One written for the purpose of outlining a small study for a master's degree may be only a few pages, and written by the postgraduate student themselves with some guidance from their supervisor.

Whatever the context, however, the proposal will certainly include a section on each of the stages of the research process outlined in Box 2.1. It will also include a section detailing the ethical issues raised by the research, and how the researcher will ensure confidentiality, informed consent, and other ethical principles are respected. Chapter 3 discusses these issues in more detail. It is usual to include a table or Gantt chart showing the timescale of the project. Table 2.1 shows such a chart for a complex evaluation study involving a survey, documentary analysis, case studies and focus groups. It is also helpful to identify milestones, stating the date by which each stage of the research will be completed, though this is obviously subject to change as the inevitable obstacles and delays come into play. It is customary to include a breakdown of resources required and a justification of why they are needed.

Clearly, the research proposal cannot be written until the researcher has thought through all the stages of the research process in some detail. However, the proposal is of necessity one of the early stages in the process, as it is impossible to proceed without one.

Gaining access to the data

Because of the sensitivity of much of the research that takes place in health care, and the vulnerability of many of its subjects, a complex system of governance has been developed to ensure all research is approved for its ethical soundness, scientific quality and legal propriety. NHS Trusts are also concerned to ensure that all research that takes place within the trust is properly funded and insured against liability. A system of ethical regulation via Multicentre (MRECs) and Local Research Ethics Committees (LRECs) has been in place for the last decade, whereby researchers working in an NHS context must submit their proposals to a committee for approval before beginning the study (*www.corec.org.uk*). Since 2001 a system of research governance has also been developed to guard against research that has

Table 2.1 Example of a Gantt chart.

Timetable	Year One July 2005–June 2006						Year Two July 2006–June 2007					
Months of evaluation	2	4	6	8	10	12	14	16	18	20	22	24
Key tasks												
1. Baseline survey												
Development of survey instrument	▓											
Baseline survey data collection		▓										
Baseline survey data analysis		▓	▓									
2. Analysis of routine activity data and resource use data												
Activity and resource use data collection (after one and two years)				▓						▓		
Data analysis					▓						▓	
3. Case studies												
Pilot case study				▓								
Case study data collection					▓	▓	▓	▓	▓			
Case study analysis					▓	▓	▓	▓	▓			
4. Focus groups												
Focus groups with project co-ordinators at pre-arranged workshops × 2				▓								
Transcription and analysis of focus groups					▓	▓						
5. Dissemination												
Interim report to Regional Advisory Group						▓						
Feedback to project sites, dissemination and writing of final report for Regional Advisory Group										▓	▓	▓

not been properly scrutinised and approved, after various high profile scandals concerning NHS research (Department of Health 2001).

Chapter 10 deals with this topic in depth. Suffice it to say at this stage that the system is necessary, but rather bureaucratic and time-consuming. Depending on arrangements at your local trust, it is likely to take anything from 4 to 20 weeks from completing a research proposal to having all the required permissions in place to begin data collection.

In addition to formal permission, however, access to the data may require negotiation of a more informal nature with local personnel who act as 'gatekeepers'.

If access to patients or their records is needed, for example, it may be necessary to gain the co-operation of the appropriate consultant, practice manager, or audit department in addition to ethical and research governance committees. Access to a nursing home or school will require the permission of the appropriate senior manager. Chapter 10 also deals in more depth with this informal process of negotiating access.

Sampling

Once the research begins, the first stage is likely to be selecting the sample. Unless it is a complete census, researchers collect data from a selected group, rather than an entire population. In our earlier example involving children and teddy bears, the researcher could collect data about anxiety levels on all children newly diagnosed with diabetes in an area for several years – but this is likely to be unnecessary to answer the research question. It would also be extremely expensive on teddy bears! How are the children to be selected, and how many is enough? These questions are dealt with in detail in Chapter 12, but the answers are rarely simple, particularly about sample size.

A quantitative study involving a comparison between two groups is likely to require a *power calculation*, a statistical technique to estimate minimum sample size. This is comforting to the researcher as it gives a scientific answer to the question, but is also based on various assumptions and decisions that any statistician making the calculation will ask the researcher to make. In qualitative research samples tend to be smaller, but again there is no hard and fast rule as to how big they must be. Data saturation, or achieving the stage where no new information is being revealed by additional data collection, may be the stated goal, but it is impossible to predict beforehand when that stage may be reached.

As to the method of selection of the sample, there is a range of well-developed methods to choose from (*see* Chapter 12). The type of sampling will depend on the research design. Random sampling, and its variants, is the method of choice in traditional survey research, whereas theoretical sampling may be more appropriate for grounded theory. Whatever approach is adopted, it is essential for the validity of the research that the sample is chosen in a rigorous way, and sampling techniques adopted are adhered to closely.

The size and selection of the sample will have an effect on the timescale and cost of the research. Usually, the cost increases with sample size, although this is less significant for, say, a postal survey than for a randomised controlled trial. Similarly, in-depth interviewing and subsequent transcription of tape recordings is resource-intensive, and each increase in sample size will require significant extra resources. A realistic assessment of how quickly a particular sample size can be obtained is necessary before embarking on a piece of research – all too often patients with the relevant condition seem to disappear as soon as a research study starts recruiting!

Pilot study

It is always advisable to conduct a pilot study before embarking on the research. This may take the form of a 'dummy run' to see if the whole recruitment process works, or may simply involve testing out a data collection instrument. Questionnaires are usually piloted on a small sample of people with similar characteristics to those in the full study, to pick up questions that are misinterpreted, or items that are frequently missed out. Modifications can then be made to the questionnaire before large numbers are printed and money wasted. If interviews are to be used, a wise researcher will conduct one or two pilot interviews to test out the interview schedule, ensure technical equipment (such as a taperecorder) works satisfactorily, and to assess how long the interview is likely to take.

Data collected in a pilot study is not usually included with the main results, but may be reported separately and even published if the pilot study is a substantial one. Box 2.4 gives an example of such a pilot study.

Data collection

A wide range of data collection techniques and methods is available, and Chapters 22 to 26 describe the commonest of these. Nursing research relies heavily on interviews and questionnaires as methods of choice, but observation, clinical measurement and the use of documents as data are also appropriate methods to be considered. The stage of data collection is, in many ways, the most straightforward and rewarding stage of research. It frequently involves interaction with patients, the public or other research participants after a long stage of filling in forms and writing research proposals. At last, the researcher gets to ask the questions he or she started out with.

Data collection tools will usually have been selected at the research proposal stage. Ethical and research governance committees like to see the intended instruments, or at least to have a draft of an interview schedule or questionnaire. The instruments will need to be refined and developed ready for use, however, and practicalities of how the data will be collected, by whom and when are often done as data collection begins.

It is at this stage that the researcher needs to keep tight control over the data collection process. Failure to keep index numbers on documents, or to record the time of a clinical observation, can render data collected useless. It is also important to consider who should be involved in data collection. Using our earlier frivolous example, an employee of a company manufacturing a rival brand of teddy bear may not be the ideal person to put in charge of data collection!

All data collected needs secure storage, whether this is in hard copy (paper records or audiovisual material) or in electronic form. Paper copies and tapes need to be locked in a cabinet or drawer to preserve confidentiality, and electronic records need to be stored on a secure computer and backed up on a separate disc or server. Many researchers will preserve both paper and electronic records, as either can be destroyed or corrupted by unexpected events such as fire, theft or computer breakdown.

Data analysis

This is perhaps the most crucial phase of any research project. Once data are collected, they need to be assembled and organised in such a way that conclusions can be drawn from them. A huge spreadsheet of numbers or multiple pages of narrative cannot be disseminated to others or used in practice until some analysis has taken place. It is also the phase that is most demanding from an intellectual point of view. Whether using qualitative or quantitative methods, data analysis is hard work. Contrary to many people's expectations, computer software analysis packages such as NVivo (for qualitative analysis) and SPSS (for quantitative analysis) do not do the analysis, they simply provide practical tools to manage the data more easily. The researcher still has to manage and guide the process, and do some serious thinking about the meaning of the data.

If the data collected are qualitative, data analysis techniques such as those described in Chapter 27 can be used. The exact methods used will vary according to the qualitative methodology adopted. In practice there are few universally accepted methods of analysing qualitative data, but the researcher must make the process 'transparent' by describing in detail how the results were derived.

Quantitative data are usually analysed statistically, and Chapters 28 and 29 provide guidance on the standard techniques available. With anything other than a small project, a quantitative piece of research should include a statistician in the research team, or at least be able to access professional statistical advice.

Some research projects use 'mixed methods' that include both qualitative and quantitative approaches. Here the analysis may attempt to combine the two sets of results, perhaps using the qualitative data to provide interpretation of the quantitative results.

Dissemination of the results

Of course there is little point in conducting any research if the results are never made known to anybody except the researcher. Dissemination can take many forms. At the local level, research can be presented to colleagues at team or unit meetings, or as a more formal seminar to local professionals who may be interested. Our study of teddy bears and children with diabetes might be of interest to parents, consultants, general practitioners, pharmacists and dieticians, as well as to nurses themselves. Many nurses have access to a specialist group of health professionals in their discipline at local or national level, and this is also a suitable forum in which to disseminate the results of small- or large-scale research.

Recently new avenues for dissemination have opened up as increasing use of the internet has provided opportunities for researchers to post details of their research on a website, perhaps hosted by a NHS trust or university. This ensures that research results are widely and freely available, but, like most online resources, provides no guarantee of quality. Increasingly, however, information is being disseminated via the web, and online discussion groups are also enabling informal exchange of ideas.

Publication in written form, in academic and professional journals, remains the most widely accepted method of dissemination of research, but presentation of results at conferences, by oral presentation or by poster, is also common. All of these media enable fellow researchers and practitioners to discuss the results and provide some feedback about the usefulness of the research, and possible avenues for further studies. Chapter 30 in this book discusses methods of dissemination more thoroughly.

Implementation of the results

This topic is dealt with in depth in Chapters 31 and 32 of this book. Needless to say, the purpose of nursing research is to improve practice in some way, whether by direct application of the results of a trial, by better informing practitioners of the culture in which they are working, or by evaluating the effects of an innovation. While it is not the direct responsibility of the research community to ensure implementation of the findings of research, it is incumbent upon researchers to ensure that their findings are being shared with those who implement nursing policy and engage in clinical practice. This implies that research findings should be published in places where practitioners, managers and policymakers will read them, and taken to professional as well as academic conferences.

Ensuring rigour

Rigour refers to the strength of the research design in terms of ensuring that all procedures have been followed scrupulously, that all possible confounding factors have been eliminated, and that the user can be confident that the conclusions are dependable. Of course this is always a relative concept; social research can very rarely be said to have eliminated all possible sources of error, but the quality of the research will be judged by the extent to which this has been done.

There are two key concepts that concern the quality of research: validity and reliability. *Validity* concerns the extent to which the research measures what it purports to measure without bias or distortion. A study to assess the health effects of air pollution in a community would not be valid if it simply collected people's views about the air quality, without measuring actual levels of disease, or even mortality rates. In our earlier frivolous example, validity would be reduced if some children were given a computer game instead of a teddy bear, or if some of the control group children were secretly given a teddy by well-meaning nurses who felt sorry for them.

Reliability refers to the consistency of measurement within a study. A set of weighing scales that gave a person's weight as 52 kg at 10:00 am and 55 kg at 10:05 am could not be said to be reliable. Repeated measurement is the usual test of reliability, and can be done by second administration of a questionnaire under similar conditions, or by two researchers making the same set of observations and comparing results. Data collection tools such as quality of life scales are extensively tested for reliability before being used as a standard measure in research studies. Unreliable measurement tools will always mean that the validity of a research study is compromised, as confidence in the quality of data collection is reduced. A study might use perfectly reliable instruments, however, and still not be valid. Meticulous collection of body mass index of patients in primary care, for example, will not generate a valid measure of the prevalence of diabetes in the practice, though the two may be related.

Some qualitative researchers reject the terms validity and reliability because of the association of the terms with the quantitative research tradition, and the assumption implicit in their definition that research can be entirely objective and free from bias (Holloway & Wheeler 1996). Such researchers may prefer to use concepts such as credibility, trustworthiness, and transparency to describe the quality of the research, but the underlying concept of rigour and the use of a systematic approach remains the same. Chapters 11, 13 and 15 of this book will discuss these issues further.

Conclusion

The research process outlined in this chapter will be adapted according to the research design, the scale of the undertaking, resources available, and the context in which the research is conducted. However, all research needs to be systematic and rigorous in its approach. This chapter began by discussing the relative complexity of conducting research in a social, rather than laboratory, context. Robson (2002) sums up the situation with characteristic frankness:

> 'One of the challenges inherent in carrying out investigations in the 'real world' lies in seeking to say something sensible about a complex, relatively poorly controlled and generally 'messy' situation' (Robson 2004:4)

One of the particular complexities is the need to conduct research that involves people according to ethical principles, and this requirement frequently impinges on the design and conduct of the research process. This question is addressed in the next chapter.

References

Department of Health (2001) *Research Governance Framework for Health and Social Care.* London, Department of Health

Graziano AM, Raulin ML (2004) *Research methods: a process of inquiry,* 5th edition. Boston, Pearson

Hek G (1994) The research process. *Journal of Community Nursing* 8:6 4–6

Holloway I, Wheeler S (1996) *Qualitative Research for Nurses.* Oxford, Blackwell

Johansson I, Hildingh C, Fridlund B (2002) Coping strategies when an adult next-of-kin/ close friend is in critical care: a grounded theory analysis. *Intensive and Critical Care Nursing* 18:2 96–108

Kirk K (1996) Embarking on the research process: a guide. *Health Visitor* 69:9 370–372

Mason S, Fletcher A, McCormick S, Perrin J, Rigby A (2005) Developing assessment of emergency nurse practitioner competence: a pilot study. *Journal of Advanced Nursing* 50: 425–423

Meadows KA (2003) So you want to do research? 1: an overview of the research process. *British Journal of Community Nursing* 8:8 369–375

Parahoo K (1997) *Nursing Research: principles, process and methods.* Basingstoke, Macmillan

Robson C (2002) *Real World Research: a resource for social scientists and practitioner-researchers,* 2nd edition. Oxford, Blackwell

Salvesen KA, Morkved S (2004) Randomised controlled trial of pelvic floor muscle training during pregnancy. *British Medical Journal* 329: 378–380

Sarantakos S (1994) *Social Research.* Basingstoke, Macmillan

Websites

www.dh.gov.uk/policyandguidance/researchanddevelopment/ – Department of Health section on Research and Development, where you can find information about research funding, ethical approval and research governance

www.rdinfo.org.uk – 'Support and Help' section gives information about the research process, writing research proposals and getting approval

www.corec.org.uk – Central Office for Research Ethics Committees (COREC) gives full information about the system of ethical regulation for the NHS and social care research

3 Research Ethics

Martin Johnson and Tony Long

Key points

- The main ethical issues which require attention when planning and conducting research include the importance of respecting participants, responding to the needs of vulnerable individuals and groups, gaining consent and maintaining confidentiality.
- Strategies for conducting ethical research include balancing the potential disadvantages of participation in the research with the likely benefit to participants, minimising the risk of harm to participants and the formal ethical scrutiny of research proposals.
- When evaluating a research report consideration needs to given to the ethical conduct of the study.

The importance of ethics in research

Early nurse researchers paid scant attention to ethics as such. Nurses were assumed to be professionals with integrity and a vocation in which putting patients' interests before their own could be assumed. Even from these times, however, researchers were confronting moral dilemmas and sometimes used methods which, when made public, were seen to have infringed human rights and possibly caused harms.

More recently, because of increasing public concern that not all health professionals have behaved with complete integrity, procedures to assure ethical probity of research programmes have become increasingly rigorous, some might even say tiresome (Howarth & Kneafsey 2003; 2005). Chapter 10 examines the procedures for the formal review of research proposals in some detail. Examples of studies where the ethical issues are controversial are considered elsewhere (Johnson 2004).

In this chapter we aim to introduce basic issues that researchers need to think about in the design of their studies. We will suggest that while it is essential to keep the core principle of respect for individuals firmly in mind, it will also be necessary in most cases to focus carefully on balancing potential disadvantages of participating in the research study with the likely benefits for participants. The chapter has two main parts: issues that require the researcher's attention, and strategies that may be employed to deal adequately and ethically with these issues.

Issues for researchers to address

Respect for participants

This key principle is based on the belief that every individual matters and has the right to be treated with respect. Most adults are autonomous: that is, they have the mental ability to deliberate about issues that affect them and to make decisions (however wise, foolish or capricious) for themselves. Respecting the individual implies respecting their decisions. Many factors may conspire to limit the autonomy of an individual.

Adequate information on which to base choices

Many decisions in life would be flawed if vital elements of relevant information were not available – or even deliberately withheld. A constant concern for researchers in health care is how much information to give people (particularly about unlikely risks) without worrying them unduly. However, the key aspects of participation should be made clear to potential recruits for them to make an informed choice, together with at least the most important risks in terms of likelihood of occurrence or extent of potential impact.

Understanding and evaluating the issues involved

While most adults (and, indeed, many children) are able to understand a sufficient depth of information or detail to allow for rational decision-making, this is not the case for all. It is possible for this ability to be temporarily or permanently lost through illness, trauma, or degenerative processes of ageing or disease. Under normal circumstances, potential participants need to know what harms, if any at all, might result. However, in circumstances where this is simply not possible, and when the research results might be important, different approaches may need to be adopted (Box 3.1).

Perceived or actual coercion

Health professionals generally accept a role in persuading their patients to do what they consider to be good for them. Nurses regularly encourage and cajole people to mobilise after surgery, to take medication and to abstain from harmful behaviours. Coercion, however, involves using 'undue' pressure or leverage to engage compliance. In practice the distinction is often blurred, particularly in circumstances of increased vulnerability of the patient, when the consequences of a poor choice are potentially disastrous, or at times when staff are under strain. These pressures are easily transferred to the research arena, too.

Box 3.1   Practical ethics.

Lawton J (2000) *The Dying Process: patients' experiences of palliative care.* London, Routledge

Julia Lawton used open participant observation in order to avoid long and possibly exhausting interviews with the dying people in a hospice. In this edited extract from her excellent book she illustrates how, while attempting to get consent, wherever possible, she had to be practical.

'Formal interviews not only seemed to be too obtrusive to many patients and their families; in a substantial number of cases they were simply not viable. Some patients, for example, were heavily sedated during their stay in the hospice, whilst others experienced changes in their mental state, such as becoming very paranoid or confused. It was, of course, impossible to interview a patient in a coma.

I worked as an 'in-house' volunteer within the hospice because this particular role enabled me to have substantial and regular contact with patients and their visitors in the wards, side rooms and other communal areas within the building . . .

I often found that performing a practical task, such as making a bed, gave me an ideal excuse to enter a ward and make observations in situations when it might have been too awkward and obtrusive to have a researcher present; for instance, when one of the patients had just died. . . .

Whenever possible, patients were informed by staff about my research and given the option of 'opting out' of any observations I made. In cases where a patient was admitted in a coma, or was suffering from confusion, the consent of his or her relatives was obtained instead.'

(Lawton, 2000:30–31)

Freedom from undue social restriction

While the individual's ability to make decisions may be compromised genuinely by severe intellectual disability resulting, for example, from dementia or head injury, it may also be limited by the social diminution of status which is inherent in the stereotyping and stigmatisation of some forms of illness or disability (Johnson 1997). Health researchers therefore need to be aware that personal autonomy can become limited for both pathological and social reasons rendering the individual more vulnerable and less autonomous.

Vulnerable individuals and groups

Every recipient of health care is in some way vulnerable, but those with more limited ability to act autonomously can also be more vulnerable to the impact of research activity. For example, those whose first language is not English, notably some members of minority ethnic communities, can find it difficult to make their preferences known or to understand the issues (RCN 2004). Similar difficulties may attach to other individuals, too, such as some deaf people who use only sign language (whether using English or some other language in the written form).

Most young children are self-evidently vulnerable. In the light of several scandals in which the poor standard of care of children has led to their deaths (Department of Heath 2001), great prominence has been given recently to safeguarding children. The ability to act and decide autonomously develops with maturity, but even very young children of primary school age can be capable of holding reasoned, well-informed views on issues that affect them. When children are unable to determine what is in their best interests, parents are normally the best alternative decision-makers.

In situations where the planned research participants are children under the care of the Social Services, special care needs to be taken to be sure that decisions are made by the appropriate legal guardian. Despite the difficulties inherent in researching with children and young people, such research is essential if advances in treatment and better understanding of their needs are to be achieved (Long 2004). Without such efforts to find ways to make inclusion in a study compatible with the best interests of children and young people we risk double jeopardy by adding denial of the chance of improvement to the misfortune of suffering from a health or social problem.

It is equally tempting to assume that older people are automatically vulnerable to inappropriate clinical or research interventions. On the other hand, the majority of health care recipients *are* older people and this trend will continue. Although it may sometimes be more convenient, excluding people from research on the grounds of age alone is not equitable and constitutes ageism.

The same applies to other groups which might require extra efforts and resources to reach, but which should not be excluded inappropriately from studies. Minority ethnic populations are sometimes difficult to involve in research, especially where there are language and cultural differences. For this reason, sensitive efforts should be made to include people with such backgrounds where possible, since everyone should have the opportunity to take part in and potentially to benefit from research (Gunaratnam 2003). This applies both to individuals and to whole groups defined by ethnicity, age, or gender.

In some cases nurses care for, and may need to be involved in research with, individuals who are considered to be no longer cognitively competent to give consent. For example, some patients may have progressive dementia or they may have brain damage to a degree, which leaves them in a persistent vegetative state. Leslie Gelling (2004) discusses approaches that he and colleagues took to doing research with patients in the vegetative state and their families. Gelling carefully discusses the different degrees of loss of competence and autonomy through brain damage. He shows that research with this group and their families can help to clarify diagnosis and prognosis, and help in arriving at more appropriate plans of care and treatment. He argues that despite the complexity involved, it would be quite wrong to avoid doing research with this group of individuals who have been largely ignored by the research community.

Nurse researchers commonly wish to study their own clients, students or staff. In this context it is important to ask why these particular participants are more appropriate, given the possibility for an existing power relationship (e.g. teacher/ student) which might affect the individual's decision to participate or the outcomes of the study. Even those who are not affected by illness may become vulnerable in circumstances of power differential.

To summarise, research samples should be inclusive of, and represent the diversity of society across all relevant groupings. In particular, vulnerable people should not be excluded from participation in research except for well-justified reasons, which do not include mere convenience to the researcher. A mature approach to such cases is needed in which extra efforts are made to ensure protection of vulnerable individuals without denying them the chance to participate and potentially to benefit from the research.

Gaining consent

People who are able to consider what participation will involve should be able to decide whether or not to take part in a study. Researchers should provide full information that is easy to understand, and software is now available to evaluate the readability of such information. For example, MS Word™ for Windows XP™ features such a facility within the spelling and grammar-checking tool, while standard tests of readability based on sentence length and other criteria are also available. A number of helpful electronic resources in this area are provided at the end of this chapter. The consent of the participant should be freely given and opportunities should be provided for consent to be withdrawn at a later stage. In some studies it may be necessary to ensure continuing consent on several occasions over a long period. However, it should be noted that an excess of concern in this respect could make respondents feel that research is more harmful than it really is. It is important to establish a sense of balance here. Engaging participation in a trial of a new anti-cancer drug carries far greater dangers than a focus group to evaluate a new service. The potential harms and possible benefits are of a different order of magnitude.

Consent freely given to a research design that might have dangers does not absolve the researcher of accountability for these dangers. It has long been established that responsibility for the welfare of research participants rests with the researcher who must prioritise the best interests of participants. Perhaps less serious, but no less challenging is what to do when the researcher discovers a clear and present need, for example, for pain relief. In such cases, where demands of the research design and more immediate needs of participants conflict the researcher needs to be clear in advance what they will do. It is debatable whether or not registered nurses retain an over-riding professional duty to pursue the best interest of patients and clients when acting solely as a researcher. Such issues cannot be left until the point at which a decision is needed, but must be resolved clearly by the individual before embarking on the study.

In practice, obtaining consent should involve giving clear unambiguous information to potential respondents so that they (or their advocate) can make an
autonomous decision. An example of participant information sheet and consent
form is given in Chapter 10. Further guidance is available for nurses from the
Royal College of Nursing (RCN 2004).

Maintaining confidentiality

The collection of data, usually about people, is the principal strategy of nursing
research. Often these data include personal, biographical and demographic information which, while essential to the analysis, should normally be used for this
purpose only. In some cases, such as focus groups, research participants and
others may need to be asked to keep matters discussed confidential to the group.
This is illustrative of the need to be responsive to the nature of the data and
address issues of confidentiality accordingly. The possibilities for collecting and
holding data of a novel or non-standard nature have expanded to a large degree
to include still photography; video images and voices; computerised patient
records; paintings, sculpture, drama and other forms of expression; and human
tissues. Each of these forms of data poses different problems for the researcher,
and sometimes creative means are required for both analysis and safe storage
(Haigh & Jones 2005). However, there is nothing inherently unethical about their
use and we feel that the potential of some of these tools is insufficiently exploited
in nursing research where the semi-structured interview seems to predominate
(Long & Johnson 2002).

Collected data must be stored securely and in many cases arrangements are
made to dispose safely of data once used for their main purpose on the grounds,
some feel, that data used for one purpose should not, without permission, be used
for any other. Certainly, there is a convention that data should not normally be
put to a use which has not previously been made clear to research participants.
However, it seems to us that the value of data, suitably anonymised and carefully
stored, should never be underestimated. There is no way to know what great
benefit it may offer in the future. What is important is that generally people know
that data may be kept, and that it might be used to support research in due course.
It is wise to make clear that such data may be used on more than one occasion for
research and publication purposes. Before data is destroyed we must ask what
undertakings were made regarding storage or destruction of data, and what harm
such data could do now.

It has become traditional in much nursing and health research to assure research
participants and organisations of the confidentiality of the data collected. However,
researchers need to be aware that in a research context (as in a clinical one) they
may become privileged with information of great importance, For example, in a
criminal matter. We take the view that in an over-riding interest such as personal
safety or the protection of vulnerable people, confidentiality cannot be considered
an absolute duty. This should also, however, be made clear to participants.
Declarations by participants which suggest the potential for harm to themselves

or third parties should prompt the serious consideration of the researcher divulging the essential information to an appropriate authority or professional.

The place of anonymity

A common way of assuring confidentiality of responses is to anonymise both individuals and organisations. In large surveys this may be relatively straightforward. In smaller qualitative studies anonymising data can be much more difficult. Certainly, erring on the side of safety, it has become common to remove identifying characteristics and to assign pseudonyms to respondents and organisations in much health and social care research. However, we need to remember that in some research traditions, like nursing history, the preservation of anonymity is inappropriate and may even be contrary to respondents' interests. A historian of British nursing research would inevitably collect data from, and name, key individuals and reserve the right to evaluate their contribution critically.

The Unlinked Anonymous Prevalence Monitoring Programme (UAPMP) began in the UK in 1990 and has tested nearly eight million samples of human tissue (mostly blood) from adults since then (Health Protection Agency 2005). Much of the activity is related to genito-urinary medicine clinic attendees, and to pregnant women – both potentially vulnerable groups. Consent is not sought, but the samples are acquired through a process that removes any link to the identity of the donor. The purpose of the programme is to measure the distribution of undiagnosed infection, particularly human immunodeficiency virus (HIV), in parts of the adult population. This programme – essentially a public health data collection activity – meets with the ethical requirements laid down by the Central Office for Research Ethics Committees, the Department of Health, the Medical Research Council, and English law, and it is a prime example of large-scale data collection in which consent is not sought but otherwise the research subjects are protected by the maintenance of their anonymity.

Strategies for ethical research

Balancing risks and benefits

We would argue that, in general, decisions about health care interventions, and about research, are ones in which we weigh the possible risks and benefits in the interests of individuals and wider society. A problem with this notion of balancing risks and benefits, however, is that this implies a degree of certainty about what these may be. It suggests a calculation that cannot actually be performed. Instead, a human judgement needs to be made which accepts the disadvantages of an approach and takes account of the benefits research may bring either now or in the future.

In some forms of experimental research, the evidence for and against the planned intervention may already be substantial and can be summarised both for approval bodies and for research participants. Certainly, obvious risks (such as allergic reaction) and discomfort or pain should be made very clear to all concerned in the context of a rationale that includes the likely benefits of the research. In exploratory research, which is often qualitative, these outcomes may be less clear. Nevertheless, compared to the quite profound iatrogenic risks of much health care, serious physical or emotional harms are rare in nursing research.

Potential benefits from participation in research

Before any research project is undertaken, the possible benefits should be clear to all concerned. First among these might be a direct improvement in the health or care of individuals participating in the study. Second are longer-term benefits for others. Third, as a report by Len Doyal (2004) has argued, is the development of research skills, which is itself a legitimate aim of research. Each of these possible benefits must be carefully balanced with any likely disadvantages.

Predicting the benefits of a particular study can be difficult even with the most rigorous of experiments. In qualitative research with less foreseeable outcomes this estimation can be even harder to make. For this reason, approval committees and other gatekeepers sometimes find it difficult to approve such studies. However, the more that such studies are undertaken the greater the likelihood that some may be very beneficial and few would doubt the influence and importance of works of this kind by Barney Glaser and Anselm Strauss (1965) which drew attention to the way the dying were treated; by Felicity Stockwell (1984) who explored the inappropriate labelling of patients; and more recently by Julia Lawton (2000) who shows clearly how grim the process of dying can actually be, even in a hospice.

Minimising harm

Most patient care and treatment contains an element of risk of harm or, at the very least, discomfort. Nurses give injections, dress painful wounds and detain patients with a clear sense of proportion between the discomfort or denial of liberty and the likely future benefit. Research is little different but the level of risk depends on the nature of the research.

The trial of new products may cause harm, such as allergic reaction or worsening of the condition, to particular individuals. Other risks are less obvious, such as the possibility of upsetting people in research about sensitive subjects or inadvertently stimulating or revealing cause for conflict between participants. It is therefore important to be clear about harms and discomforts and to discuss these openly with research participants. In many cases nursing research will involve minor inconvenience at most. This should be kept to a minimum, but complete avoidance may be impossible.

Watson (1996) argues that

'the concept of a test or trial immediately raises ethical issues' (Watson 1996:7).

Above and beyond the risk of actual harm, he argues that it is almost impossible to conduct a clinical trial without a measure of deceit. For example, even though respondents know they are in a trial, they may be blinded to which, if any, intervention they are receiving. Once again, the risk of harm must be minimised, and in such cases truly informed involvement means that the subject accepts this element of potential deception.

It may be that this situation of conflict – between ensuring high-quality research that can result in positive outcomes and protecting participants – is compounded by being a health professional. It could be argued that non-professionals would feel less responsibility to rescue research subjects from minor discomforts and dangers. With the aim of minimising harm, health professional researchers now more clearly see that they should intervene to prevent or reduce harms in certain circumstances. Occasionally, the issue is potentially too serious for a nurse to ignore. Researchers learn, however, that many dilemmas are much less clear-cut, and some tolerance of standards and procedures different to one's own is part and parcel of doing research in practice settings. Such issues are best discussed with experienced research colleagues or supervisors.

Personal integrity and professional responsibility

Although there are many safeguards such as research ethics committees and NHS research governance procedures and university approval arrangements, the protection of participants' interests in matters of research still often relies on the professionalism and personal integrity of the members of the research team.

Promises to keep data safely should be kept, and research processes should be carried out rigorously. Research approval processes increasingly have a brief reporting procedure, but sadly this can hardly be relied upon to assure quality and proper adherence to high standards of research conduct. Perhaps more reliable, although far from foolproof, is effective training of researchers and accountability to departmental or unit-based supervisors. Being overseen by a steering committee which contains suitably briefed representatives of the population being studied and a genuine peer review process are also usually of great help, if time-consuming. Additional guidance on personal responsibility for nurses in research is provided by the Royal College of Nursing (2004).

The ethical evaluation of research studies

The methodological literature in nursing research is expanding, but it is clear that despite the current fashion in the UK for procedural control of research in an attempt to prevent problems, little exists by way of ethical evaluation of the nursing research literature. An edited collection of essays (de Raeve 1996) examines some dilemmas and legal problems that researchers have faced themselves but there is a general reluctance to debate the issues and problems faced by others. Matthews and Venables (1998) offer areas or criteria that might be used to such a purpose such as the degree to which participation was voluntary, whether

Box 3.2 Questions to ask about research conduct.

For each question the reviewer ought to consider: Did this exert any impact on the worth of the findings?

- What were the aims of the study? How important were they and why?
- Who undertook the study and how did their background prepare them?
- Who supervised or monitored the study?
- What sort of ethical approval was given, if any?
- What information were participants given and how readable and accurate was this?
- What checks were made to ensure that consent was given and remained in force?
- What opportunities were given for participants to withdraw?
- How were issues of power between researcher and respondents dealt with?
- Were any social groups excluded, and if so how powerful was the justification?
- Were participants deprived of a known helpful intervention? If so on what grounds?
- What risks/harms were associated with the study? Were these acceptable in the context of the potential benefits?
- What benefits were thought possible to arise from the study? Who was likely to benefit?
- Did the effort made to disseminate the study outcomes to all concerned match the promises made?

informed consent was achieved and the risk–benefit ratio. Unfortunately, they shrink from identifying genuine studies to illustrate their use of this approach. Instead they offer four brief hypothetical examples. Their general intention is sound, however.

It is important that as part of the reader's and especially the advanced student's evaluation of any research report they give thought to its ethical conduct. Achieving this may sometimes require the reader to dig a little deeper than the published article, since not all authors are equally robust in reporting the mistakes made and problems encountered while undertaking research. In Box 3.2 we offer a list of questions, which might be asked about studies being reviewed or developed. It would be useful if more attention were given to these issues in the review of literature than has been customary in the past. It is possible to bring moral theory such as consequentialism, duty, and 'ethics of care' to bear on these discussions (Johnson 1992), but much can be achieved generally by critical debate of the issues raised by these questions.

Conclusion

Despite the developing bureaucracy which is meant, at least in part, to assure ethical conduct of research, much will continue to rely on the integrity and training of the researchers themselves and their supervisors. They should try not to be intimidated from undertaking an important study by myths that the proposed study may be unethical. Such myths include the involvement of children or the very ill as participants, and the use of technology to record data. The ethical approval mechanisms should really review what, if any, real harm might result, and, in balance with this, what benefits might accrue. Provided that these are addressed clearly in the proposal, and the approach defended with rigour and obvious integrity it should be possible to negotiate the bureaucracy.

Of course, for those who are less experienced, it is wise to work with a supervisor to design a study, which is realistic and avoids putting the approval mechanisms, and the researcher, under too much strain. Reading widely, and considering some of the more difficult issues that we can refer to only briefly here can also help. Certainly, novice researchers should try to develop the skill of identifying the ethical issues in every study they read or hear about, but they should also maintain a realistic sense of proportion.

References

de Raeve L (ed) (1996) *Nursing Research: an ethical and legal appraisal*. London, Baillière Tindall

Department of Health (2001) *The Royal Liverpool Children's Inquiry Report*. London, The Stationery Office

Doyal L (2004) *The Ethical Governance and Regulation of Student Projects: a draft proposal*. Working group on ethical review of student research in the NHS, Chair: Professor Len Doyal

Gelling L (2004) Researching patients in the vegetative state: difficulties of studying this patient group. *NT Research* 9:1 7–17

Glaser BG, Strauss AL (1965) *Awareness of Dying*. Chicago, Aldine

Gunaratnam Y (2003) *Researching 'race' and ethnicity*. London, Sage

Haigh C, Jones N (2005) An overview of the ethics of cyber-space research and the implications for nurse educators. *Nurse Education Today* 25: 3–8

Health Protection Agency (2005) *The Unlinked Anonymous Prevalence Monitoring Programme*. HPA *www.hpa.org.uk/infections/topics_az/hiv_and_sti/hiv/epidemiology/ua.htm*

Howarth ML, Kneafsey R (2003) Research governance: what future for nursing research? *Nurse Education Today* 23: 81–82

Howarth ML, Kneafsey R (2005) The impact of research governance in healthcare and higher education organisations. *Journal of Advanced Nursing* 49: 1–9

Johnson M (1992) A silent conspiracy? Some ethical issues of participant observation in nursing research. *International Journal of Nursing Studies* 29: 213–223

Johnson M (1997) *Nursing Power and Social Judgement*. Aldershot, Ashgate

Johnson M (2004) Real world ethics and nursing research. *NT Research* 9: 251–261

Lawton J (2000) *The Dying Process: patients' experiences of palliative care*. London, Routledge

Long T (2004) *Excessive Crying in Infancy*. London, Whurr Publishing Ltd

Long T, Johnson M (2002) Research in *Nurse Education Today*: do we meet our aims and scope? (paper commissioned for Special Issue 2002). *Nurse Education Today* 22:1 85–93

Matthews L, Venables A (1998) Critiquing ethical issues in published research. In Crookes P, Davies S (eds) *Research Into Practice*. Edinburgh, Baillière Tindall

Royal College of Nursing (2004) *Research Ethics: RCN guidance for nurses*. London, RCN

Stockwell F (1972, 1984) *The Unpopular Patient*. London, Croom Helm

Watson R (1996) Product testing on trial. In de Raeve L (1996) *Nursing Research: an ethical and legal appraisal*. London, Baillière Tindall pp3–17

Websites

www.corec.org.uk – UK Central Office for Research Ethics Committees (COREC) offers comprehensive guidance to researchers

The websites of the relevant government departments in the four countries of the UK contain relevant information for researchers:

www.dh.gov.uk/policyandguidance/researchanddevelopment/fs/en – England

www.dhsspsni.gov.uk – Northern Ireland

www.show.scot.nhs.uk/cso/ – Scotland

www.wales.gov.uk –Wales

www.invo.org.uk/ – INVOLVE is a national advisory group, funded by the Department of Health, which aims to promote and support active public involvement in NHS, public health and social care research.

www.hpa.org.uk/infections/topics_az/hiv_and_sti/hiv/epidemiology/ua.htm – details of the Unlinked Anonymous Prevalence Monitoring Programme (UAPMP), an example of a major survey undertaken without consent from participants

Sources of standard tests for readability:

www.literacytrust.org.uk/campaign/SMOG.html

www.tasc.ac.uk/depart/media/staff/ls/modules/MED1140/Fog.htm

www.usingenglish.com/glossary/readability-test.html

www.sharedlearning.org.uk/fog_index.htm (helpful for those with English as a second language)

4 Sources of Funding and Support for Research

Senga Bond and Anne Lacey

Key points

- Research activity is enhanced by access to sources of human and financial support.
- Appropriate educational preparation to conduct research is essential.
- Advice and supervision is also essential for the new researcher.
- Nursing research can attract funding from a wide variety of sources.

Introduction

This chapter is devoted to sources of support, human and financial, for those who wish to begin to carry out research. Of course, research efforts extend from large-scale multi-disciplinary, multi-centre projects involving major financial and man-power resources, to those which can be done by an individual requiring little more than a notebook and pencil, or perhaps a computer, and lots of time. It is well nigh impossible, however, for anyone to carry out good research without support. Different forms of assistance are appropriate for all types of research, and all research workers, whatever the stage of their research career. However for those at the earlier stages, it is of the utmost importance to obtain good advice as well as the means to support the research.

Let us assume you have the motivation, interest, and a bright idea and want to embark on research but lack the knowledge of where to begin. The fact that you are reading this book would suggest that you are on the right track! Books like this are a useful source of ideas but because they are not interactive in the same way as people, they are at best only a partial answer. Doing research is an intellectual craft activity and no one learns their craft out of books. If we posed the question, 'Why do I want help?' it might be answered in a number of ways including:

- education for research
- supervision
- advice about practical or methodological aspects of a specific project
- kindred spirits to provide emotional sustenance
- financial support
- information resources

Education for research

An introduction to basic concepts in research and evidence-based practice is generally included as a component of most diploma and degree level nursing courses. In addition, there are many short 'research appreciation' courses, as well as longer forms of research preparation at diploma, masters, and doctorate levels. While you may have had some introduction to research ideas and to research studies in your professional training, it may be worth considering extended research training at master's level or above. Courses in research methods are available in many higher educational institutions as well as by distance or online learning. It is generally easier to obtain time off work for a part-time day/evening course, but it is often more beneficial to be able to concentrate on full-time study if it can be arranged. The calendars and websites of universities and colleges should provide details of whether suitable courses are available, and their entry requirements. It may be that research does not feature in the course title, (for example MSc Health Sciences) and so course content needs to be examined carefully. Appropriate courses may be found in nursing departments, in social sciences, public health or in health services research departments.

A traditional way to obtain research education is to register for a higher degree after having secured a good quality first degree. Depending on the level of research education in the first degree, it may be advantageous to combine a Master or Doctor of Philosophy (MPhil/ PhD) with some formal research teaching within a masters or similar level of taught course. For those who are serious about pursuing a career that includes doing research, doctoral training is now almost mandatory and is better obtained at the earliest opportunity.

Information about local courses and study opportunities should be available from the Research and Development (R&D) manager in your local NHS trust, or from your local school of nursing and midwifery. Staff in the R&D office may know people who have attended courses and are able to offer some insight into what they offer. Some NHS trust R&D departments may also be able to provide help with fees for approved courses. Online information about research training courses nationwide is available from the Research and Development Learning website (*www.rdlearning.org.uk*). Many universities advertise research study opportunities in the professional press (for example *Health Services Journal*) or the national press (for example *The Guardian* and *The Times Higher Education Supplement*).

Rather than embark on formal research training you may be guided in the direction of a 'research appreciation' course. These are no preparation for those with a serious intention to do research and are oriented more for 'consumers' and 'participants' in research to raise awareness and interest. One advantage of doing a formal research methods course is to assist those who have found research interesting in an undergraduate programme to decide whether they have the motivation and ability to proceed to carry out original research. While taking a higher degree may delay the start of an interesting project, it is essential in laying down a good foundation from which to proceed. It is for this reason that students embarking on a higher degree by research are advised to participate in a general methods course first (or as part of their higher degree), so that, as well as learning through a project using a particular method, they can extend their knowledge to other methods and techniques used in research.

Advanced research training at postdoctoral level is also advised for those whose career intentions include research. This means that it can take up to 10 years of academic training to get on to the first rung of the research ladder to generate research income from peer-reviewed sources. Research training fellowships are designed to support people who want to embark on a research career, or advance further once started. Fellowships include an award to cover course fees and expenses and, usually, full salary for a period of several years. They are available from the Department of Health (*www.dh.gov.uk*), the Research Councils such as the Medical Research Council (*www.mrc.ac.uk*), and many voluntary and charitable sources such as The Health Foundation (*www.health.org.uk*). In Scotland, training fellowships are available through the Chief Scientist Office (*www.show.scot.nhs.uk/cso/*). In addition, monies are currently ringfenced to develop research capacity and capability within the nursing, midwifery and allied health professions (NMAHP) through three consortia of Scottish Higher Education Institutions and NHS Scotland. These consortia are supported by the Scottish Executive, NHS Education for Scotland and Scottish Higher Education Funding Council (SHEFC) and details of the consortia can be found in *Making Choices, Facing Challenges* (*www.nes.scot.nhs.uk/nmapresearch/index.htm*).

Postdoctoral fellowships are available through the Nursing Midwifery and Allied Health Professions Research Training Scheme (*www.nmahpresearch-training.ac.uk/index.htm*).

A comprehensive overview of doctoral and postdoctoral fellowships available to candidates in Scotland is provided on the website of the Scottish School for Primary Care (*www.show.scot.nhs.uk/sspc/training/training_opps.html*).

In Northern Ireland, research fellowships are administered through the R&D office located with a Central Services Agency. Here there is a nurse appointed to facilitate the development of R&D within the nursing and allied health professions throughout the country (*www.centralservicesagency.com/display/rdo*).

Such fellowships are, however, highly sought after and application processes are very competitive. More discussion of these and other funding options can be found later in this chapter, and in the discussion on national research policy in Chapters 1 and 33.

Supervision

Those who embark on a formal research education course will be allocated one or more supervisors. It is very important that supervision relates to the methodological aspects of the study, the practical aspects of planning and conducting the research as well as to its subject matter. There is usually also need for supervision in the substantive topic – from a nutritionist, psychologist or nurse expert in the subject. Supervisors are there to discuss, challenge, guide and offer advice, not to do the project themselves. They need to be asked for help and are encouraged when students have done preparation and thought through the problems of conducting the research at theoretical, methodological and practical levels.

Most supervisors, especially if they are good and hence popular, will have heavy demands on their time. However if they are faced with a keen student who is well prepared, then demands are more likely to be met. Most higher educational institutions now prepare guidance for students and supervisors in managing projects and the supervision process. They are expected to set clear work targets and meet them. Choosing your supervisor wisely can make all the difference in benefiting from research training. Supervisors should themselves have substantial research experience before taking on supervision. It is wise to check their credentials, publications and the experiences of previous students before making your selection.

Advice about a specific project

Of course the need for advice could be at any stage of the research process. Initially, advice may be needed to help turn an unformed idea into a researchable question, as described in Chapter 6 of this book. Thereafter advice might be required at any stage from writing the proposal through to data analysis and publication. In general terms the earlier advice is sought the better, but it is also advisable to go to the right source of advice at each point. Many NHS R&D offices can offer general advice and guidance at the earliest stages of developing a research project. Staff in the R&D office should have a sufficiently broad overview of research to enable you to refine your ideas and begin to formulate possible directions for the project. The office may also be able to put you in touch with more experienced researchers in the trust, or in a local university, who can help you, or who may be able to include you in their research programme. For those working in primary or social care, it may be necessary to go to a local research consortium or network, as some health and social care organisations are too small to support an R&D office that has substantial practical research expertise.

Furthermore, some larger NHS trusts now employ a research advisory nurse, whose specific remit it is to develop nursing research capacity. It is important to bear in mind that it is not possible for any one individual to have detailed knowledge of every research problem with which they are faced, but nurses in research advisory roles should be able to assist you sufficiently to enable you to prepare to consult with someone with more specialist knowledge if this is warranted.

At a national level, the Department of Health National Co-ordinating Centre for Research Capacity Development (NCCRCD) funds a network of Research and Development Support Units (RDSUs) across England, and the Welsh Office has three in Wales. These units are usually located within university departments and have a range of capacity building functions including research training, individual advice and support, developing research networks and providing information resources for research. The RDSU network is a multidisciplinary one, but advice specific to nursing research is also available within many of the units. More information about your local unit is available from the Department of Health website under R&D research capacity development (look for research infrastructure section), or from your local health library. Trent RDSU (*www.trentrdsu.org.uk*) is the largest of these organisations in England and provides a comprehensive service including research training, research support and advice, and a primary care research network. In Scotland and Northern Ireland specific research units and networks have been created for nurses and allied health professionals to cover the whole of the country and to offer advice to those wishing to conduct health-related research. Sometimes specific research advisory mechanisms have been developed for nurses to assist them to get a toehold into research.

These local resources may not be specifically for nurses nor are they provided by nurses themselves and can come from a diverse range of scientific backgrounds. Whatever their background, personal recommendation of someone who is helpful is by far the best way of securing useful contacts. The message is to begin where you are and to use whatever talent is available locally before proceeding further. It is always appreciated if you arrive with well thought out questions and having prepared your material for the meeting.

Kindred spirits to provide emotional sustenance

Another type of support, which is rather different from specific advice or supervision for your project, is to find like-minded individuals who are carrying out research and facing similar problems. It is probably a universal finding that research workers at some point in developing or carrying out a project feel isolated, dejected, and ready to give up. At such times it is useful to share your experience with someone who may have gone through, or be in the process of facing the same distress. This is when membership of an informal or formal research group may be useful. There may be a local research interest group near you and these serve several functions. One of their strengths is bringing together people who have a general interest in learning about and supporting research. On the whole you are likely to find others with research interests very willing to help and listen, and offer support of different kinds. In this regard, the research networks in Scotland serve a useful function in bringing together people from a range of backgrounds and interests.

Other benefits to be gained from membership of a local research group are in hearing of current developments in research, nationally as well as locally, learning how others have gone about research and how they have attempted to overcome their particular difficulties. By providing an informal setting to discuss research issues generally, research meetings can be very positive occasions for those planning to begin, or already engaged in, research. Less formal get-togethers of nurses involved in research are also useful. Sometimes an informal lunchtime gathering of fellow students and new researchers is sufficient to air a difficulty and regain vital energies that may be dwindling.

At a national level the conferences organised by nursing organisations including the RCN annual international nursing research conference (*www.man.ac.uk/rcn/*) or specific clinical groups provide occasions for hearing research workers talk about their work. This is most effectively done at conferences that arrange opportunities for networking as well as hearing about recent developments and where special interest groups can meet to discuss particular issues. The RCN Research Society has both national and regional research networks as well as a PhD network specifically geared to supporting doctoral students. The RCN also supports a number of specialist research interest groups, e.g. research in child health (RICH) that operate at national and/or regional level, and provide e-mail communications at regular intervals.

The other kind of group or association worth considering joining are those with a more specific focus of interest; examples would be the Society for Tissue Viability, the British Society of Gerontology, the Society for Research in Rehabilitation, and the Society for Social Medicine. While their interests are not confined to research, a major part of their business is the discussion of current research and methods in their respective fields. These groups are of major importance in keeping abreast of developments that are broader than nursing and maintaining current awareness of findings and methods. Membership of such a group will bring you into contact with others who share an interest in a narrower substantive field. Gradually professional nursing groups like the RCN professional forums have developed research-oriented themes in their conferences and professional meetings so that they are a focal point for researchers and clinical practitioners alike.

Financial support

Financial assistance may be sought for research education or for funding a specific project. The opportunities available for research education described above may also carry remuneration with them.

Funding for research education and training

The funds apportioned to research education within the health service are highly variable, though should gradually become standardised through the Workforce Development Confederations in each Strategic Health Authority. At present there is a variable system of bursaries available for taught research courses at masters level, and national systems of fellowships for doctoral and postdoctoral level research. The Department of Health, in England, has now integrated its awards schemes for different professional group into one, while in Scotland the Chief

Scientist Office and the Nursing Midwifery and Allied Health Professions Research (NMAHP) Training Scheme provides training fellowships specifically for nurses, midwives and allied health professions. Similarly in Northern Ireland research training fellowships are being offered through the R&D Office.

Many charitable organisations such as The Health Foundation offer fellowships that are open to nurses along with other health professions and some, such as those given by the Smith & Nephew Foundation, are open only to nurses. Such fellowships are highly competitive, but once awarded provide a unique form of support for the individual wishing to advance in a research career, with salary, training and research expenses paid over a number of years.

Many nurses will also be able to access partial or full funding for research education through their employer, via a clinical directorate, or NHS R&D office.

Funding for individual projects

In financial terms, far more money is available for funding individual projects than for research training. In nursing the problem to date is not that there is not the funding but that there is a shortfall in the number of nurses with the experience needed to attract it from the most competitive sources. Grant awarding bodies are unlikely to fund research proposed by an inexperienced would-be researcher with no evidence of their capability of managing a research project. It is naïve to expect funding without a track record so how does one ever get a foot in the door?

There are no short answers. Traditionally individuals build up research credibility by publishing findings, working with experienced researchers and learning the craft from them. By so doing one gradually develops a reputation sufficient to enable grants to be awarded on the basis of sound proposals. Research funding is available to nurses in some of the health-related charities as well as central government research funds, the NHS Health Technology Assessment (HTA) Programme and the Research Councils. The Department of Health's Service Delivery and Organisation (SDO) Programme now has a specific funding stream in which calls are made periodically for proposals on nursing related issues (see Box 2.1 in Chapter 2 for an example). Researchers responding to such calls do not themselves have to be nurses, but are likely to benefit from having a nurse as a member of the research team. Such calls are, however, ideal opportunities for experienced nurse researchers to become lead applicants or principal investigators.

Most research funds are not earmarked for nurses but are open to competition on the basis of the quality of the proposal. In some ways, nurses are disadvantaged by the membership of many funding bodies being medically rather than health oriented and with a preference for particular approaches to research. However this is changing, as qualitative as well as quantitative methods become more widely accepted, and nursing research becomes increasingly sophisticated in both its range of methodological approaches and in presenting its case, and as multi-disciplinary applied research becomes more valued.

Many research funding sources operate in 'response mode' – that is, they will respond to proposals originating from the applicants. Increasingly, however, priority areas are being identified and proposals invited in line with specified topics. This is not a bar to nurses applying for funding so long as their proposals are in line with what is requested. It is important, therefore, to know what the priorities of different funding agencies are, what the policy imperatives behind research questions are, and to ensure that proposals are appropriately targeted.

Funding at local level

To assist novices, some larger NHS trusts and research capacity building organisations make small amounts of money available for small grants (for example £5000–10 000) to local researchers, which do not have to go through such a stringent peer-review process for those new to research. To obtain a small grant the project being prepared often has to be seen as pilot work leading to a more substantial, externally funded, research project. It may be available to assist in funding higher degree work, but will not be awarded unless what is being prepared is of high quality and feasible within the resources being asked for. Additionally, NHS trusts are expected to put forward cohesive programmes of research in particular priority areas, e.g. care of older people, diabetes, and your small project will stand a better chance of being funded if it fits into an existing local priority.

Searching for funding sources

The first port of call for sources of research funding should probably be the website RDInfo (*www.rdinfo.org.uk*) run by Leeds University. This website has a search facility that enables you to request a list of funding sources by topic or keyword, by closing date, or by size of grant requested. Having found a possible source of funding, the website will then provide a link through to the webpage of the funding body itself, so that you can read more about the conditions of the award. Application forms are often then available online, or on request by telephone or e-mail. This useful website includes a wide range of health-related research grants, in both subject area and size of grant, and from major programme grants to grants for small pieces of equipment or for travel. RDInfo also carries a range of practical guides to doing research, available by clicking on the appropriate buttons of the opening webpage.

A directory of charities is available online at (*www.charitychoice.co.uk/*). Although not specifically for nursing or health-related charities, the online directory is searchable by category (e.g. 'health' or 'medical research'), and many of these organisations provide small amounts of money for educational purposes but some also indicate a willingness to finance research projects. Other sources of availability of grants for research are listed at the end of the chapter.

Finance for research may also be attracted from industry and commerce, particularly the pharmaceutical companies and those devoted to other health products. Some companies like 3M, Smith & Nephew and Nutricia annually award scholarships, but *ad hoc* projects may also be funded. Commercial concerns could probably be more widely used than they are but sometimes ethical considerations intervene. It is wise to ensure, if accepting research funding from a commercial source, that you will be free to publish and disseminate the results in your own name, regardless of the findings. The issue of 'intellectual property' is a complex legal one, and advice should be sought from your employing organisation if you have any concerns.

Chapter 9 in this volume deals with writing a proposal, which is only one facet of attracting research money, but a crucial one. The proposal, irrespective of its scientific merits, must prove sufficiently appealing to attract sponsorship and there is an art in preparing such a submission. Research proposals need to be carefully targeted at appropriate funding agencies. Novices typically would be advised to gain some experience of working as a member of an established research team before bidding for substantial research funds as a lead researcher.

Information resources

While information resources have been placed last, they are by no means least in importance. Anyone wishing to carry out research will need to know what has already been published on the topic. For this reason libraries and other information services are integral to research development. Chapter 7 describes major sources of research information that are largely accessible through on-line and electronic facilities.

While using these abstracting and indexing sources is important for individuals to keep abreast of current literature, group efforts to share knowledge and reading can be stimulating and beneficial. In some clinical and academic departments, journal clubs meet on a regular basis to discuss recent important publications and to inform participants of useful papers and books. By allocating particular journals to members and sharing the reading, an enormous amount of scanning can be shared and useful items located which might otherwise have been missed. Journal clubs have the added advantage of encouraging discussion, learning how others regard methods and findings, and generally sharpening research awareness. An active journal club demonstrates to others the importance placed on knowing what is happening nationally and internationally. They are, therefore, as important for 'users' as for 'doers' of research.

Conclusion

No matter who you are, or the degree of development in your research career, support is necessary to carry out research. This chapter has done little more than indicate some of the sources of such support in getting started and moving towards a research career. It would be easy to consider support purely in financial terms; for research education or to fund a project to buy staff time or materials. This is only part of the story. Just as important are sources of support that are sustaining in both intellectual and emotional terms. One has only to read the acknowledgements section of any thesis to find reference to the assistance given by supervisors and colleagues, not to mention long-suffering family and patients. Often it is the generosity of others in terms of their time, intellectual application, listening ability and advice, as well as their skills in motivating and encouraging others to write proposals and reports, which enable research to succeed.

The research community itself is perhaps the most important supportive agency. Researchers, by their willingness to give the same encouragement and assistance to others that they themselves have received, are an important source of mutual support. Used wisely they are of incalculable benefit.

Further reading

Leonard D (2001) *A Woman's Guide to Doctoral Studies*. Buckingham, Open University Press

Phillips EM, Pugh DS (2001) *How to get a PhD*. Buckingham, Open University Press

Websites

www.man.ac.uk/rcn/ – the RCN's research co-ordinating centre is probably the single most useful source of and access to relevant information. This site offers links not only to information about research activities in the RCN but to R&D in all of the areas of England, Northern Ireland, Wales and Scotland. It provides details of local research networks, funding opportunities, training and support units. There are also links to the National Research Register of completed and ongoing research projects funded by the Department of Health, to the main NHS research programmes and to the web pages of some research organisations. Accessing this site offers a very quick route into a great deal of useful information

(*www.rdinfo.org.uk*) – RDInfo provides a comprehensive and searchable database of funding sources for research. This is not specific to nursing research but includes many funding opportunities to which nurses can apply. The website also has general research advice and information about research ethics and governance procedures

www.fons.org/ – the Foundation of Nursing Studies is a useful organisation for those who are interested more in the application of research in practice. They offer courses and funding for research implementation projects.

www.charitychoice.co.uk/ – searchable directory of grant-giving charities

www.rdlearning.org.uk/ – RDLearning is a website, associated with RDInfo, which details health-related research training courses available throughout the UK. A search facility is available to locate courses specific to your needs

www.rddirect.org.uk/ – general research advice and an opportunity for healthcare researchers to e-mail or telephone for individualised advice

www.dh.gov.uk/ – the Department of Health website has a section devoted to research and development where you can find details of the main government-funded research programmes, the research capacity development programme, and government priorities for research

www.nccrcd.nhs.uk/ – the National Co-ordinating Centre for Research Capacity Building website lists the RDSUs and other sources of research support

5 User Involvement in Research

Gordon Grant and Paul Ramcharan

Key points

- User involvement has emerged in the context of new research approaches, in the political move towards consumerism, the public service orientation and localisation of services and within a policy and practice context that recognises that those best placed to inform service development are those on the receiving end of such services.
- User involvement in research ranges on a continuum from consultation with users, through partnerships in a collaborative model, to complete user control. Each of these may apply to different parts of the research process.
- User control tends to be equated with a commitment to emancipatory principles and therefore with political actions to improve the lives of service users through the removal of barriers to their health, social inclusion, and citizenship.
- More work is required in the development of user involvement in research and in making judgements about different approaches. Involvement itself should be seen as being fit for purpose and not an end in itself. Attention should be paid to the inclusion of groups that have been marginalised, hard-to-find or lacking in capacity.

Introduction

Recent government endorsement of the importance of the user voice has served to strengthen a growing commitment to user involvement in nursing research from many quarters; charitable trusts that fund research, user organisations and activists, as well as advocacy organisations and the wider research community. Evidence has been accumulating about the engagement of service users in different parts of the research process (INVOLVE 2004) but many first-hand accounts by users themselves remain anecdotal. The rhetoric of user involvement in research has, however, encountered methodological and other challenges in its practical implementation.

In this chapter, we therefore consider:

- why user involvement in health and social care research has become popular
- how user involvement in research has been depicted
- some experiences of user involvement in research

- ethical and methodological questions associated with a commitment to user involvement in research

A brief history of user involvement in research

User involvement in research has a rich and long history and extends at least as far back as the genesis of action research (*see* for example Lees & Smith 1975) and the early forays into community development research commonly associated with developing countries (*see* for example, Freire 1968; Richards 1985). Within social science circles the 1980s saw major questions raised about Grand Theory (i.e. those social theories designed to understand the whole of society and human action), a move to localisation and user involvement in health and social care (Hadley & Hatch 1981) and the emergence of participatory politics (Richardson 1983). The problem was, and remains, how ordinary citizens are best involved in decisions about how public services affect their lives.

The political response in the UK in the 1970s and 1980s under Margaret Thatcher and then later under John Major was the marketisation of health and social welfare and consumerism such as that represented by the *Citizen's Charter* (1991). This 'public service orientation' (Clarke & Stewart 1987) involved promoting:

- closeness to the customer and citizen
- listening to the public
- access for the public
- service from the public's point of view
- the views, suggestions and complaints of users
- the public's right to know
- an emphasis on service quality
- public opinion as a test of quality

Recognition of the importance of the user voice quickly found its way into national policy. Over 20 years ago it featured in the innovative All Wales Strategy for the Development of Services for Mentally Handicapped People (*sic*) (Welsh Office 1983) that emphasised the right of service users and their families to be involved in the planning, management, delivery and review of services. The primacy of public and user involvement is now firmly embedded within the NHS Plan (Department of Health 2000a), in research and development policy (Department of Health 2000b), in the National Service Frameworks, and in the White Paper *Valuing People* (Department of Health 2001a) in which people with learning disabilities helped to shape policy itself under the banner of 'nothing about us without us' (People First London *et al.* 2000).

It is easy for researchers to claim that users are involved in research, but in conventional forms of research this typically means that users are passive or compliant subjects with no hand in prioritising, commissioning, planning, undertaking, disseminating or utilising research. More recently users have been challenging this position, the disability movement being particularly vocal and effective in this respect (Moore *et al.* 1998). For some years now leading research funding bodies like the Joseph Rowntree Foundation and the National Lottery Charities Board (now the Big Lottery Fund) have been exceptions in adopting a more open and inclusive approach to research that includes service users, especially those who are vulnerable. INVOLVE, formerly Consumers in NHS Research, has been established and officially sanctioned by the government to promote good practice in research committed to user involvement, but with a remit extending to social care as well as health care research. INVOLVE (2004) suggest user involvement in research may be valuable because people who use services:

- will offer different perspectives
- can help to make sure that research priorities are important to them
- can help to ensure that money and resources are not wasted on research that has little or no relevance
- can ensure that research does not just measure outcomes that others (academics and professionals) consider important
- can recruit their peers for research projects
- are better placed to access people who are often marginalised (i.e. 'hard-to-reach' groups in research terms)
- can help with the dissemination and implementation of research findings
- can be empowered through taking part
- are involved in the increasing political priority of involving consumers around the services they receive

So what does this growing experience add up to? Are assumptions about the value of user involvement in research, such as those identified by INVOLVE, mirrored in practice? In order to address such questions we need to be rather more discriminating in how we account for user involvement in research.

Mapping user involvement in nursing and nursing-related research

A cursory glance at the nursing and nursing-related research literature now shows growing evidence of user involvement, for example learning disabilities (Ham *et al.* 2004; Richardson 2002), mental health (Trivedi & Wykes 2002), forensic mental health (Faulkner & Morris 2003; Simpson *et al.* 2003), elder care (Tetley & Hanson 2000; Tetley *et al.* 2003), cancer and palliative care (Seymour & Skilbeck 2002; Maslin-Prothero 2003), primary care (Thornton *et al.* 2003) and back pain care (Ong & Hooper 2003). Box 5.1 provides an example of user involvement.

The Faulkner and Morris report (Box 5.1) is singularly applied to the field of forensic mental health. Consider your own practice field. How far has user involvement in research gone?

> **Box 5.1**   User involvement in mental health research.
>
> Faulkner A, Morris B (2003) *User Involvement in Forensic Mental Health Research and Development*. Liverpool, NHS National Programme on Mental Health Research and Development
>
> In this expert paper the authors report that user involvement in forensic mental health research is currently limited to small-scale consultations and audits. Issues associated with the need to maintain security, confidentiality and the protection of individuals appear to be challenging user involvement in research as well as in services. At the present time there is thought to be no magic formula, implying therefore that it is necessary to continue testing and evaluating different ways of involving users in research. Based on evidence assembled the report suggests principles, encompassing procedures and ethics, that may be helpful in guiding good practice.

In describing the range of activity conducted under the banner of user involvement in research there has been a tendency to adopt one or both of two extremes, i.e. user control versus researcher control. Similarly the Consumers in NHS Research Group (2001) suggest that involvement may entail:

- *consultation* – where consumers are consulted with no sharing of power in the decision-making
- *collaboration* – that involves an active ongoing partnership with consumers in the research process
- *user control* – where consumers design, undertake, and disseminate the results of a research project

There are advantages and disadvantages associated with each of these levels of involvement. We briefly examine these in relation to a case study (Box 5.2) provided by Rodgers (1999).

Consultation

The main advantage of a *consultation* approach is that it is simple. It enables people to express their views without a commitment to act upon them, and it can feel safe when people have not been involved before. The disadvantages are that involvement without action can lead to frustration; consultation fatigue can set in; and ideas may be constrained by the agenda of those in power, so some people may not see it as worthwhile unless they are full partners. The case study shows that there was consultation involved in establishing the research interest and in various parts of the research process. It also indicates that the development of the research idea was not purely an unencumbered product of the users' interests. However, the gatekeeping role of ethics committees and services tended not to confer as high a value on the user voice independent of those of 'professionals'.

> **Box 5.2** Case study 1: involving people with learning disabilities in research.
>
> Rodgers J (1999) Trying to get it right: undertaking research involving people with learning difficulties. *Disability and Society* 14:4 421–433
>
> Rodgers aimed to examine the health of 30 people with learning difficulties from their own point of view. The research interest was partly prompted by a consultation with a group of women with learning difficulties who raised issues about health and medical care. However, it also reflected the interests of both the researcher and the local health services. Rodgers had to gain permission for the research from several quarters (ethics committees, GPs, parents and services) as well as from the research participants. People with learning disabilities were employed as consultants to the study and developed research questions that gave new insights into health from their point of view. They also helped in developing plain language findings summaries, and took part in the interviewing with the main researcher. However, Rodgers found it hard to include them in the analysis of data.

Collaboration

In a *collaborative* approach there are more likely to be outcome measures, assessment criteria and forms of evaluation relevant to consumers; as collaborators consumers can help to recruit research participants; in dealing with consent issues; and consumers can feel a greater sense of ownership. The disadvantages appear to be related to the heightened user commitment, associated issues of time and cost, the supports that may be needed to sustain commitment, and the problematical nature of power sharing. In the case study article, Rodgers reports that although people with learning difficulties were supposed to be interviewers they seldom took a lead role.

User control

Finally in the *user control* approach, the main advantages are tied to the greater likelihood of being able to address questions not thought of by academic researchers; prospects of revealing evidence missed by other researchers; an even higher sense of ownership and therefore a fuller commitment to research dissemination. There are also raised prospects for the empowerment of service users. Disadvantages relate to the relative lack of experience and expertise of users in the conduct of the research; higher research costs; the lack of evidence about what constitutes good research facilitation and support for user researchers; and therefore some fears that user-controlled research may not be as independent as it seems.

Rodgers reports in the case study article that analysis continued as the research took place so that subsequent interviews could reflect emergent issues, but she adds that:

> 'I found it hard to contemplate how methodological considerations that I found challenging could be made more accessible to people with learning difficulties.' (Rodgers 1999: 431)

Rodgers does claim that there was success in turning complex ideas into plain language in reporting the findings and that this could not have been done without the co-researchers. However, despite her best efforts, the research was commissioned neither by people with learning difficulties nor their allies; it was not wholly controlled by people with learning difficulties; and it was greatly affected in its orientation by other stakeholders from service, professional and governance sectors. In short, user control of research is not an easy ideal to accomplish.

We can see in the case study an implicit reliance on understanding levels of involvement alongside different parts of the research process, a position formalised by Faulkner and Morris (2003) and summarised in Figure 5.1. However, while providing a framework for understanding, Figure 5.1 does not directly address what value should be placed on each combination of activities, and whether any are meaningful and relevant to service users. One way of approaching this last question is to ask about the values and principles that should be attached to user involvement in research.

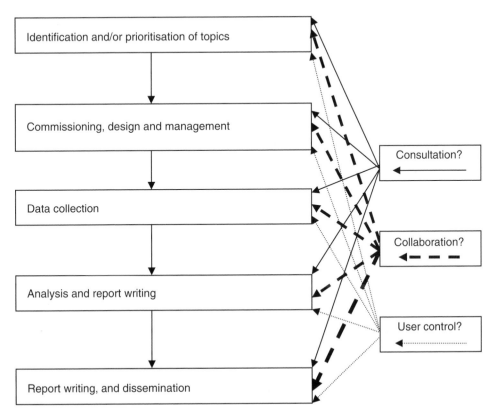

Figure 5.1 Possible levels of involvement at different stages of the research process.

In a consensus study Telford *et al.* (2004) developed a series of principles and indicators about the successful involvement of consumers in research. Consensus was reached among a wide range of research participants on eight principles. The principles are worth listing (adapted from Telford *et al.* 2004).

- Research roles of consumers and researchers are agreed.
- Budgets should include all costs of consumer involvement in research.
- Researchers respect the differing skills, knowledge and experience of consumers.
- Consumers are offered training and personal support, to aid their research involvement.
- Researchers ensure that they have the necessary skills to involve consumers in the research process.
- Consumers are involved in decisions about how participants are both recruited and kept informed about the progress of the research.
- Consumer involvement is described in research reports.
- Research findings are made available to consumers, in formats and in language they can easily understand.

Consensus-based principles have an instant appeal but, as the authors themselves suggest, the value and utility of these principles have yet to be established with reference to different research methodologies and models of consumer involvement.

The application of general principles like these may well have rather limited utility when considered against forms of participatory or participatory-action and emancipatory research. This may become clearer when we consider how these forms of research differ in their stated purposes, philosophy and methods, and therefore in terms of the roles and allegiances required of users. These are summarised in Box 5.3.

It is important to say that Box 5.3 is very much a simplification of broad categories of research.

Traditional research as used here refers to those forms of scholarly endeavour that are based on careful hypothesis testing, coupled with testing of the generalisability of findings. Experimental designs, randomised controlled design studies, population sample surveys, and many kinds of service evaluation studies fall within this broad category and generally require high technical expertise.

Participatory research is another very broad category. For Cocks and Cockram (1995:32), participatory research involves a research question being brought to the attention of (disabled) people; (disabled) people and researchers working together to achieve a collective analysis; and alliances formed between (disabled) people and others to make changes following research. The potential methods of research have been suggested as discussion groups, public meetings, the establishment of investigative research teams, community seminars, factfinding tours, the collective production of educational material, the use of popular theatre and educational camps or retreats.

Box 5.3 Parameters of traditional, participatory and emancipatory research.

Parameter	Traditional	Participatory	Emancipatory
Ownership of research	Held by academic researchers	Joint/shared	Held by service users
Values	Value-neutral	Shared/negotiated	Political, partisan, reflecting user interests
Accountability	To academic peers, host organisation, funding agency	To research group, host organisation, funding agency	To co-researchers (service users), host organisation, funding agency
Focus of enterprise	Science and accumulation of generalisable knowledge; an emphasis on limited forms of research dissemination	Articulation of user voice; an emphasis on research dissemination and utilisation	Orientation towards changing or improving people's lives and opportunities; an emphasis on research utilisation to bring about change in people's everyday lives
Locus of control for change	External	Internal and external	Internal, generated by service user research group
Concepts, methodology	Imposed	Product of process, evolutionary	Product of process, evolutionary
Research dissemination	Written for academic audiences, therefore likely to be published in academic journals	Could be written for a multiplicity of audiences, therefore found in academic and popular outlets, and grey literature	Likely to be written mostly for user audiences, often located in grey literature and on user organisation websites
Costliness	Can be costly	Can be costly	Expensive
Sources of funding	Widespread	Growing	Very limited; still constrained by lack of official backing for putting evidence into practice

Emancipatory research, on the other hand, represents the overt politicisation of research in which the researcher struggles for *transformative change* (Barnes 2003) as a direct product of the research experience. Chappell (2000), reviewing the contributions of Zarb, Morris and Oliver, points to key features of emancipatory research as:

- being a tool for improving people's lives
- providing opportunities for (disabled) people to be researchers themselves
- involving a more reflexive stance
- being commissioned by democratic organisations of (disabled) people
- having an accountability to democratic organisations of (disabled) people

Yet Chappell argues that very little emancipatory research has been funded by or accountable to organisations of (disabled) people. Of course a possible reason for this is that few such organisations are in the financial position to fund programmes of research. The difficulties of accomplishing such an approach are also clear in our consideration of the earlier case study.

Taking *traditional, participatory and emancipatory* research as points of reference allows us to pose rather more discriminating questions about the status of user involvement, as well as emergent good practice.

In the case of *traditional* research it would be wrong to assume that user involvement does not have an important place. The new research governance and ethics arrangements (Department of Health 2001b), should at least ensure that inclusion/exclusion criteria, and consent and capacity issues affecting users, are accorded their proper status much as with any kind of research. Hence the right to participate in research, but also the accompanying rights to protection and well-being, are to be afforded to everyone. However some categories of service users are frequently excluded from traditional research, possibly on spurious grounds. For example, in the earlier case study Rodgers was instructed to 'seek permission' from both the GP and family carer of each interviewee in the research and this affected who was finally recruited. People with serious mental health problems, people with severe learning disabilities, and others where capacity to consent may be an issue are often subject to exclusion. Policy guidance on this matter is unfortunately rather confused at this time. It asserts that the presumption of capacity, while stating that:

> 'It is not appropriate to carry out research on adults who cannot give consent for themselves, if the research can instead be carried out on adults who are able to give or withhold consent. The only exception to this rule would be where clinicians believe that it is in the person's best interests to be involved in research'(Department of Health 2001c:15).

Given the contradictions and ambiguities, it is easy for researchers to 'play safe' by excluding people in these categories. The wider research ethics issues involved are discussed more fully in Chapter 3.

Most published evidence about user involvement concerns *participatory* research. By its very nature participatory research is predicated on strong alliances and partnerships between those involved. In principle potentially all the stages of the research process are shared. In practice this is much less the case. As the example from Ong and Hooper's study (Box 5.4) indicates, there is no guarantee of a strong alliance between people who share particular symptoms. There are also potential variations between what constitute such alliances dependent upon the user groups themselves. People with learning disabilities, for example, are likely to experience a lifetime to form their alliances. In contrast pregnant women or those with treatable critical illnesses may only be users over a short period. The concept and meaning of alliances may therefore differ substantially between different user groups.

Moreover it is not uncommon for academic researchers to go looking for user organisations as partners, pre-armed with research questions where the research interest was a product of several competing interests such as in the case of Rodgers (Box 5.2: case study 1). Participatory research can also be a messy business: power relations between those involved having to be tested and retested; accommodations required between the various partner organisations that fund the research, employ workers or support users; with research methods being worked out as things proceed. The rhetoric of participation sounds very rosy; the reality on the other hand can be quite different (Walmsley & Johnson 2003).

Emancipatory research, much of it tied to social model thinking within the disability field (Barnes 2003), seeks to address and deal with social, political and environmental factors that perpetuate forms of exclusion or oppression in people's lives and, given a paucity of research using its principles, remains largely aspirational. It takes a particular kind of person to commit themselves to this kind of research, and resilience to see things through to the end, particularly in the later

---

Box 5.4   Case Study 2: involving users in low back pain research.

Ong BN, Hooper H (2003) Involving users in low back pain research. *Health Expectations*, 6: 332–341

The aim of this study was to determine how patient and professional perceptions of low back pain and its treatment relate to the use of healthcare and to subsequent outcomes. Focus groups were held with GPs, other healthcare practitioners and low back pain sufferers. Tensions arose between involving patients (users) as co-researchers both in designing research tools and in sharing their experiences of low back pain. However, sharing experiences became a problem over emotive issues with some contributors seeking to place an emphasis on areas relating to their own experiences over those of others. It was therefore considered that agreeing a certain distance from personal experiences may be a prerequisite for formulating a research agenda, especially when discussing emotive issues and that this kind of dilemma might be the product of the focus group process.

action stages. As the example in Box 5.4 also demonstrates, there are often 'structural impediments' such as lack of funding through user organisations, lack of support from services and professionals, and with ethical and governance issues that make such research difficult to accomplish in practice.

Challenges for user involvement in nursing and nursing-related research

The practicalities of user involvement in research still leave some important unanswered questions that are illustrated below.

Fitness for purpose

As has been illustrated, different kinds of research require different commitments from users, their supporters, researchers and others. It is useful to think of user involvement strategies being informed and led by the purposes and goals of individual research projects, that is they need to be *fit for purpose*. To involve people as an 'end in itself' can lead to tokenism where there is no role to be played by users and no clear gain for either side. There are as yet no published criteria against which to measure fitness for purpose in relation to traditional, participatory and emancipatory research.

Questions remain about why user involvement in some parts of the research process has been more likely than others. INVOLVE's website reveals a database of 181 projects at the time of writing. These confirm that users are involved to varying extents in key stages of the projects listed (*see* Table 5.1). Early stages of the process, especially prioritising research topic areas and planning research, appear to have quite high proportions of users involved. Writing publications and implementing action appear to involve users least of all. Why users appear to be less involved in writing publications is less clear at this time, although collabora-

Table 5.1 Summary of user involvement in research projects listed on the INVOLVE website.*

Stage of involvement	Number of projects	%
Prioritising research topic areas	120	66
Planning research	139	77
Managing research	91	50
Designing research instruments	131	72
Undertaking research	94	52
Analysing research	85	47
Writing publications	61	34
Disseminating	101	56
Implementing action	63	35

*As at December 2004

tive writing, especially when directed towards academic publishing, can generate tensions between user and academic researchers. More accounts are required about how these issues are best addressed.

User involvement and excluded groups

As suggested in relation to traditional forms of research it is easy to exclude categories of people on grounds of mental capacity. Unfortunately, people can be excluded for other reasons too. People may be 'invisible', meaning that they can be 'lost' in service systems through poor case records; lost 'outside the service system' because they have lost contact with services (many people with mild learning disabilities for example); or they may 'lack voice' or articulacy (following stroke, head injury or the onset of dementia for example). Those who are marginalised may pose researcher–user translation problems both at a cultural and language level especially where there are no assistive technologies for communication. Indeed, Rodgers in Box 5.2 above notes that,

'The inclusion of people with more severe impairments meant that there were times when I was not able to talk directly with the person concerned.' (Rodgers 1999: 427)

This forced her to rely instead on carers or advocates who knew the person well. The roles that advocates, proxies and guardians play here as spokespersons or enablers for such users in research are matters warranting closer study.

The indications are that articulate service users or those closely connected to user organisations are most likely to be involved in participatory and emancipatory research. If this is indeed the case it raises further issues about whose voices are being represented in such research, and whether this matters.

Weighing user experiences – learning disability as a case example

In this light, user views and experiences also prove complex. Such experiences are seldom unitary. For example, in a review of the views and experiences of people with learning disabilities Ramcharan and Grant (2001) point to a range of research products: 'testaments of life' (e.g. life histories, narrative accounts); 'user movement media' incorporating materials published by self-advocacy groups and those available on the web; and 'research-based studies' in which a range of experiences are collected from people with learning disabilities. In these varied accounts there are issues relating to how best to judge:

- the extent to which non-disabled researchers have set the agenda of experiences from which to draw

- the difficulties of translation that are often required to bring the voices to a wider audience
- the representativeness of the voices heard relating their experiences
- the power of users in the research process

As part of our own work as academic co-ordinators of the Department of Health Learning Disability Research Initiative (LDRI) linked to the implementation of Valuing People (Department of Health 2001a), we have involved people with learning disabilities in commissioning a nationally-funded research initiative as well as advising on dissemination strategies. Service users were paid accepted consultancy rates and involved as:

- members of the research commissioning group
- reviewers whose expert knowledge was used in assessing proposals against criteria relating to the involvement of people with learning disabilities in the funded research projects and whether the research was likely to change the lives of people for the better

Research applicants were asked to provide easy-to-read as well as technical research proposals so that judgments could be made about the capacity of research-ers to produce information in accessible formats. Dissemination at three annual research seminars has brought together service users with academics, managers and civil servants. Newsletters about the LDRI have incorporated plain language summaries to reach user as well as academic and policy audiences. The final project to be commissioned under the initiative is a user-led study, supported by INVOLVE and Values into Action (VIA), which is evaluating the arrangements for user involvement in the remaining 12 projects.

Comments from participants have suggested that involvement was welcomed though the practice related to implementation was not seen by users as unprob-lematic. Among the issues they raised were more time for their personal assistants to 'talk them through' their allocated proposals, prior training, feedback to know where the funding was allocated and quicker financial reimbursement. Users on the research commissioning group felt that people listened to them, and that their views made a real difference to decision-making, though they would have liked more service users to be members of the group.

In cancer care research it has similarly been shown that there are creative avenues for involving consumers in regional and local forums where research priority setting and commissioning takes place, for example, in the North Trent Cancer Research Network (NTRCN) (Stevens et al. 2003). In the NTRCN consum-ers have an equal say in deciding what research ideas should be developed and funded, in identifying topics of particular interest to themselves, and in being part of a recruitment panel that appoints researchers. In addition, sponsored confer-ences for consumers have added to this voice. Dimensions of this experience are being independently evaluated.

Conclusion

Above we have considered how and why user involvement has become popular. We have shown how it might be categorised in terms of the level of involvement i.e. via consultation, collaboration or control. Categorisations emerging from theoretical research perspectives have been outlined, i.e. the consumer involvement, participatory and emancipatory models. We have sought to examine how each of these categorisations might be used in understanding the place of users within the research process; and, most importantly, we have pointed out using a case study that there remain a substantial number of issues still to be addressed in the field of user involvement in research.

There is much potential to the involvement of users in research but this potential remains to be more fully demonstrated and substantiated. The survival of the approach is therefore at a critical point in its history.

References

Barnes C (2003) What a difference a decade makes: reflections on doing 'emancipatory' disability research. *Disability and Society* 18: 3–17

Chappell AL (2000) Emergence of participatory methodology in learning disability research: understanding the context. *British Journal of Learning Disabilities* 28: 38–43

Clarke M, Stewart J (1987) The public service orientation: issues and dilemmas. *Public Administration* 65: 161–177

Citizen's Charter (1991) Cm. 1599. London, HMSO

Cocks E, Cockram J (1995) The participatory research paradigm and intellectual disability. *Mental Handicap Research* 8:1 25–37

Consumers in NHS Research (2001) *Getting Involved in Research: a guide for consumers.* Eastleigh, Consumers in NHS Research

Department of Health (2000a) *The NHS Plan: a plan for investment, a plan for reform.* Cm. 4818. London, Stationery Office

Department of Health (2000b) *Research and Development for a First Class Service: R&D funding in the new NHS.* London, Department of Health

Department of Health (2001a) *Valuing People: a new strategy for learning disability for the 21st century.* Cm. 5085. London, Stationery Office

Department of Health (2001b) *Research Governance Framework for Health and Social Care.* London, Department of Health

Department of Health (2001c) *Seeking Consent: working with people with learning disabilities.* London, Stationery Office

Faulkner A, Morris B (2003) *User Involvement in Forensic Mental Health Research.* Liverpool, NHS National Programme on Forensic Mental Health Research and Development

Freire P (1968) *Pedagogy of the Oppressed.* New York, Seabury Press

Hadley R, Hatch S (1981) *Social Welfare and the Failure of the State: centralized social services and participatory alternatives.* London, Allen and Unwin

Ham M, Jones N, Mansell I, Northway R, Price L, Walker G (2004) 'I'm a researcher!' Working together to gain ethical approval for a participatory research study. *Journal of Learning Disabilities* 8:4 397–407

INVOLVE (2004) *Involving the Public in NHS, Public Health, and Social Care Research: briefing notes for researchers*. Eastleigh, INVOLVE

Lees R, Smith G (1975) *Action-Research in Community Development*. London, Routledge and Kegan Paul

Maslin-Prothero S (2003) Developing user involvement in research. *Journal of Clinical Nursing* 12: 412–421

Moore M, Beazley S, Maelzer J (1998) *Researching Disability Issues*. Buckingham, Open University Press

Ong BN, Hooper H (2003) Involving users in low back pain research. *Health Expectations* 6: 332–341

People First London, Change, Speaking Up in Cambridge and Royal Mencap (2000) *Nothing About Us Without Us: The Learning Disability Strategy:* The User Group Report. London, Department of Health

Ramcharan P, Grant G (2001) Views and experiences of people with intellectual disabilities and their families 1: the user perspective. *Journal of Applied Research in Intellectual Disabilities* 14: 348–63

Richards H (1985) The *Evaluation of Cultural Action: An evaluation study of the parents and children's program*. London, The Macmillan Press

Richardson M (2002) Involving people in the analysis: listening, reflecting, discounting nothing. *Journal of Learning Disabilities* 6:1 47–60

Richardson A (1983) *Participation*. London, Routledge

Rodgers J (1999) Trying to get it right: undertaking research involving people with learning difficulties. *Disability and Society* 14:4 421–433

Seymour J, Skilbeck J (2002) Ethical considerations in researching user views. *European Journal of Cancer Care* 11:3 215–219

Simpson EL, Barkham M, Gilbody S, House A. (2003) Involving service users as researchers for the evaluation of adult statutory mental health services. (Protocol) *The Cochrane Database of Systematic Reviews* 2003, Issue 4.

Stevens T, Wilde D, Hunt J, Ahmedzai SH (2003) Overcoming the challenges of consumer involvement in cancer research, *Health Expectations* 6: 81–88

Telford R, Boote JD, Cooper CL (2004) What does it mean to involve consumers successfully in research? A consensus study. *Health Expectations* 7: 209–220

Tetley J, Haynes L, Hawthorne M, Odeyemi J, Skinner J, Smith D, Wilson V (2003) Older people and research partnerships. *Quality in Ageing* 4:4 18–23

Tetley J, Hanson E (2000) Participatory research. *Nurse Researcher* 8:1 69–88

Thornton H, Edwards A, Elwyn G (2003) Evolving the multiple roles of 'patients' in health-care research: reflections after involvement in a trial of shared decision-making. *Health Expectations* 6: 189–197

Trivedi P, Wykes T (2002) From passive subjects to equal partners: qualitative review of user involvement in research. *British Journal of Psychiatry* 181: 468–472

Walmsley J, Johnson K (2003) *Inclusive Research with People with Learning Disabilities: past, present and futures*. London, Jessica Kingsley

Welsh Office (1983) *All Wales Strategy for the Development of Services for Mentally Handicapped People*. Cardiff, Welsh Office

Zarb G (1992) On the road to Damascus: first steps towards changing the relations of disability research production. *Disability, Handicap and Society* 7: 125–138

Further reading

Morris J (1991) *Pride Against Prejudice: transforming attitudes to disability*. London, Women's Press

Oliver M (1997) Emancipatory research: realistic goal or impossible dream? In Barnes C, Mercer G (eds) *Doing Disability Research*. Leeds, Disability Press pp15–31

Ramcharan P, Grant G, Flynn M (2004) Emancipatory and participatory research: how far have we come? In Emerson E, Hatton C, Thompson T, Parmenter TR (eds) *The International Handbook of Applied Research in Intellectual Disabilities*. Chichester, John Wiley

Websites

www.qrd.alzheimers.org.uk/ – Alzheimer's Association Quality Research in Dementia Programme (QRD) provides information for member and prospective members of the QRD consumer network and researchers

www.biglotteryfund.org.uk/ – details of funding programmes to support research involving users.

www.ceres.org.uk/ – Consumers for Ethics in Research (CERES), independent charity set up to promote informed debate about research and help users of health services to develop and publicise their views on health research

www.invo.org.uk/ – INVOLVE is a national advisory group, funded by the Department of Health, which aims to promote and support active public involvement in NHS, public health and social care research

www.scmh.org.uk/ – the Sainsbury Centre for Mental Health is a charity that works to improve the quality of life for people with severe mental health problems. It carries out research, development and training work to influence policy and practice in health and social care

Section 2
Preparing the Ground

At the beginning of any research enterprise, a considerable amount of work needs to be undertaken before the active stages of data collection and analysis. This section deals with five major issues that require attention in the early stages of any research project, leading on to research design that will be the subject of Section 3.

First of all, a clear research question is required. Chapter 6 traces the development of a research question from its origin in clinical practice or health care policy, through stages of refinement when aims, objectives and hypotheses are clarified, to links with methodology and ethical issues.

Chapters 7 and 8 are linked together, and form a major new strand in this edition of *The Research Process in Nursing*, which draws upon the new discipline of information science. Chapter 7 takes the reader through the essential preparatory stage of reviewing existing evidence in the field of interest for research. This process is now much more systematised than previously, with the widespread availability of computers, information databases and the internet. Chapter 8 builds upon this base, introducing the now well-established science of critical appraisal, and equipping the reader with tools with which to test the validity and applicability of published research to their own situation. It is impossible to overstate the importance of this preparatory stage in research; unless new knowledge is developed from the sound base of previous well-validated evidence, the credibility of nursing research will be called into question.

The last two chapters in this section are concerned with practical issues of preparing to undertake a specific project. Chapter 9 guides the reader through the formal process of writing a research proposal, whether for an academic dissertation or in response to a national funding call from a leading charity or government organisation. Getting the proposal right is likely to make the difference between getting funding or approval for the project or not, but also helps to clarify the researcher's thinking and requires decisions to be made about the research question and design.

Chapter 10 reflects significant changes in the regulation of research in health and social care. Formal ethical scrutiny of research proposals has been in place for some years in the NHS, but it has been considerably standardised and extended in recent years. Research governance is a new system of regulation that has been introduced in response to some high profile abuses in health care research, and has had considerable impact upon the amount of bureaucracy that accompanies the research process. This chapter makes a valuable and up-to-date contribution to assisting a new researcher through the complex processes of research ethics and governance regulations.

6 Asking the Right Question

Gill Hek

Key points

- Research studies usually define a precise research question, though sometimes this is expressed as an aim, objective, purpose, or a hypothesis.
- Research questions can be derived from clinical experience, professional practice, theoretical issues, or from policy imperatives.
- Choice of research methodology follows from the clarification of the research question.
- Feasibility and ethical issues are important considerations in selecting a research question.

Introduction

Some key components of the research question are shown in Figure 6.1. However, the term 'research question' can be misleading. It does not necessarily mean a sentence structured as a question although it can be expressed in this way. Sometimes it is expressed as a statement of purpose or research aim. For example, a research study about wound healing may have the following research questions:

Does patient mobility have an effect on the rate of healing in patients with lower limb burns?

To what extent does mobility affect the rate of wound healing in patients with lower limb burns?

Alternatively it could be expressed as a statement of purpose or research aim:

The purpose of this study is to examine the effect of patient mobility on the rate of wound healing in patients with lower limb burns.

Some studies do not report the research question, rather they will identify aims and objectives, and, in some types of research, a hypothesis. A good research question (Box 6.1) is one that is clearly expressed and focused on a researchable problem. A statement of purpose or research aim (Box 6.2) is a broader statement

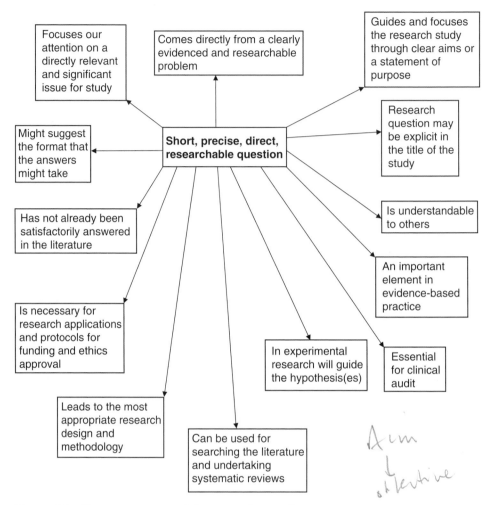

Figure 6.1   Key components of the research question.

that often uses words such as *examine, describe, explore,* etc. Research objectives (Box 6.2) are a way of breaking down and detailing a research aim or statement of purpose into more manageable pieces. A hypothesis (Box 6.3) is used instead of a research question in certain types of research to attempt to answer a question and predict an outcome. These terms will be discussed in more detail later in this chapter.

Research questions in published studies

Box 6.4 shows ten published studies that have been identified to demonstrate the ways in which authors use research questions, research aims, statements of

Box 6.1   Example of a study with a research aim and specific research questions.

Hoffman K, Donoghue J, Duffield C (2004) Decision-making in clinical nursing: investigating contributing factors. *Journal of Advanced Nursing* 45: 53–62

This Australian study investigates the contextual factors that influence clinical decision-making.

Aim: To determine if occupational orientation, educational level, experience, area of practice, level of appointment and age are related to clinical decision-making in a sample of Australian nurses.

Four specific research questions were asked:

Question one: To what extent do nurses participate in clinical decision-making and to what extent do they want to participate?

Question two: What occupational orientations (role values) do nurses working in an Australian acute care context hold?

Question three: Are there any significant relationships between occupational orientation (role value), educational level, experience, age, level of appointment and area of clinical practice and frequency of clinical decision-making?

Question four: Which variables are the strongest predictors of clinical decision-making?

The design of the study was a one-group prospective correlational postal survey of a convenience sample of registered nurses' perceptions of their participation in clinical decision-making. Multiple regression was used to model and weigh the relative influence of a number of factors on decision-making. A response rate of 58% was achieved with 96 questionnaires out of 174 being returned.

Results indicated that education and experience were not significantly related to decision-making. The most important factor that accounted for the greatest variability of clinical decision-making was holding a professional occupational orientation. The authors concluded by highlighting the importance of holding a professional orientation to work and developing a professional outlook in all practising nurses, including students.

purpose, research objectives and hypotheses. In all cases the author's exact words are used. In addition to the aims and research questions (when provided), the title of the article is given to demonstrate how they link together.

It can be seen from these examples that some studies clearly express what the research is trying to discover, whereas others are not so obvious. Furthermore, some titles of published articles are nearly the same as the research questions, whereas in others they differ. In some cases there is also an indication of the research methodology adopted, such as Reilly *et al.* (2004), which includes 'A controlled trial' in the title.

Developing a research question can be aided by building up the question with the key elements and then moving them around so that they make sense. The earlier example given in this chapter includes 'rate of wound healing', 'mobility' and 'patients with lower limb burns'. For some types of research, the

Box 6.2   Example of a study with specific research aims.

Chan S, Wai Yu I (2004) Quality of life of clients with schizophrenia. *Journal of Advanced Nursing* 45: 72–83

This study describes the quality of life and related factors in clients with schizophrenia in the Hong Kong Chinese population. The study had an overall aim and three specific aims:

Overall aim: to investigate the Quality of Life (QoL) of clients with schizophrenia who resided in the community in Hong Kong

Specific aim one: to provide a profile of QoL in clients with schizophrenia

Specific aim two: to examine relationships between QoL and socio-demographic factors, such as gender, age, marital status, employment status and level of education

Specific aim three: to examine relationships between QoL and clinical factors such as mental status, number of hospitalisations and duration of illness

A convenience sample of adults attending a psychiatric outpatient department was recruited over a seven month period. Face-to-face interviews were conducted using a semi-structured interview schedule that included two rating scales to assess clients' mental condition, and to assess quality of life.

The results indicated that women reported less satisfaction with their quality of life than men, and unemployed people were the least satisfied. Most participants were least satisfied with their psychological health, financial situation, life enjoyment and sexual satisfaction. Although not generalisable, the authors concluded that the findings suggest a need to strengthen social and vocational rehabilitation for people with schizophrenia in Hong Kong.

research question can be expressed in a particular way so that the methodological approach is indicated within the research question. The question could be expressed as:

Wound healing in patients with lower limb burns: a randomised controlled trial of mobilisation strategies

What is the lived experience of patients who are beginning to mobilise after suffering from lower limb burns?

The effectiveness of different types of mobilisation techniques on wound healing in patients with lower limb burns: a systematic review

---

Box 6.3   Example of a study with a hypothesis.

Reilley S, Graham-Jones S, Gaulton E, Davidson E (2004) Can a health advocate for home-less families reduce workload for primary healthcare team? a controlled trial. *Health and Social Care in the Community* 12: 63–74

This British quasi-experimental controlled trial took place in an inner-city health centre. Four hundred homeless people registered at the health centre were entered into a 'three-arm' trial in a systematic (non-randomised) manner. The control group received usual care from the health centre and the two intervention groups were offered either health advocacy with a family health worker at the health centre when they registered, or outreach advocacy through visits to hostels and bed and breakfast hotels before they registered. The three groups had similar demographic profiles and no significant differences in morbidity at baseline.

   The *hypothesis* tested was that a dedicated health advocacy service for homeless people can reduce the workload of GPs and other health workers. The hypothesis was supported as the results indicated that outreach health advocacy successfully reduced the workload for primary care staff. Furthermore, health advocacy can alter patterns of help-seeking by home-less people, and can address psychosocial issues at no extra cost.

How do patients with lower limb burns move around, and how does this affect the rate of wound healing?

How do community nurses help patients mobilise after burns injuries? an ethno-graphic study of family and nurse interactions.

Research questions are not always clearly stated in published literature. It is more common to find aims and objectives identified, or a hypothesis may be presented. This may be because authors try to be succinct in their writing. However, research questions are essential to guide the whole research process. Furthermore, the research question will be one of the first things that needs to be identified in a research protocol.

Sources of research questions

There are many potential research topics of interest to nurses arising from both professional and personal experience. The most likely sources of topics are those that arise from problems and questions identified through clinical practice (*see* Box 6.5).

Box 6.4 Examples of research questions in recent published literature.

Research question, aim or hypothesis	Title of published article	Authors
Aim: to investigate Swedish undergraduate nursing students' attitudes and awareness of research and development within nursing, and to illuminate factors that may have an impact on their attitudes and awareness	Swedish nursing students' attitudes to and awareness of research and development in nursing	Bjorkstrom *et al.* (2003)
Aim: evaluate the Breast Care Nursing Service from the patients' perspective *Question one*: how do patients with breast cancer experience the Breast Care Nursing Service? *Question two*: what are the strengths and weaknesses of the Breast Care Nursing Service from the patients' perspective?	A patient-focused evaluation of breast care nursing specialist services in North Wales	Carnwell & Baker (2003)
Aim: to determine if occupational orientation, educational level, experience, area of practice, level of appointment and age are related to clinical decision-making in a sample of Australian nurses *Question one*: to what extent do nurses participate in clinical decision-making and to what extent do they want to participate? *Question two*: What occupational orientations (role values) do nurses working in an Australian acute care context hold? *Question three*: Are there any significant relationships between occupational orientation (role value), educational level, experience, age, level of appointment and area of clinical practice and frequency of clinical decision-making? *Question four*: Which variables are the strongest predictors of clinical decision-making?	Decision-making in clinical nursing: investigating contributing factors	Hoffman *et al.* (2004)
Overall aim: to investigate the quality of life (QoL) of clients with schizophrenia who resided in the community in Hong Kong *Specific aim one*: to provide a profile of QoL in clients with schizophrenia	Quality of life of clients with schizophrenia	Chan & Wai Yu (2004)

Specific aim two: to examine relationships between QoL and sociodemographic factors, such as gender, age, marital status, employment status and level of education

Specific aim three: to examine relationships between QoL and clinical factors such as mental status, number of hospitalisations and duration of illness

Objective: to determine whether provision of health advocacy for homeless patients would reduce the burden of care for a primary healthcare team

Hypothesis: that a dedicated health advocacy service for homeless patients can reduce the workload of GPs and other health workers

Can a health advocate for homeless families reduce workload for the primary healthcare team? A controlled trial — Reilly *et al.* (2004)

The **aim** of the evaluation was to provide case studies of families and their key supporting agency members' perceptions and experiences of the PATCH service

Evaluation of the PATCH nursing service: partnership and training supporting children with complex needs at home — Runciman & McIntosh (2003)

A study that was undertaken to *investigate* newly recruited student nurses' attitudes to gender and nursing stereotypes and pinpoint any change of attitude from 1992–2002

Angel, handmaiden, battleaxe or whore? A study which examines changes in newly recruited student nurses' attitudes to gender and nursing stereotypes — Jinks & Bradley (2004)

Aim: whether cognitive behavioural therapy would promote behavioural change on fluid consumption due to increased awareness and acknowledgement of the impact

Question: Can cognitive behavioural therapy (CBT) reduce interdialactic weight gain?

Can cognitive behaviour therapy assist adherence to fluid restriction with dialysis patients? a case series — Ekers and Kingdon (2003)

Aim one: to elicit the views of consultants, GPs and patients on the idea of copying GP referral letters to patients

Aim two: to describe the experiences of a smaller group of GPs and patients actually involved in copying and receiving copies of referral letters

Copying GP referral letters to patients: the benefits and practical implications — Jelley *et al.* (2003)

Aim: to understand how general practitioners conceptualise binge eating disorder

Binge eating disorder: general practitioners' constructs of an ambiguous pathology — Henderson *et al.* (2003)

Box 6.5 Sources of research questions.

Clinical experience
Why do some patients seem reluctant to take their medication?
Why is methicillin-resistant *Staphylococcus Aureus* (MRSA) more prevalent on some wards than others?
More patients appear to be discharged on Fridays than any other day – what effect does this have on transfer to the community?

Professional development
What is the best way of retaining student nurses?
What are the educational needs of modern matrons?
Are there benefits of nurses learning together with doctors and social workers?

Theoretical frameworks
Validation of a post-operative pain assessment tool for young children
Testing a Finnish care dependency scale in British nursing homes
Evaluating the validity, reliability and readability of a critical care family needs assessment tool.

Other sources
Unusual or unanticipated events e.g. BSE crises, new phenomena, radiation leak, violent event, natural disasters such as floods and storms
What are the long-term health needs of survivors of an earthquake?
The impact of contaminated food products on mothers' attitudes to breastfeeding

Policy imperatives
What is the effect of policy changes on the health needs of asylum seekers?
What staff training needs are required by the introduction of a National Service Framework?

Clinical experience

Clinical experience is a key source of research questions that interest nurses because it is based on every-day work experience, for example:

Why are particular patients reluctant to take their medication?

What is the best way to break bad news to carers?

Male surgical patients seem to mobilise more quickly than females – why is this?

Each of these questions, and many others, would be an appropriate starting point for research. Research questions are also required for evidence-based practice, in which case the question will be asked of the available literature on the subject.

Professional issues

Professional issues may also be a rich source of topics:

- Does interprofessional learning result in enhanced patient care?
- Is e-learning as effective as lectures in terms of developing student knowledge?
- To what extent does a nursing degree influence career opportunity?

Attending a conference on a particular topic such as cancer nursing will expose nurses to cutting edge research, and at the end of a presentation researchers may identify new research questions to be answered. Likewise, many published research studies will identify further research questions. These can be very useful, as they come directly from research that is topical and has a good foundation in evidence.

Most local NHS trusts support particular research programmes related to their specific care provision. For example, an acute trust with a regional oncology centre is likely to support a programme of research related to the care of people with cancer. Local R&D departments may be able to identify specific research questions that need investigating and help to build up expertise in a particular area as well as support the research.

Theoretical issues

Some researchers are interested in developing theory in a particular area. The research questions they seek to answer might be about testing or developing theory. The theories may have arisen from the work of other disciplines such as sociology or psychology, but may need to be tested in nursing practice. This may entail validating a particular data collection tool to ensure that it measures the phenomena accurately, reliably and without bias. Or it may be about testing a previously validated tool such the BARRIERS to research implementation utilisation scale (Funk *et al.* 1991) with a different sample. Replication studies may use the same research questions, and the same or a similar sample at different points in time.

Research questions might also be developed from events that are unpredicted or accidental. The bovine spongiform encephalopathy (BSE) crises might have led to nurses in rural areas exploring the impact of such an event on the mental health of farmers, or the effects of salmonella outbreak in a small community might interest school nurses and public health nurses.

Policy imperatives

Research questions may also derive from policy imperatives associated with nursing policy or health and social care policy. In these cases, an organisation such as the Department of Health or the Royal College of Nursing may advertise that they want research undertaken in particular areas, and suggest research questions that need to be answered. This is called 'an invitation to tender', and can be highly competitive. For example, the Department of Health Research Programmes that are driven by policy imperatives have recently commissioned research about inpatient discharge procedures, information needs of patients and urban community hospitals. The NHS Service Delivery and Organisation R&D programme, a national programme established to develop the evidence base on the organisation, management and delivery of health care services, has recently invited research about the impact of changing workforce programmes on patient care, new forensic services for people with personality disorder and the dynamics of organisational culture change.

The questions identified are developed as a result of changes in policy where the Government wants to consider what effect these policies may have had. These could be related to issues such as modernising services, changes in the workforce, such as expansion and diversity in the workforce, turnover of staff, etc., all of which are the focus of new policies that could affect nurses and nursing practice. They are usually posted on relevant websites (*see* Websites at the end of this chapter).

National Service Frameworks and clinical guidelines

National Service Frameworks (NSFs) might also identify questions that need researching. Recent NSFs have identified new roles for nurses, and key priorities that need actions that will require evaluating to see if they are effective. For example, the recent NSF for children has a priority of reducing teenage pregnancy; research studies arising from this may seek to answer research questions such as:

Does a dedicated teenage sexual health service provided by school nurses reduce pregnancy?

What do teenage boys think about love and relationships?

Likewise clinical guidelines such as those produced by NICE (National Institute for Health and Clinical Excellence) are likely to identify areas where further research is needed because they have found minimal evidence. For example, the pressure ulcer prevention guideline (NICE 2003) which focuses on how to prevent pressure ulcers in both primary and secondary care settings, identifies the following recommendations for further research:

The effectiveness of repositioning patients

A need for data on patient comfort in different positions

For novice researchers looking for a topic to research, clinical guidelines produce a rich source of ideas that are topical and have a sound basis in a systematic literature review of previous research. Consensus activities can also lead to new areas that need researching. A recent Delphi study about career pathways in nursing (Beattie *et al.* 2004) identified that there is still uncertainty about whether nursing should become an all-graduate profession. They recommend further research to identify exactly what level of education is required for a nurse today.

Questions, aims, objectives and hypotheses

Researchers need to be able to clearly express the research question(s), and may identify aims and/or objectives as well. A good research question is clear and focused and is based on a researchable problem. Background information and previous research that identifies the problem, and an underlying rationale as to why it is an important question to answer, will support the research question. It can be difficult to phrase the question appropriately. There needs to be a balance between being succinct and being precise. Figure 6.2 suggests a number of stages in developing research questions, and research aims and objectives.

Having identified sources of research problems, the problem needs to be clearly articulated. The research problem should be significant for nursing and be clearly outlined with a narrow scope. It is then used to develop the aims of the research. In order to identify overall research aims or a statement of purpose, it is necessary to consider the feasibility of undertaking the research. A common problem when trying to prepare aims is to think 'too big' and try to do too much. Research aims and statements of purpose are often quite broad and will summarise the overall goal of the research and maybe identify key variables (*see* later in this chapter). The research question, however, is narrow and focused. Consider the difference between a question 'Does mobility influence wound healing in patients with lower limb burns?' compared with 'In young people 12–16 years old, what is the effect of a supported walking programme for 30 minutes per day on the rate of wound infection of lower limb burns?'

When preparing research aims and ultimately research questions, it helps to consider the feasibility of the study in terms of the amount of time available, the experience and expertise needed, and the support available. The involvement of others, including service users, to help shape the research questions and ethical issues also need to be considered at this stage.

Identifying overall aims, or a statement of purpose can be aided by using words such as *describe, explore, reduce,* etc. It is also useful to define specific terms such as the type of problem (lower limb burns and healing), population or sample (young people 12–16 years of age), outcome (rate of wound infection or increased healing rate). If the study is looking at a particular intervention, then this will need to be defined (supported walking programme of 30 minutes per day).

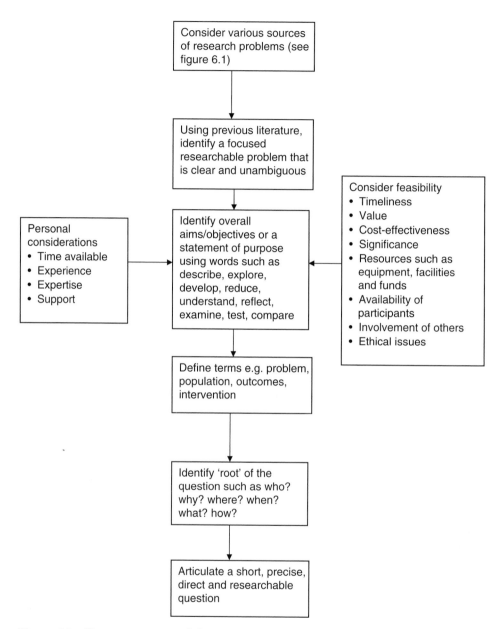

Figure 6.2 Key components of the research question.

Another activity that can help with framing research questions is to consider words such as *who? why? where? when? how?* and *what?* These can be extended to phrases such as: *to what extent . . .? how do . . .? what are . . .?* This is particularly useful in qualitative research, which by its nature has a more open and holistic approach in its methods.

Prioritising research questions

Research questions may need to be prioritised. This can help in determining what is the most important thing to study, and can also aid the novice researcher who is undertaking a time-limited project. The following criteria may help to prioritise:

- of importance to patients', clients' or participants' well-being
- most feasible to answer in the time available
- most interesting question
- most likely to be a recurring problem in practice
- of importance to nursing
- most likely to produce implementable recommendations

Other factors such as cost, ethical issues, or policy imperatives may need to be taken into consideration.

Research objectives

Although objectives normally provide greater detail in relation to a research aim, the term objective is sometimes used interchangeably with aim. In Box 6.4, the study by Reilly *et al.* (2004) had an objective 'To determine whether provision of health advocacy for homeless patients would reduce the burden of care for a primary health care team' and some readers would see this as an aim rather than an objective. In reality, a research study will usually have a broad statement of purpose expressed as an aim and then some more specific statements, expressed as objectives or research questions, which address different aspects of the aim. The examples in Box 6.4 show the considerable variability amongst aims, questions and objectives. Rather than debate the difference between aims, objectives and questions, what is important is that there are clear research questions that are short, precise, direct, researchable, and that drive the study. The boxed examples provide more detail about how research aims, research questions and hypotheses are used in specific studies.

Defining the variables

A variable is a characteristic that varies between individuals and can be measured, such as weight, age, and gender. Some examples of variables are given earlier, such as wound healing rates or, mobilisation strategies. Variables can change or be changed depending on the design of the study and can be studied in isolation or in combination. During the course of a study a new variable may arise which could affect the data collected. Variables are used in different types of research including experimental designs, surveys, correlational studies and epidemiological research. As noted earlier, it is important to define the specific terms including variables that are to be included in a study, and express them precisely in the research question, aims or objectives.

Hypotheses

In some types of research, a hypothesis or hypotheses are used to drive the research. These are normally studies that take a quantitative approach and most commonly, but not exclusively, will be experimental studies. A hypothesis goes further than a research question in that it predicts an outcome. It is a statement about the relationship between two or more variables. The hypothesis will predict the relationship between variables, and through testing the hypothesis, may or may not support the theory.

There are two types of variables used in hypotheses – independent and dependent variables. Independent variables are those seen as a 'cause', which might be an intervention or treatment, and dependent variables are seen as the 'effect' or outcome. This is commonly called a cause and effect relationship.

Using the earlier examples, the independent variable (or intervention) would be 'supported walking for 30 minutes' and the dependent variable (or outcome) would be 'the rate of infection'. Hypotheses should be expressed clearly with all the variables identified explicitly, for example:

> Young people aged 12–16 years with more than 20% lower limb burns who have a supported walking programme of 30 minutes per day will have a reduced wound size within 10 days of injury than those that are placed on bedrest for 10 days following injury.

In this example, the supported walking programme and bedrest are the independent variables (cause/intervention) and wound size (effect/outcome) is the dependent variable.

A hypothesis can also be stated as a 'null' hypothesis, which begins 'there is no difference . . .' The null hypothesis states that there is no relationship between the independent and dependent variables. It is used predominantly in research where there are to be tests of statistical significance (*see* Chapter 29). Hypotheses are never 'proved' or 'disproved', rather they are supported or unsupported, accepted or rejected by the data. Chapter 16 provides more detail about how hypotheses and null hypotheses are used in experimental studies.

Feasibility

As stated earlier and as can be seen from Figure 6.2, it is essential at this early stage of the research process to consider the feasibility of the proposed study at the same time as identifying the research questions. The proposed study needs to be timely. It must be self-evident that the research questions have not already been answered and that they are relevant. At the same time, it must be clear that it is of value to try to answer the questions through the proposed study, that it will be cost-effective, and that resources are available. An important consideration is the availability of research participants; there is no point posing a research question, if participants cannot be recruited successfully. As pointed out in Chapter 5, it can be beneficial to involve service users in preparing the research question. Nurses may think it is an important question to try to answer through research, but patients and/or carers may have different priorities that need to be considered.

Ethical issues

Chapter 3 provides an overview of the ethical principles that need to be considered when identifying the research questions. Of particular importance are the principles of doing no harm, and respect for autonomy of participants in gaining consent.

An NHS Research Ethics Committee (REC) will require an application to clearly set out the main research question and any other secondary research questions. The research question should express the 'knowledge gap' that the research is designed to fill. The committee will expect clearly articulated questions that are based on a comprehensive justification that demonstrates why the research is worth doing and what will be gained from undertaking it. The research question is thus crucial. Depending on the type of research being undertaken, the committee may also expect to see the null and any alternative hypothesis(es). Chapter 10 discusses the requirements of research ethics committees in more detail. Research funders will have similar expectations regarding the clarity of research questions. Members of the public may be involved in reviewing proposals for funding bodies and research ethics committees: research questions therefore need to be phrased so that lay people can understand them.

Research questions and methodology

Research questions should inform decisions about the research methodology to be selected. The earlier example of a hypothesis relating to the effects of a supported walking programme would suggest an experimental design such as a randomised controlled trial comparing different types of mobilisation (bed-rest or walking for 30 minutes). A research question such as 'What is the lived experience of mobilising after lower limbs burns?' might suggest a phenomenological study.

The research may be influenced by the particular beliefs of the researcher, and may lead to research questions that will be answered by a particular research approach. For example, a researcher with a scientific background might pose a research question that leads to the prediction of a specific outcome (a hypothesis) and an experimental study. Conversely, a researcher influenced by interpretivism might pose a research question that suggests a qualitative methodology. Chapter 11 of this book discusses these different perspectives.

Conclusion

This chapter has focused on identifying the right research question at the beginning of the research process, and then designing an appropriate study to answer the question or fulfil the aims of the study. Although the background, experience and expertise of the researcher are clearly important, it is the research question that should drive decisions about the research design.

Figure 6.1 identified the key components that are influenced by the research question. The research question identifies a gap in knowledge or a problem and focuses attention on directly relevant and significant issues that need to be researched. It guides and focuses the research study and will lead to an appropriate research design. Nurses who are facilitating evidence-based practice will also find that the research question is a key component when searching for evidence, developing clinical guidelines and implementing evidence in practice.

References

Beattie A, Hek G, Galvin K, Ross K (2004) What are the future career pathways in nursing and midwifery? A Delphi survey of nurses and midwives in the south west of England. *NT Research* 9: 348–364

Bjorkstrom EA, Johansson IS, Hamrin EK, Athlin EE (2003) Swedish nursing students' attitudes to and awareness of research and development within nursing. *Journal of Advanced Nursing* 41: 393–402

Carnwell R, Baker SA (2003) A patient-focused evaluation of breast care specialist services in North Wales. *Clinical Effectiveness in Nursing* 7:1 18–29

Chan S, Wai Yu I (2004) Quality of life of clients with schizophrenia. *Journal of Advanced Nursing* 45: 72–83

Ekers D, Kingdon D (2003) Can cognitive behaviour therapy assist adherence to fluid restriction with dialysis patients? a case series. *Clinical Effectiveness in Nursing* 7:1 15–17

Funk SG, Champagne MT, Wiese RA, Tornquist EM (1991) BARRIERS: the barriers to utilization scale. *Applied Nursing Research* 4:1 39–45

Henderson E, May C, Chew-Graham CA (2003) Binge eating disorder: general practitioners' constructs of an ambiguous pathology. *Primary Health Care Research and Development* 4: 301–306

Hoffman K, Donoghue J, Duffield C (2004) Decision-making in clinical nursing: investigating contributing factors *Journal of Advanced Nursing* 45: 53–62

Jelley D, Scott D, van Zwanenberg T (2003) Copying GP referral letters to patients: the benefits and practical implications. *Primary Health Care Research and Development* 4: 319–328

Jinks AM, Bradley E (2004) Angel, handmaiden, battleaxe or whore? A study which examines changes in newly recruited student nurses' attitudes to gender and nursing stereotypes. *Nurse Education Today* 24: 73–156

National Institute for Clinical Excellence (2003) *Pressure Ulcer Prevention.* London, NICE

Reilly S, Graham-Jones S, Gaulton E, Davidson E (2004) Can a health advocate for homeless families reduce workload for primary healthcare team? a controlled trial. *Health and Social Care in the Community* 12: 63–74

Runciman P, McIntosh J (2003) Evaluation of the PATCH nursing service: partnership and training supporting children with complex needs at home. *Primary Health Care Research and Development* 4: 307–318

Websites

www.NICE.org.uk/ – the National Institute for Health and Clinical Excellence (NICE) gives details of published clinical guidelines and those in progress, and how to develop guidelines

www.rdinfo.org.uk/ – RD Info provides guidance on how to start a research project including a flow chart that guides the reader through turning an idea into a research question

www.sdo.lshtm.ac.uk/ – details of the NHS Service Delivery and Organisation research programme. Also available is a checklist for researchers who are preparing proposals, with a section on research questions and research objectives

www.dh.gov.uk/ – details of research funded by the Department of Health, and invitations to tender for new projects

7 Finding the Evidence

Claire Beecroft, Angie Rees and Andrew Booth

Key points

- Effective literature searching is an essential skill for research, audit, and practice development in nursing.
- The research literature consists of journals, reports, theses, conference proceedings, government publications and web-based resources.
- Much literature searching now uses electronic databases and the internet.
- A focused question is important in developing a good literature search.
- New sources of evidence include systematic reviews and evidence syntheses.
- Reference management skills are important for literature review report writing.

Introduction

As the nursing and health care literature grows, so does the need for individuals to acquire and maintain the skills to search it effectively. While databases such as CINAHL (the Cumulative Index to Nursing and Allied Health Literature) continue to be key for those seeking to access the nursing and health care literature, newer resources such as the Cochrane Library and Clinical Evidence now complement traditional information sources.

The nursing literature is expanding rapidly as more nurses become involved in research (Bird 2003). Searching the literature is also essential when developing policy, evaluating practice or attempting to implement change. When auditing a service, up-to-date high-quality evidence on which to base the proposed standards is required. So, even if you feel you do not need conventional 'research skills' consider the ability to search the literature as a skill to support you throughout your career and one to enhance your lifelong learning.

Electronic information sources and the internet

Recent years have seen dramatic increases in access to the internet by health care staff. It is now recognised that all staff need to be able to access the necessary resources if they are to obtain timely, quality information to support clinical effectiveness and evidence-based practice. For example, most NHS staff have work-based access to the internet and to a host of specialist resources developed to meet their needs via a National Library for Health (NLH) (Marriott & Gibbens 2004). Such resources underpin the use of high-quality research. It is of paramount importance that any research undertaken begins with a systematic search of the literature to identify previous studies that are similar or identical to the proposed study.

In this chapter the 'internet' is not considered as an information source in itself; strictly speaking it is primarily a means of delivering access to information. The internet, while undoubtedly useful, is unsystematic and provides materials of variable quality. However once a useful report or journal article has been identified it is worth checking to see whether the internet provides access to this specific item.

The research literature

We have already referred to the 'research literature', but it is important to be aware of the full range of literature available to support research and practice. Increasingly the word 'evidence' is used to describe the information on which to base clinical decisions, and this evidence comes from a variety of sources (McKibbon & Marks 1998). Below we shall consider some key forms of 'evidence'.

Journals and journal articles

Journals and journal articles perhaps come first to mind when thinking of the 'research literature'. Journals not only contain research (such as clinical trials) but also opinion, editorials, letters, case studies and reports. All contribute evidence to support practice and research. However, background questions, such as general information on a disease or condition, may best be answered from a current text-book. Knowledge in journal articles tends to be specialised rather than general.

Electronic access to journals has developed in two main ways: first, many librar-ies pay for access to electronic journals that are simply an electronic version of the traditional printed journal. Additionally, as electronic databases such as Medline and CINAHL have developed, so access to full-text articles has grown. These databases now offer increasing numbers of articles electronically as full text. With a few clicks of a mouse you can move from the database results to the full version of the article. This potentially saves a visit to the library and the effort of photo-copying articles that have been identified.

Books

While books will not always be sufficiently up-to-date to support research, they can provide useful background information to assist in developing a research question. Many library users enjoy browsing the shelves to find books of interest, but electronic library catalogues now feature in most health libraries. These enable relevant books to be identified much more efficiently.

Reports

In addition to research published in journals, some research findings are published as reports. Research reports may yield useful facts and figures such as statistics and cost data and thus complement information from books and journals. Bear in mind that some research that has not been successful in achieving publication in the journal literature may be published as a report as a 'last resort', so quality may be variable. However, reports are often not included in major databases such as Medline. It is possible to identify reports using specialist databases such as the Health Management Information Consortium (HMIC) database or by searching appropriate internet sites.

Theses

Theses are usually the output from research degrees both at master's and doctoral level. They provide an extensive record of a student's research project and are therefore considerably longer than most journal articles. To identify relevant theses, major databases and specialised sources such as *Dissertation Abstracts* (an electronic database of abstracts for theses) need to be searched. Most university libraries hold an extensive collection of theses by their own students so will be a good place to look.

Conference proceedings

Papers presented by speakers at a conference are often collected together and published either in print or electronic form as 'Conference Proceedings'. This allows those not at the conference to read through the papers that were presented. Conferences are frequently used as a forum for presenting the results of ongoing or recently completed research. They can therefore provide up-to-date information if proceedings are published soon after the conference has closed. Not all papers presented at a conference are necessarily included in the proceedings – sometimes a peer-review process will approve those papers to be included. Conference proceedings are often referenced in the main databases, and health libraries may have a small collection of printed conference proceedings. Finally, to find the proceedings of a particular conference, it might be worth searching the internet to see if the conference has a website as proceedings are sometimes published this way.

Government circulars

Government circulars are published by governmental departments, groups and committees. Such documents are usually available via the relevant government department's website, though again, a health library may have a small print collection.

Grey literature

'Grey literature' describes literature, ranging from pamphlets and leaflets to governmental or health service documents, which is often not collected by libraries and is frequently not referenced in electronic databases (Conn *et al.* 2003). The key characteristic of this literature is that it is elusive and fugitive. Again, the internet has made such literature easier to identify and obtain. Specialist databases, such as HMIC, offer access to selected grey literature. Local health library staff will be able to identify available resources to locate grey literature.

Accessing the literature

The internet has led to major changes in not only how the literature is accessed but also where it can be accessed from, be that in the workplace or at home. Many resources discussed earlier can now be accessed in electronic format. Clearly, information technology skills are an important factor in how an individual searches the available literature, so both traditional and modern methods will be examined.

Finding the nearest/best library

Most health organisations run their own libraries and additionally many have 'access agreements' with local libraries to complement their own resources. However certain services, such as printing, borrowing materials or photocopying may either be unavailable or only available on a fee-paying basis. If you are unsure of what services are available, enquire at the nearest hospital-based library. Training is usually provided in the use of electronic resources, either as hands-on sessions, lectures or on an individual basis.

Going further afield

As mentioned above resources may need to be accessed that a local library cannot provide. The three main things to consider when accessing services other than at a local library are:

- Can the cost of the services such as photocopying and printing be met if they are not provided free?
- How feasible is it to travel to use the library?
- How can the best use be made of libraries that are not nearby?
- Making sure that the resources you are looking for further afield are not available locally will prevent wasting valuable time.

National/international electronic resources

Many public health care systems fund access to major electronic databases, journals and books. For example, the National Library for Health (*www.nlh.nhs.uk*) offers access to a variety of databases that match the needs of staff in the NHS. Also bear in mind that some nursing organisations provide access to databases and/or electronic journals. For instance, the Royal College of Nursing provides electronic access to a core collection of nursing and health-related journals to its members. Key international databases include:

- AMED: an allied and complementary medicine database with references from over 400 journals.
- CINAHL: the Cumulative Index to Nursing and Allied Health has references to almost all English language journals in the nursing and allied health literature, plus conference proceedings and reports. It is the most comprehensive nursing database of its kind.
- MEDLINE: a major medical database of over 12 million records with references from over 4600 journals covering a broad and expanding range of medical specialities. It also contains some references to conference proceedings.
- Embase: similar to MEDLINE but has an emphasis on drugs and pharmacology and has better coverage of European publications. It has references from over 4600 journals and a total of over 10 million records. It also has some references to books and conference proceedings.
- PsycInfo: this is a specialised database covering psychology and allied fields. It has references from over 1900 journals plus books, reports, etc.
- CAREDATA: this database abstracts social work and social care literature. It contains over 75 000 references to books, journal articles, government reports, etc. The database covers English language publications from the UK, North America and beyond.
- The above list of databases is by no means definitive (Conn *et al.* 2003). Information about access to other databases, e-journals and e-books can be obtained from a local health library.

Access to PCs

With much money being invested in information technology equipment, most nurses should be able to access a personal computer (PC) that is connected to the internet. Ward computers are not always available for literature searching, so alternatives should be investigated. A senior member of staff with their own PC may be willing to let others use it. Alternatively, PCs are normally available in libraries or ask at the local R&D office or postgraduate education centre. Booking in advance is wise as it may save a wasted trip. If using a personal computer from home, make sure that you register for any necessary passwords.

Planning a literature search

Planning a literature search is vital and yet this stage is often neglected. It is tempting to head straight for the major databases as soon as you have a research idea in your head. However, you can save much time and effort by planning a search strategy before you begin searching. This will also dramatically improve the quality of the search.

The importance of a focused search question

A focused search question is crucial when searching the literature (Flemming 1998). If the question is not sufficiently focused you will find yourself wrestling with large sets of mostly irrelevant search results. A focused question helps to ensure that the search is precise and accurate and that you are able to manage the volume of literature rather than drowning in it (McKibbon & Marks 2001).

The anatomy of a question

It is helpful to develop a focused question using one of the available models (*see* the PICO or SPICE models below). These will assist you in planning the search strategy.

PICO

The PICO model is an acronym made up as follows (Ask an Expert 2002):

- Patient/problem (e.g. common cold)
- Intervention/exposure (e.g. vitamin C supplements)
- Comparison (e.g. no vitamin C supplements)
- Outcome (e.g. reduced incidence of common cold)

PICO works well for questions about health care interventions. Once the four elements to the question have been identified, the next step is to make a list of all the words and phrases needed to search for each PICO element. Remember to think of synonyms, alternative spellings and plurals. Box 7.1 provides an illustration of the PICO model.

There will be many additional terms so Box 7.1 is a simplified version. Under the 'comparison' heading the term 'placebo' (i.e. vitamin C is being compared with no treatment) is provided as a suggestion. The 'comparison' element of PICO may sometimes be implicit and it may be possible to obtain a good set of results by simply identifying the other elements and then combining them.

Box 7.1 Illustration of the PICO model.

Patient/Problem	Intervention/Exposure	Comparison	Outcome
Cold/s Common cold/s	Vitamin C Ascorbic acid	Placebo	Prevention Prevents Preventative Incidence

Box 7.2 Illustration of the SPICE model.

Setting	Perspective	Intervention	Comparison	Evaluation
General practice Primary care Family practice	Smokers Smoking	Advice Support Counselling	No terms required	Motivation? Selection? Reason? Choice?

SPICE

The SPICE model is a useful alternative to the PICO model for questions that relate to qualitative methodologies or the social sciences. Working in the same way as PICO, the SPICE model breaks a search question down into:

- Setting (e.g. general practice)
- Perspective (e.g. smokers)
- Intervention (e.g. smoking cessation advice)
- Comparison (e.g. variation from patient to patient)
- Evaluation (e.g. reasons for giving/not giving advice)

As Box 7.2 illustrates, it is not necessary to identify terms for all aspects of the SPICE model to produce a useful list of terms and a search strategy. In this example it might be sufficient to combine the terms in the 'S' 'P' and 'I' sections to find relevant articles. Adding additional terms from the 'E' section might help to identify papers that investigate how GPs decide to provide or not provide smoking cessation advice to smokers. A search using just the 'S' 'P' and 'I' sections of this strategy finds the article from Medline shown in Box 7.3.

Clearly, analysing the search using these models helps to produce a more accurate set of results. Once the PICO or SPICE model has been developed, each element should be searched *separately* and then each search statement is combined to produce a smaller set of results using Boolean operators.

Box 7.3   Example of a MEDLINE abstract.

Authors
Coleman T, Cheater F, Murphy E

Institution
School of Community **Health** Sciences, Division of General **Practice**, University Hospital, Queen's Medical Centre, Nottingham NG7 2UH, UK. tim.coleman@nottingham.ac.uk

Title
Qualitative study investigating the process of giving anti-**smoking advic**e in general **practice**.

Source
Patient Education & Counselling 52(2):159–63, 2004 Feb.

Abstract
General practitioners' (GPs') anti-**smoking advic**e promotes patients' **smoking** cessation but little is known about how GPs use their short consultations to give **advic**e. We used semi-structured interviews with 27 UK GPs to investigate how GPs believe they should **advi**se smokers to stop and the reasons underpinning these beliefs. GPs reported a limited repertoire of techniques for dealing with smokers who were not motivated to stop. They also reported using confrontational **advic**e-giving styles with patients who continued to smoke despite suffering from **smoking**-related illnesses. GPs might find it easier and more rewarding to discuss **smoking** with patients if they possessed a greater range of skills for dealing with non-motivated smokers.

Boolean operators

Although their name sounds frighteningly complicated, Boolean operators are simply the words 'and', 'or' and 'not' that are used to combine searches. Box 7.4 shows how they work in the example given earlier.

Box 7.4   Example of Boolean operators.

Patient/Problem	Intervention/Exposure	Comparison	Outcome
cold/s **or** common cold/s **and**	Vitamin C **or** Ascorbic acid **and**	placebo **and**	prevention **or** prevents **or** preventative **or** incidence

When using the 'or' operator you are asking the database to identify papers that feature either of the terms you have searched. In the example above the 'patient' element will look for papers that use the word 'cold' or the phrase 'common cold', as both could be relevant. Similarly for the 'intervention', 'ascorbic acid' is a synonym for 'vitamin C', so 'or' is used to find papers that feature either term. When combining across PICO elements the 'and' operator is used. When combining the Patient and Intervention columns we are instructing the database to find papers featuring the terms 'cold' or 'common cold' and also the terms 'vitamin c' or 'ascorbic acid' within the same paper.

Searching the literature

Electronic searching

Many people feel that searching electronic databases, while undoubtedly useful, is bewilderingly complicated. While it does take practice to become proficient at searching electronic resources, it is within the reach of anyone who is willing to learn. Whereas databases differ, key techniques are common to many different databases, so once you have learned these techniques the task will get much easier (Poynton 2003).

Free-text searching

Most databases allow you to type in words and phrases and search for references that feature those terms in the title, abstract, authors, journal name, etc. This is how most people instinctively search databases, but it has its drawbacks. As mentioned above, you need to be able to think of all the synonyms and alternative spellings for the terms to be sure not to miss anything important. One technique which saves time when typing in variations of a word is truncation. Most databases allow you to enter a truncation mark (often a $ or a *) after a word stem. For instance, if you want to search for:

prevent

prevents

prevention

preventative

You can simply enter:

Prevent$ (or Prevent* depending on the database) to find all the above words.

It is important to note that searching this way will generate numerous results that make a fleeting reference to the search term but are not fundamentally about that subject. The abstract in Box 7.5, found by searching MEDLINE for the free-text terms 'vitamin C' and 'cold', illustrates this. Although vitamin C and cold are mentioned in the abstract, this paper is not about these subjects but is using an analogy about how regulation of telemedicine is as annoying as a common cold!

Box 7.5   An example of a retrieval error from MEDLINE.

Journal of Medical Practice Management. 2003 May–Jun;18(6):289–94.

Telemedicine: laws still need a dose of efficiency.
Bilimoria NM.

Ever have a **cold** that just won't go away? You try lozenges, **vitamin C**, and a humidifier. Nothing seems to work. Telemedicine still has the same **cold** today in the form of laws and regulations that make the practice of telemedicine onerous. The best a health practitioner can do today is weather the **cold** that plagues telemedicine and make the best of it until legislators and regulators work on solutions to remove the barriers to effective telemedicine practice. This article provides a view of the landscape of telemedicine law today, outlines the barriers to the effective practice of telemedicine, and offers strategic concerns for health care providers to consider before entering into telemedicine arrangements.

Subject headings

Due to the limitations of free-text searching, it may be necessary to search for subject headings that relate to the topic. Subject headings are standardised terms used to describe the content of an article. They enable searchers to avoid typing multiple terms for the same subject, as a single subject heading is assigned to replace them all. For instance, to carry out a free text search for papers about 'vitamin C', all of the following terms (and possibly others) would need to be entered:

- vitamin C
- ascorbic acid
- hybrin
- l-ascorbic acid

However, a single subject heading 'ascorbic acid' is assigned to describe all papers about this subject, regardless of which terminology the authors use. Once a paper has been read and a list of subject headings created for it, a few of these are emphasised as 'major subject headings', and these are the terms that describe the main subjects of the paper. There are several subject heading systems that are used by health-related databases. One of the most well known is MeSH (Medical Subject Headings), which are used by the US National Library of Medicine for the MEDLINE database.

Limiting searches

Most databases allow you to limit the search once the free-text and subject heading searches have been completed. Typical limits are:

Age: restricts the search to patients within certain age groups

Language: enables the search to be restricted to publications in a specified language

Date range: useful to identify papers that have been published in the last few years or if historical articles are required.

Full text: restricts the search to papers that are available in full to print or download

Limits are a useful way of making the results set more focused and smaller, but should be used with caution to ensure that relevant material is not missed.

Grey literature

A good starting point for health-related grey literature is to go to the homepage of a national governmental health department, such as the Department of Health (*www.dh.gov.uk*) in England or the United States Department of Health and Human Services (*www.hhs.gov*). In terms of electronic databases, in addition to HMIC (mentioned earlier), there are UKOP, the UK official publication database, and the SIGLE (System for Information on Grey Literature in Europe) database. Ask at your local health library about access to these databases or for any others that they can recommend.

Manual searching

Some techniques used for manually searching the literature have been mentioned earlier in this chapter. These are particularly useful when searching for grey literature which often 'slips through the net' of the major electronic databases.

Journal indexes

Many journals produce an annual printed index to help users find the articles they need. This is either published as a separate volume or is sometimes published in the back of the last issue of a volume or year. The index usually enables a search to be made by author and keyword. These indexes are useful if you want to browse a key journal in a subject area, but do not want to go through each table of contents individually.

Reference lists

It can be useful to search through the lists of references of any relevant articles that you have found. When a useful reference has been identified this way, it is worth checking the entry on the databases that have already been searched to try to identify why it has not been found by the search strategies. This will also allow you to read the abstract for the paper and will help you to decide whether the paper is worth obtaining.

Tables of contents

For journals that do not produce an annual index, the next best thing is to browse tables of contents. This can be a lengthy process, so target the key journals in your subject area and simply read through the titles in the table of contents of each issue to find relevant articles.

Grey literature

Manual searching of grey literature can be a lengthy process. Most libraries will stock a collection of reports, statistics, and pamphlets, etc. that form a 'grey' literature collection, so ask the librarian for help as they know their collection well. Even if these resources can be identified via the library catalogue, and thus speed up the searching, it may also be necessary to browse the shelves. It is important to seek help when searching this type of literature to avoid wasting time.

Further help with literature searching

Literature searching is an important skill for nurses to develop, and while this chapter has attempted to introduce the key concepts and methods, further assistance may need to be sought. Always remember to ask for help from your local health library or the research support facilities in your area. In the UK the Research and Development Support Unit (RDSU) networks provide a range of support services to NHS staff wishing to become research-active, including training and support for literature searching. The Trust' Research and Development Office should be able to provide information about available support.

Specialist information sources

'New' forms of evidence: reviews and syntheses

While there is a wealth of literature available to help nurses answer clinical questions it is often difficult and time-consuming to wade through the enormous quantities of studies published. One approach is to limit a search to a particular type of study design (Barroso *et al.* 2003; Littleton *et al.* 2004). However even within one type of study design the quality of studies will vary considerably due to such factors as poor resourcing, inappropriate methodology, etc. The need to provide health care professionals with reliable evidence on which to base decisions has led to the increasing importance of published reviews (Docherty 2003). Reviews aim to bring together a body of research on a subject and to find common themes in the results, enabling the reviewer to draw conclusions for their proposed research question. Broadly speaking there are two different types of review, 'traditional' and 'systematic'.

Traditional reviews can take a number of forms, but they are usually highly selective in the literature that is reviewed. For instance, in a literature review, a reviewer may restrict the literature that they review to papers published in the last year, or which are published in certain key journals. Reviews such as this are a useful way of keeping up-to-date and managing the volume of literature in a subject area, as they provide a brief summing up of several papers in a single article.

Systematic reviews are the focus of Chapter 21. They have become the 'gold standard' research method for reviewing the literature on effectiveness in health care. As such they aim to approach the review process with the same rigour and discipline as primary research, leaving a reproducible audit trail of methods. Systematic reviews are often, though not always, characterised by the presence of 'meta-analysis': a combination of statistical techniques enabling the reviewer to produce an overall estimate of the results of the individual studies. They are mentioned here because they will often provide an invaluable starting point for your own research.

Cochrane Library

The Cochrane Library is produced by the Cochrane Collaboration, an international organisation made up of numerous subject-specific groups conducting systematic reviews in their topic areas. The Cochrane Library comprises seven different databases. The most prominent of these is the Cochrane Database of Systematic Reviews (CDSR), which contains reviews undertaken by the Cochrane Collaboration. The other databases include the Cochrane Central Register of Controlled Trials (CENTRAL) containing randomised controlled trials used in Cochrane systematic reviews. CENTRAL is now considered the single best source of information on controlled trials of quality. The Cochrane Library also includes a database of appraised reviews *not* produced by the Cochrane Collaboration, the Database of Abstracts of Reviews of Effects (DARE).

Evidence-based journals

The number of journals devoted to publishing reviews has grown significantly in recent years. The BMJ Publishing Group alone numbers three such titles, *Evidence-Based Medicine, Evidence-Based Mental Health* and *Evidence-Based Nursing.* Digests of systematic reviews, reviews and meta-analysis such as *Bandolier* (*www.ebandolier.com*) and *Effective Healthcare* (*www.york.ac.uk/inst/crd*) make the findings from research even more accessible. Other titles of interest to nurses include: *Evidence-based Healthcare & Public Health* and *Worldviews on Evidence-Based Nursing.*

Evidence summaries

Clinical Evidence (*www.clinicalevidence.com*) is aimed at UK clinicians and summarises the evidence of the effectiveness of health care interventions. Arranged alphabetically by condition, it enables the health care practitioner to make decisions about patient care based on up-to-date evidence about treatments. Similar resources are available via the internet and are easily accessible.

Writing a literature review

Once the literature search is completed and papers are identified to answer the search question, the next stage is to write a review. There are three key stages:

- *Sorting the 'wheat from the chaff'* – this involves examining retrieved papers critically to decide whether they meet the criteria for the review and whether they really help to answer the question. Chapter 8 considers this in more detail.
- *Identifying key points, results and themes* – this involves interpreting research findings and applying them to your own questions (Greenhalgh 2001).
- *Writing up your findings* – this involves using a clearly structured approach. It may be helpful to look at a couple of reviews or digests to get a feel for the different ways of presenting the results.

Managing references

Why you need to record and manage your search results

When the electronic and manual searches are completed it is important to document the search strategies. First, providing examples of search strategies demonstrates the quality and efficacy of the search effort; second, it may later be necessary to update the searches or to re-run them. Searches can be recorded manually (by printing out the search strategies) or electronically. Many bibliographic databases now permit users to store their search strategies online for later recall. This is particularly useful if you need to conduct the searches again or modify them, saving you the time-consuming task of having to retype the search terms. The databases that have been used should also be noted together with the dates on which they were searched.

Consideration should also be given to using a system to manage all the references as they are obtained (Nicoll 2003). Using an organised system to manage these will help you when obtaining copies of papers and appraising them. It will also prove valuable when you come to write up your work and need to produce bibliographies, footnotes, etc.

Electronic reference management software

Several software packages exist to help researchers manage their references. Popular commercial examples include Procite, Reference Manager, and Endnote. Other products are available to download free of charge from the internet. A principal advantage of using an electronic method is that most forms of software allow you to produce bibliographies in various formats very efficiently. Many also interact with wordprocessing software to enable references to be inserted directly into the text. References can also be individually annotated and keywords identified as they are imported into the software. This allows subgroups of different records to be kept within the database.

Figure 7.1 shows a screen-shot for a popular reference management software package called 'Reference Manager'. Individual references are displayed at the top of the screen and a full list of references appears below. This makes browsing and checking references simple and speedy. If you prefer the idea of managing references electronically, but do not wish to learn a new software package, consider using spreadsheet or word processing software.

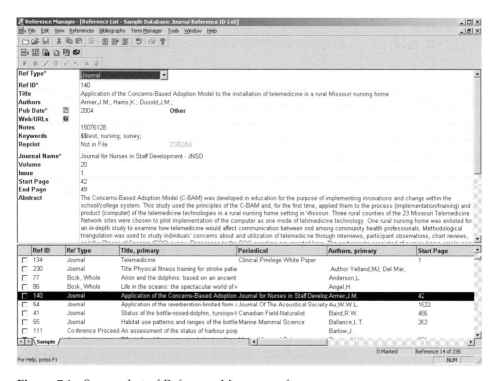

Figure 7.1   Screen shot of Reference Manager software.

Manual methods

Manual methods still have their advantages. They will likely be cheaper and simpler to manage without requiring special training. One method is to maintain a simple card index. A manual handwritten index card might look like Box 7.6.

Box 7.6 A manual index card.

Author/s: Smith, A, Jones B
Title: Manual Reference Cards versus Reference Management Software: a review of
             the literature
Source: International Journal of Reference Management
Year: 2001
Volume: 52
Part: 3
Pages: 79–93
Notes: mentioned in footnote 2

Whichever method you choose, it is important to get into the habit of recording references as they are obtained. This will help to prevent references 'slipping through the net' and becoming lost. Managing references effectively as the search progresses will save much hard work at the end!

Conclusion

This chapter has examined the importance of focusing a search question and planning the search to save both time and frustration. Consideration has also been given to the various methods of searching and using the literature. Here are a few key points to remember:

- First, focus your question and plan your search strategy. Make notes on paper and do not be tempted to go straight to the computers to start searching.
- Get to know your local health library and the librarians who work there. They are a valuable resource for your research and can save you time and effort.
- Get to know the resources that are most relevant to you by regular browsing.
- Try to practise your searching as frequently as you can. Repeated searching is the best way to hone your search skills.

Finally, remember that the skills of searching and using the literature are not just useful for research, they will support you throughout your professional career. Taking the time to gain these skills now will pay great dividends both immediately and for many years to come.

References

Ask an Expert (2002) Popping the (PICO) question in research and evidence-based practice. *Applied Nursing Research* 15: 197–198

Barroso J, Gollop CJ, Sandelowski M, Meynell J, Pearce PF, Collins LJ (2003) The challenges of searching for and retrieving qualitative studies. *Western Journal of Nursing Research* 25: 153–178

Bird D (2003) Discovering the literature of nursing: a guide for beginners. *Nurse Researcher* 11: 56–70

Conn VS, Isaramalai S, Rath S, Jantarakupt P, Wadhawan R, Dash Y (2003) Beyond MEDLINE for literature searches. *Journal of Nursing Scholarship* 35: 177–182

Docherty B (2003) How to access online research reviews to inform nursing practice. *Professional Nurse* 19:1 53–55

Flemming K (1998) EBN notebook. Asking answerable questions. *Evidence-Based Nursing* 1:2 36–37

Greenhalgh T (2001) *How to Read a Paper: the basics of evidence based medicine.* London, BMJ Publishing

Littleton D, Marsalis S, Bliss DZ (2004) Searching the literature by design. *Western Journal of Nursing Research* 26: 891–908

Marriott R, Gibbens S (2004) The changing role of libraries. The changing role of NHS libraries: how you can access the new services. *NT Research* 9: 143–149

McKibbon K, Marks S (1998) EBN notebook. Searching for the best evidence. Part 1: where to look. *Evidence-Based Nursing* 1:3 68–70

McKibbon KA, Marks S (2001) Posing clinical questions: framing the question for scientific inquiry. AACN Clinical Issues: *Advanced Practice in Acute and Critical Care* 12: 477–481

Nicoll LH (2003) A practical way to create a library in a bibliography database manager: using electronic sources to make it easy. *CIN: Computers, Informatics, Nursing* 21:1 48–54

Poynton MR (2003) Information technology and the clinical nurse specialist. Recall to precision: retrieving clinical information with MEDLINE. *Clinical Nurse Specialist* 17:4 182–184

Further reading

Guyatt G, Drummond R (eds) (2001) *Users' Guides to the Medical Literature: essentials of evidence-based clinical practice.* Chicago, AMA Press

Hart C (1998) *Doing a Literature Review: releasing the social science research imagination.* London, Sage

Hart C (2001) *Doing a Literature Search: a comprehensive guide for the social sciences.* London, Sage

Websites

www.nlh.nhs.uk – National Library for Health has a wide range of electronic health resources intended as a source of evidence and best practice to support health care and research

www.shef.ac.uk/scharr/ir/netting – Netting the Evidence provides access to learning resources, such as an evidence-based virtual library, software and journals

www.national-rdsu.org.uk/ – the network of Research and Development Support Units (RDSUs) in England

8 Critical Appraisal of the Evidence

Andrew Booth

Key points

- Critical appraisal is needed for researchers and practitioners to assess the validity of a research study or group of studies, and whether their results can be applied to a particular situation.
- Three concepts are of key importance to critical appraisal: validity, reliability and applicability.
- Checklists are available to assist with critical appraisal of both quantitative and qualitative research, and for systematic reviews.
- Ready-made critically appraised products are now available in some areas and in evidence-based health care journals.

Introduction

Critical appraisal focuses on the practical application of research, whether it be in applying the findings of research to clinical or managerial practice or in establishing an evidence base to which our own research will add a distinctive contribution.

Critical appraisal skills enable us to assess whether an individual study has particular value for us. Equally they help us to reconcile dissonant, even conflicting, messages from different research studies. For example, one study conducted in a very selective population may show that a treatment works. A similar study in a general population may show less favourable results. Critical appraisal helps us to understand reasons for such differences and to decide which study, if any, we will use to inform our practice. Critical appraisal is equally valuable whether we have to start from scratch ourselves in assessing a research study for a new treatment or whether we seek to interpret the appraisals of others such as systematic literature reviews, guidelines or critically appraised topics (CATs) (Guyatt et al. 2000).

For a profession with a justifiable reputation for challenging 'nursing ritual' critical appraisal is a key skill. Critical appraisal of relevant research helps us to cease ineffective procedures and put a brake on unquestioning acceptance of novel or fashionable technologies. For example, after critically appraising evidence supporting vitamin C in the healing of pressure sores, a dietician and information specialist were able to challenge textbook recommendations based on a 20-year-old flawed study. They were thus able to:

'encourage disinvestment from an ineffective, although non-harmful, treatment in favour of spending resources on treatments for which there is at least sufficient proof of benefit' (North & Booth 1999:243)

What is critical appraisal?

Critical appraisal is:

'the process of assessing and interpreting evidence by systematically considering its validity, results and relevance' (Parkes *et al*. 2001:10)

This definition not only values the technical skills of 'assessing evidence', understanding study design and research quality, but also the contextual knowledge of 'interpreting evidence', based on clinical experience. This combination of skills and knowledge, while recognising the values and preferences of the individual patient, constitutes evidence-based practice.

A key principle of critical appraisal is that a good study usually provides enough information to help a researcher to judge that it is a good study. Unfortunately, the reverse is not necessarily true – the IMRAD (Introduction, Methods, Results and Discussion) structure used to present published research may make research appear superficially plausible. To help 'scratch beneath the surface' you typically use a published checklist. Many such checklists exist for different audiences or different types of study. However checklists should focus on the actual quality of the methods and not merely on how well the study is reported. Avoid checklists that focus on factors that are external to the study itself such as 'Have you heard of the author? What qualifications do the authors have? Is the journal peer-reviewed?' The study should speak for itself! A useful critical appraisal checklist focuses on the validity, reliability and applicability of a study. These three associated concepts are central to all critical appraisal, regardless of whether the research being appraised is quantitative or qualitative or whether it is a primary study (e.g. a randomised controlled trial) or a secondary study (e.g. a guideline or systematic review). Each concept will be considered in turn.

Validity (are the results of the study valid?)

Suppose that you were to stand in the work area with a clipboard. What effect might this have on patients or colleagues? Given that even the smallest observational study can, like a pebble in a lake, disturb the 'real world', what might we expect if we design a large and complex experimental study? Clearly we want limitations arising from our chosen research method to be outweighed by the 'trueness' of the findings. If we suspect that the picture obtained by the research no longer relates to the 'world' that we are investigating then the study is invalid. The researchers may have based their study on flawed assumptions, there may be some inherent weakness in the study design they have chosen (bias) or they may have failed to take into account an important complicating factor (confounding).

Reliability (what are the results?)

All research results are subject to the possible effects of chance. When we measure outcomes we want to be sure that the results are reliable. If we were to measure the same outcomes repeatedly would we still obtain the same results? Statistical measures allow us to interpret whether the results fall within the bounds of reasonable expectation. Finally when the variability of results from repeated measurements is taken into account we want to be able to judge whether we would make the same decision based on the best possible result as we would when faced with the worst possible result.

Once we have established that the results are reliable we want to ascertain whether an effect is meaningful – is it large enough to be clinically significant? For example, a study may demonstrate a change of five points on a pain scale. However you may know from experience that a change of less than ten points makes no difference at all to how a patient is feeling. A change of 5 points may be *statistically significant* but a change of 10 points or more is *clinically significant*.

Applicability (will the results help locally?)

If the study is well designed and shows a reliable enough result, we need to consider its implications for both current clinical practice and for future research. It is helpful to separate the strength of the evidence (in terms of validity and reliability) from the strength of recommendations or action (in terms of applicability). Most practitioners will broadly agree whether a study has been designed well or a result is meaningful. However, when they come to determining whether the results can be applied locally they will take into account available resources, the skills of involved staff and local policies and politics.

The need for critical appraisal

Critical appraisal has become increasingly important for several reasons. First, the sheer volume of information available, in printed form or via the internet, has meant that any aspiring researcher needs to filter out unreliable lower quality studies. Second, even the best journals can publish poor or misleading information. Even where information is of good quality delays of up to ten years may occur before research findings become standard practice in textbooks (Antman *et al.* 1992).

Researchers need to judge whether the study design used to conduct research makes the findings either potentially useful or unusable. If an inferior study design has been used, you may be able to examine the same research question with a more robust design. If a robust design has been used and the findings are still open to doubt you may wish to repeat the study with a larger sample size. Finally, if the research has been conducted well and has conclusive results you are free to concentrate on other aspects that need to be researched. Critical appraisal skills are required throughout a research career and are thus skills for lifelong learning.

Any research study is prone to two potential flaws: bias and confounding.

'Bias is a systematic tendency to underestimate or overestimate the parameter of interest because of a deficiency in the design or execution of a study' (Coggon *et al.* 2003:21)

For example, when patients self-report whether they have given up smoking some may convey a more positive image than is truthful. Whereas self-report is open to bias, biochemical confirmation of nicotine in their blood or saliva would be a more objective (less biased) way of establishing the facts. Confounding is where you cannot ascertain whether an effect is caused by the variable you are interested in or by another variable. For example, a study may demonstrate a link between alcohol consumption and lung cancer. However alcohol consumption is commonly associated with smoking. Smoking is therefore a potential confounder for your study. Ideally a researcher identifies potential confounders before they begin and then adjusts their results accordingly in the analysis. Common confounding variables are age, sex, ethnicity and co-morbidity.

Validity of research designs

An optimal research design minimises bias and anticipates confounding. The researcher therefore has the responsibility to choose the best research design to answer the question that they are asking. This choice is limited by ethical or practical considerations (Roberts & Di Censo 1999; Ploeg 1999). For example, if a researcher believes that keeping pigeons causes bird-fanciers' lung it is not ethical to randomise subjects to keep pigeons or not within a randomised controlled trial. The strongest available design would be an observational study that simply observes what the population chooses to do. A researcher selects the most appropriate research design from within a so-called 'hierarchy of evidence' (Sackett 1986) (Box 8.1).

This hierarchical approach has several limitations. By emphasising the study design over the features of an individual study it gives the false impression that a poor randomised trial is better than a good observational study. Neither can it handle conflict between the findings of several observational studies and a single randomised controlled trial, or a situation where randomised controlled trials are split in favour and against the same intervention. It is more important to trade-off

---

Box 8.1   The hierarchy of evidence.

1. Systematic reviews and meta-analyses
2. Well-designed randomised trials
3. Well-designed trials without randomisation (e.g. single-group pre-post, cohort, time-series or matched case-controlled studies)
4. Well-designed non-experimental studies from more than one centre
5. Opinions of respected authorities based on clinical evidence, descriptive studies or reports of expert committees

---

the strength of a paper's findings against the weaknesses of its methodology than slavishly follow a hierarchy of evidence (Edwards *et al.* 1998).

How to appraise quantitative research studies

As a researcher you will encounter many checklists that claim to be useful when appraising different types of quantitative study. A useful checklist will only include criteria that are relevant for a given paper. For example, a clinical trial should demonstrate that it has avoided selection and observer bias and that the large majority of subjects (80% or more) are accounted for by the results. We also want to ensure that the outcomes chosen measure the right thing over the right time period. Finally quantitative studies need large enough numbers of patients, to avoid being wrong because of the random play of chance. In summary, then, for a quantitative paper to provide strong evidence, it must be high-quality, valid and well-powered.

For an individual researcher, checklists provide a framework for analysing a published article. Similarly, for the reviewer producing a systematic review or a clinical guideline, a checklist provides a standardised, explicit tool for consistently examining all articles being considered. Two main sources for checklists are the Critical Appraisal Skills Programme and the influential Users' Guides to the Medical Literature (Box 8.2).

Box 8.2   Sources of critical appraisal checklists.

Critical Appraisal Skills Programme: *www.phru.nhs.uk/casp/*
Evidence Based Medicine Tool Kit: *www.med.ualberta.ca/ebm/ebm.htm*
Users' Guides to Evidence-Based Practice: *www.cche.net/usersguides/main.asp*
Guyatt G, Rennie D (eds) (2001) *Users' Guides to the Medical Literature: A Manual for Evidence-Based Clinical Practice*. Chicago, AMA Press
Guyatt G, Rennie D (eds) (2002) *Users' Guides to the Medical Literature: Essentials of Evidence-Based Clinical Practice*. Chicago, AMA Press

Getting started

While every quantitative article is different, LoBiondo-Wood *et al.* (2002) suggest that critical reading falls into four stages:

- *preliminary understanding* – skimming or quickly reading to gain familiarity with the content and layout of the paper
- *comprehensive understanding* – increasing understanding of concepts and research terms
- *analysis understanding* – breaking the study into parts and seeking to understand each part
- *synthesis understanding* – pulling the above steps together to make a (new) whole, making sense of it and explaining relationships

Experience confirms that several practical strategies prove useful when appraising a research article. First, briefly read the abstract. Increasingly articles use a structured abstract to make it easier to identify the study design, the participants and the intervention being studied. Pay particular attention to the main outcome measures – most studies contain multiple measurements but you should isolate the outcome measures of importance. If the study is a randomised controlled trial you should look for a table describing the baseline characteristics. This enables you to assess whether the experimental and controlled groups are similar at the beginning of the study. Having established a 'level playing field', you can look for a detailed description of the study design.

While the Introduction, Discussion and Conclusions may inform an understanding of the issue it is the Methods section that enables you to decide whether or not it is a good study. The Methods and Results sections should command most attention. Increasingly randomised controlled trials present a flowchart which shows how withdrawals and dropouts are handled within the study – an outcome of the CONSORT agreement among journal editors (Begg *et al.* 1996) which dictates clearer standards of trial reporting. You should also focus on results that are considered significant (i.e. that have a p value of 0.05 or less) as these are where the research team has demonstrated a measurable (and possibly important) difference.

Examples of published checklists include those for randomised controlled trials (Box 8.3), those for surveys (Box 8.4) and those for observational and epidemiological studies. Box 8.5 gives a sample critical appraisal of a survey.

How to appraise qualitative research studies

While critical appraisal of quantitative research studies is relatively well-established and uncontroversial, appraisal of qualitative studies is less widely

---

Box 8.3   Questions for critical appraisal of a randomised controlled trial.

A.   Are the results valid?
1.   Did the study address a clearly focused issue?
     Are you able to describe the study participants, the intervention under study, the outcomes being measured and the comparison(s) being made?
2.   Was the assignment of subjects to treatments randomised?
3.   Were all the subjects who entered the trial properly accounted for at its conclusion?
4.   Blinding: Were the subjects, workers, study personnel 'blind to the treatment'?
5.   Were the groups similar at the start of the trial?
6.   Aside from the experimental intervention, were the groups treated equally?

B.   What are the results?
7.   How large was the difference between the two groups? (consider what outcomes were recorded, and how the differences between the groups were expressed?)
8.   How precise was the estimate of the treatment effects? (*hint:* look for confidence intervals)

C.   Will the results help locally?
9.   Can the results be applied to your work? (*or* how different are the subjects in the study to the population you are interested in?)
10.   Were all the important outcomes considered? (would you make a different decision if other important outcomes had been included?)
11.   Are the benefits worth the harms and costs?

---

accepted. Appraisal of qualitative studies seems more intuitive and less deductive – less of a science and more of an art (Booth & O'Rourke 2001). In addition, tools used for data collection (such as interviews and focus groups) seem more prone to the influence and bias of the observer. Indeed some argue that such research does not seek a result that is replicable, and hence generalisable, but rather to provide a valid observation of an individual phenomenon.

Recent research into the use of checklists in appraising qualitative research suggests that it is neither desirable nor practical to select a single instrument or tool (Barbour 2001). With so many different approaches to qualitative research one checklist might privilege, for example, grounded theory, while another might be more appropriate for ethnographic studies. Nevertheless qualitative research should still demonstrate:

- a clear aim for the project
- an appropriate methodology
- justification for the sampling strategy, i.e. who was and who was not included.

Box 8.4 Questions for critical appraisal of a survey.

A. Are the results valid?
1. Objectives and hypotheses
    - Are the objectives of the study clearly stated?
2. Design
    - Is the study design suitable for the objectives?
    - Who/what was studied?
    - Was this the right sample to answer the objectives?
    - Did the subject represent the full spectrum of the population of interest?
    - Is the study large enough to achieve its objectives? Have sample size estimates been performed?
    - Were all subjects accounted for?
    - Were all appropriate outcomes considered?
    - Has ethical approval been obtained if appropriate?
    - What measures were made to contact non-responders?
    - What was the response rate?
3. Measurement and observation
    - Is it clear what was measured, how it was measured and what the outcomes were?
    - Are the measurements valid?
    - Are the measurements reliable?
    - Are the measurements reproducible?

B. What are the results?
4. Presentation of results
    - Are the basic data adequately described?
    - Are the results presented clearly, objectively and in sufficient detail to enable readers to make their own judgement?
    - Are the results internally consistent, i.e. do the numbers add up properly?
5. Analysis
    - Are the data suitable for analysis? Are the methods appropriate to the data? Are any statistics correctly performed and interpreted?

C. Will the results help locally?
6. Discussion
    - Are the results discussed in relation to existing knowledge on the subject and study objectives?
    - Is the discussion biased?
    - Can the results be generalised?
7. Interpretation
    - Are the authors' conclusions justified by the data? Does this paper help me answer my problem?
8. Implementation
    - Can any necessary change be implemented in practice? What are the enablers/barriers to implementation?

Box 8.5   Sample critical appraisal of a survey.

Question: What are the perceptions of paediatric nurses with regard to barriers to their use of research?
McCleary L, Brown GT (2003) Barriers to paediatric nurses' research utilization. *Journal of Advanced Nursing* 42: 364–372

Aim
The objective of the research reported here was to investigate barriers to research utilisation and relationships between those barriers and participation in research, self-reported research utilisation and education among paediatric nurses.

Design and setting
A survey of all nurses in a paediatric teaching hospital. There is reason to suppose that *respondents in a paediatric teaching hospital are not typical of the more general paediatric nursing population* (either within non-teaching hospitals or within a community setting)

Methods
Two standardised measures were used, the Barriers Scale and the Edmonton Research Orientation Scale. Measures used are *well-established* and have been *previously validated.*

Results
176 nurses (33.3%) responded. While not untypical of survey response rates, this is a *low rate of response. No characteristics of non-responders* are given and it is difficult to assess *how representative respondents are of the complete population.* Lack of time to read research was the most frequently cited barrier to using research and administrator resistance to implementation was least frequently cited. Characteristics of the communication and of the setting were more likely to be cited as barriers to research use than characteristics of the nurse. Nurses who reported that they use research more frequently were slightly less likely to see themselves as barriers. Those who had taken a course about reading or using research were more likely to see the organisation as a barrier. Barriers to research use were not associated with whether or not nurses reported that they had a good understanding of research.

Conclusions
These results confirm that implementing research in practice is a complex process. Individual nurses' knowledge about research may not be as important as the process by which organisations implement research. However, the Barriers Scale measures general perceptions about barriers to research utilisation and not specific barriers to implementing particular research.

In addition qualitative research should be reflexive on the possible effect that the relationship between investigators and subjects might have had upon interpretation of the phenomenon. Ironically, given general mistrust of subjectivity in qualitative research, approaches to handling bias in quantitative research appear crude and formulaic by comparison.

While much is made of differences between quantitative and qualitative research both should essentially pose and answer the same three questions:

What is the message?

Can I believe it?

Can I generalise?

The recent growth in so-called mixed methods research has made it more necessary to establish a common approach between both types of research (Johnstone 2004).

While it is clear that qualitative research has an important and expanding role within nursing research, the researcher should be aware that there remains much opposition to criteria-based approaches to appraisal. In an attempt to sidestep such objections Dixon-Woods *et al.* (2004) have proposed a minimal set of prompts which have been designed to stimulate appraisal of different dimensions of qualitative research but are explicitly methodology neutral. They argue that any approaches to critical appraisal of qualitative studies should recognise the importance of distinctive study designs and theoretical perspectives within qualitative research. They conclude that any such approach should distinguish fatal flaws from minor errors. They further assert that:

'the more important and interesting aspects of qualitative research may remain very difficult to measure except through the subjective judgement of experienced qualitative researchers' (Dixon-Woods *et al.* 2004:225)

Boxes 8.6 and 8.7 show examples of how a qualitative research article might be appraised.

How to appraise systematic reviews, practice guidelines and economic analysis

Up to this point we have focused on single research studies, either quantitative or qualitative. Nevertheless basing research plans on the results of a single research study in isolation may prove misleading. As a researcher you will need to examine the entire body of evidence as captured by a systematic review (overview). Typically this provides a rigorous summary of all the research evidence that relates to a specific question; be it causation, diagnosis, prognosis, effectiveness or patient views (Ciliska *et al.* 2001).

Box 8.6   Critical appraisal checklist for a qualitative research article.

A. **Are the results of the study valid?**
1.   Was there a clear statement of the aims of the research?
     Why is it important?
2.   Is a qualitative method appropriate?
3.   Sampling strategy
     (includes selection and purpose of sample, who was selected and why, how they were selected and why, whether the sample size is justified and why some participants may have chosen not to take part)
     Was the sampling strategy appropriate to address the aims?
4.   Data collection
     (includes whether it is clear why the setting was chosen, how the data were collected and why (e.g. focus group, structured interview, etc.), how the data were recorded and why (e.g. tape recording, note taking, etc.) and if the methods were modified during the process and why.
     Were the data collected in a way that addresses the research issue?
5.   Data analysis
     (includes a description of the analysis, how categories and themes were derived from the data, whether the findings have been evaluated for credibility and whether we can be confident that data have not been overlooked)
     Was the data analysis sufficiently rigorous?
6.   Research partnership relations
     (includes whether the researchers examined their own role, the setting in which data was collected and how the research was explained to participants)
     Has the relationship between researchers and participants been adequately considered?

B. **What are the results?**
7.   Findings
     Is there a clear statement of the findings?
8.   Justification of data interpretation
     (includes whether sufficient data are presented to sustain the findings and how the data used in the paper were selected from the original sample)
     Do the researchers indicate the links between the data presented and their own findings on what the data contain?

C. **Will the results help locally?**
9.   Transferability
     Are the findings of this study transferable to a wider population?
10. Relevance and usefulness
     (includes whether the research is important and relevant in addressing the research aim, in contributing new insights and in suggesting implications for research, policy and practice)
     Are the findings of this relevant and important to your patients or problems?
11. Eliciting your patient's preferences and values
     Do you and your patient have a clear assessment of their values and preferences?
12. Meeting your patient's preferences and values
     Are they met by this regimen and its consequences?

Box 8.7 Sample critical appraisal of a qualitative research study.

Question: What are the perceptions of patients with co-morbidities in relation to the quality of acute care services?
Williams A (2004) Patients with co-morbidities: perceptions of acute care services. *Journal of Advanced Nursing* 46: 13–22.

Design and setting
Qualitative descriptive design conducted in a large metropolitan private hospital in Melbourne, Australia.

Patients
A purposive sample of 12 patients of 18 years or older with one or more chronic conditions (mean 6 chronic conditions) for approximately five years, requiring an acute care stay for greater than four days. The sample comprised 50% males and 50% females.

Methods
Individual semi-structured interviews were conducted within 14 days of hospital discharge minimising the possibility of *recall bias*. Data collection and analysis were ongoing until *theoretical saturation* was reached (i.e. until no new major themes emerged). Analysis used *multiple data sources* (verbatim transcripts, field notes, and patient medical histories). Template analysis was used to develop themes. Strengths of the study were that *themes were confirmed by a second, independent data analysis* and *patients were able to verify interpretations* from a summary of the main findings.

Main findings
Three themes emerged:

1. *Poor continuity in the care of co-morbidities*
2. *Something always goes wrong in hospital*
3. *Chronic conditions persist after discharge*

Conclusions
Patients with co-morbidities highlighted the need for comprehensive discharge planning and described poor continuity in care of their co-morbidities, the inevitability of something going wrong during acute care, and chronic conditions persisting after discharge. *Generalisations cannot be drawn because a purposive sample was used.*

Systematic reviews make strenuous attempts to overcome possible biases. They follow a rigorous methodology of search, retrieval, appraisal, data extraction, data synthesis, and interpretation. To protect against possible bias, explicit, preset inclusion criteria are used in selecting studies for inclusion. Similar protections are used when producing clinical guidelines. Much time and resources are expended in assuring the quality of the process by using more than one reviewer to independently select studies and by recording explicit details of methods used at every stage.

Systematic reviews focus on high-quality primary research reports in attempting to summarise research-based knowledge on a topic. Nevertheless, not every systematic review is of high-quality and critical appraisal remains essential. Box 8.8 gives guidelines on appraising a review article.

Systematic reviews are one type of research synthesis (Cook *et al* 1997). Other examples include practice guidelines and economic evaluations. These integrative studies frequently draw upon the results of systematic reviews and so share common principles for critical appraisal. Economic evaluations compare costs and consequences of different strategies with consequences and the values attached to them frequently being generated from systematic reviews.

Box 8.8   How to critically appraise review articles.

A.   Are the results of this systematic review valid?
1. Is this a systematic review of randomised trials?
2. Does the systematic review include a description of the strategies used to find all relevant trials?
3. Does the systematic review include a description of how the validity of individual studies was assessed?
4. Were the results consistent from study to study?
5. Were individual patient data or aggregate data used in the analysis?

B.   What are the results?
6. How large was the treatment effect?
7. How precise is the estimate of treatment effect?

C.   Will the results help locally?
8. Are my patients so different from those in the study that the results do not apply?
9. Is the treatment feasible in our setting?
10. Were all clinically important outcomes (harms as well as benefits) considered?
11. What are my patient's values and preferences for both the outcome we are trying to prevent and the side effects that may arise?

Applying the results of critical appraisal

Reading, appraising and applying the results from research articles is a time-consuming concern. While the evidence-based health care movement originally aspired for all practitioners to locate and appraise their own evidence recent years have seen the lowering of this bar (Guyatt *et al.* 2000). Now proponents suggest all practitioners should learn the skills of critical appraisal primarily to enable them to use other people's products of critical appraisal with confidence. Such products fall into one of two categories: article-based and topical-based.

Article-based critical appraisal is represented by a plethora of evidence-based journals such as *Evidence-Based Nursing, Evidence-Based Medicine, Evidence-Based Healthcare*, etc. These present the cream of current journal articles in single-page summaries that give the main methodological features of each study and appraise them for likely quality. Each summary is arranged under an indicative title that captures the study's principal result in a clinically relevant 'bottom line'. Similarly, databases such as those from the NHS Centre for Reviews and Dissemination (CSD) at the University of York provide free internet access to article-based summaries of particular types of research synthesis, notably systematic reviews (the Database of Abstracts of Reviews of Effects – DARE) and economic evaluations (the NHS Economic Evaluations Database – NEED).

Topical-based critical appraisal is question driven, rather than literature driven. Important questions from clinical practice are identified and specialist staff or volunteer clinicians search for answers from the research literature. Results identified from the literature are summarised and presented in a concise and meaningful summary, for example as a Critically Appraised Topic (CAT). Alternatively this process may contribute to some wider publishing enterprise such as the clinical handbook, *Clinical Evidence* published by BMJ Publishing Group or results posted on a website as with the Manchester-based *BestBETS* initiative. Concern has been expressed over the quality of CATS – not with regard to appraisal, which is largely found to be satisfactory, but because search procedures have frequently failed to identify the most relevant items to address the clinical question (Coomarasamy *et al.* 2001). Clearly the value of appraisal depends on first finding the most appropriate research study.

Successful application of appraisal results also assumes that the study population is similar enough to the local population. Questions such as those below are key when deciding whether we need to replicate research carried out elsewhere or simply to extrapolate findings from already existing research.

Can I apply results from a study that only includes patients between 70 and 80 years old to those in the 65 to 70 age group?

What about relatively fit and 'biologically young' 81-year-olds?

Can the results of studies conducted in Edmonton, Alberta be extrapolated to Edmonton, North London?

Are rural practices in Finland different to those in Wales?

For the researcher the value of pre-appraised products is twofold. First, they provide a quality-fortified environment for assessing key research studies that contribute to knowledge within a particular topic area (for example, hospital infection or handwashing). Second, and more important, studies critically appraised by experienced researchers provide a useful benchmark against which you, as a less experienced researcher, can chart your progress as you become more aware of methodological issues.

Conclusion

This chapter demonstrates that critical appraisal has become increasingly important. It can be used by the researcher as a quality control tool to assess individual studies. Alternatively, if the researcher is reviewing multiple studies, it provides a standardised approach for producing systematic reviews and clinical guidelines. The key concepts of validity, reliability and applicability have been emphasised together with the usefulness of a checklist-led approach. Notwithstanding essential differences between quantitative and qualitative research, this chapter demonstrates the value of a common approach. Above all, the take-home message is that critical appraisal is not simply a pure academic skill – it is an ongoing strategy to help you in your continuing clinical and research career.

References

Antman EM, Lau J, Kupelnick B, Mosteller F, Chalmers TC (1992) A comparison of results of meta-analysis of randomised controlled trials and the recommendations of experts. *Journal of the American Medical Association* 268: 240–248

Barbour RS (2001) Checklists for improving rigour in qualitative research: a case of the tail wagging the dog? *British Medical Journal* 322: 1115–1117

Begg C, Cho M, Eastwood S, Horton R, Moher D, Olkin I *et al.* (1996) Improving the quality of reporting of randomized controlled trials. The CONSORT statement. *Journal of the American Medical Association* 276: 637–639

Booth A, O'Rourke AJ (2001) *Critical appraisal and using the literature.* www.shef.ac.uk/scharr/ir/units/critapp/appqual.htm

Ciliska D, Cullum N, Marks S (2001) Evaluation of systematic reviews of treatment or prevention interventions. *Evidence-Based Nursing* 4: 100–104

Coggon D, Rose G, Barker DJP (2003) *Epidemiology for the Uninitiated,* 5th edition. London, BMJ Publishing

Cook DJ, Mulrow CD, Haynes RB (1997) Systematic reviews: synthesis of best evidence for clinical decisions. *Annals of Internal Medicine* 126: 376–380

Coomarasamy A, Latthe P, Papaioannou S, Publicover M, Gee H, Khan KS (2001) Critical appraisal in clinical practice: sometimes irrelevant, occasionally invalid. *Journal of the Royal Society of Medicine* 94: 573–577

Dixon-Woods M, Shaw RL, Agarwal S, Smith JA (2004) The problem of appraising qualitative research. *Quality and Safety in Health Care* 13: 223–225

Edwards AG, Russell IT, Stott NC (1998) Signal versus noise in the evidence base for medicine: an alternative to hierarchies of evidence? *Family Practice* 15: 319–322

Guyatt GH, Meade MO, Jaeschke RZ, Cook DJ, Haynes RB (2000) Practitioners of evidence-based care. Not all clinicians need to appraise evidence from scratch but all need some skills. *British Medical Journal* 320: 954–955

Johnstone PL (2004) Mixed methods, mixed methodology health services research in practice. *Qualitative Health Research* 14: 259–271

LoBiondo-Wood G, Haber J, Krainovich-Miller B (2002) Critical reading strategies: overview of the research process. Chapter 2. In LoBiondo-Wood G, Haber J (eds), *Nursing Research: methods, critical appraisal, and utilization,* 5th edition. St Louis, Mosby

McCleary L, Brown GT (2003) Barriers to paediatric nurses' research utilization. *Journal of Advanced Nursing* 42: 364–72

North G, Booth A (1999) Why appraise the evidence? a case study of Vitamin C and the healing of pressure sores. *Journal of Human Nutrition and Dietetics* 12: 237–244

Parkes J, Hyde C, Deeks J, Milne R (2001) Teaching critical appraisal skills in health care settings. *The Cochrane Database of Systematic Reviews* 2001, Issue 3.

Ploeg J (1999) Identifying the best research design to fit the question, Part 2: qualitative designs. *Evidence-Based Nursing 2:* 36–37

Roberts J, DiCenso A (1999) Identifying the best research design to fit the question, Part 1: quantitative designs (editorial). *Evidence-Based Nursing* 2: 4–6

Sackett DL (1986) Rules of evidence and clinical recommendations on the use of antithrombotic agents. *Archives of Internal Medicine* 146: 464–465

Williams A (2004) Patients with co-morbidities: perceptions of acute care services. *Journal of Advanced Nursing* 46: 13–22

Further reading

Ajetunmobi O (2002) *Making Sense of Critical Appraisal*. London, Arnold

Cullum N (2000) Evaluation of studies of treatment or prevention interventions (editorial). *Evidence-Based Nursing* 3: 100–102

Cullum N (2001) Evaluation of studies of treatment or prevention interventions, Part 2: applying the results of studies to your patients. *Evidence-Based Nursing* 4: 7–8

Greenhalgh T (2000) *How to Read a Paper: the basics of evidence based medicine*, 2nd edition. London, BMJ Publishing

Website

www.phru.nhs.uk/casp/ – Critical Appraisal Skills Programme (CASP)

9 Preparing a Research Proposal

Senga Bond and Kate Gerrish

Key points

- A research proposal assists researchers clarify their intentions and communicate these to funding bodies and committees granting ethical or research governance approval.
- A research proposal should present a reasoned argument about the need for the proposed study on theoretical or practical grounds and provide explicit details of how it will be carried out.
- A clear statement of the rationale for the proposed study, the research questions, details of the methods to be used to answer to the questions, the resources required to undertake the study and the methods of dissemination should be included.
- The precise format of the proposal will depend on the reason for writing it: universities and funding organisations often produce guidance about the different sections within which information should be provided.

Introduction

Research proposals may be written for several reasons: to obtain funding, to present to a higher degrees committee in a university, for research governance or ethical approval or as an academic exercise as part of a research course. This chapter focuses on general principles in preparing a proposal but will emphasise the first of these since obtaining funding often precedes other reasons.

Preparing a research proposal will be addressed in two ways. The first is to provide novice researchers with some guidance about possible structure and content. The second is to suggest some ways of making a proposal more appealing and thus more likely to be funded.

The most important function of research proposals is to make explicit a reasoned argument about the need for the proposed study on practical and/or theoretical grounds and how it will be carried out. The very act of writing a proposal assists in identifying the strengths and weaknesses of a study. This is achieved through the process of setting down a clear statement of the question(s) that the study proposes to answer, the methods that will be used to find the answer and the resources required to do it. Information should also be provided about how the study findings will be disseminated and any products likely to arise. The particular form that a proposal takes will depend on the reason for writing it:

funding organisations, universities, and increasingly health care organisations produce special forms giving guidance about the different sections within which information should be provided. It is essential that these directions are followed. The general guidance about preparing a proposal provided here may be amended to suit the requirements of a particular case.

Typical content of a research proposal

It is useful to have a checklist of the main topics to be included. Such a list would contain the following:

- title of project
- summary
- justification for the study
- related research
- aims and objectives
- plan of investigation
- project management
- ethical considerations
- products arising from the project
- dissemination
- resources
- budget
- curriculum vitae

   This chapter will consider each of these headings in turn and give some pointers to the kind of information within each one.

Title of project

Research projects become known by their title so it is important to make the title explicit and relatively brief while describing the proposed study. Sometimes studies change in direction during their evolution while the subject matter remains essentially the same. An experiment may collapse or the nature of the variables being considered in a survey may be altered on the basis of pilot work. The title should be able to override these changes while still conveying the essence of the study. The use of words like 'evaluation' and 'survey' are helpful in alerting readers to the approach the study will take. It is more informative to call a study 'An evaluation of counselling for patients who have had a mastectomy' than to call it 'Caring for mastectomy patients' even if the design or counselling methods change as the project evolves.

Summary

In practice the summary is usually written after the main body of the proposal has been put together since it requires to be succinct yet state clearly the objectives of the study and how it will be carried out. It should contain only the most relevant information. The space allocated to it or word length specified means that every word is important and it is an art to describe a major project in a paragraph.

Because it appears early, the summary, like the title, alerts the reader as to what to expect in the subsequent text. The summary is an important indication of the quality of the remainder of the proposal and so it requires careful consideration and probably several drafts to ensure all of the main points are included.

Justification for the study

The statement of the problem that opens the main body of the proposal must convince the reader that the proposed study is important. It needs to introduce the research questions and put them into a context that indicates the importance of the problem, its costs and consequences. It should identify how the proposed study will add to previous work and build on theory. In nursing studies there are likely to be practical implications of the research so that, as well as having value in contributing to knowledge, its utility value for education or practice needs to be stressed. There may be methodological gains, for example, in developing a new research instrument, which would have future applications.

In developing the problem statement, avoid making claims for the study that are either too grandiose or too general. Novices often express research as setting out to *prove* something, for example that parents prefer booked home visits from health visitors, rather than as an open question of their response to different systems of visiting, or stating a well-reasoned formal hypothesis of preference. There is also a tendency to be over ambitious when enthusiasm for the topic overrides their judgement about delivering the project. A key piece of advice therefore is *to focus on the manageable*.

Related research

Next, it is important to demonstrate a command of the current state of the field and how this study would move it forward. To achieve this, the key studies that provide the basis for the proposed project should be included. Indicate in language for non-specialists how they are relevant to the proposed study and how this study moves beyond them. This review should relate both to substantive concerns and methods, and be provided in sufficient detail to inform the reader of its relevance. It may also be useful to include knowledge of ongoing studies as a reflection of the author's competence in keeping abreast of developments, as well as point out how they differ from the study being proposed. Some funders of research, for example government agencies, commission research to address their policy concerns. In such circumstances it is important to demonstrate a familiarity with current policy documents and show how the proposed research relates to these concerns.

The theoretical aspects of the study and the firmness of the theoretical base should be described. This information can be extremely influential in demonstrating the applicant's grasp of complex issues and in showing that the study is well grounded and has more than practical implications.

The development of the literature base is a major feature of the research process described in Chapters 7 and 8 and it is equally an important feature of developing the research proposal. If the literature search and the literature section of the proposal is an afterthought, it will shine through by virtue of its unrelatedness to the remainder of the proposal.

Aims and objectives

Any reviewer of proposals likes to see objectives that are clear, specific, concrete and achievable. List and number them in order of importance in a clear sequence, taking only a sentence or two for each.

The remainder of the proposal will be judged in relation to the stated aims. Therefore, avoid vague terminology and generalities; define criteria as specifically as possible. Do not leave it up to the reader to have to do the guesswork about what the objectives are or their order of priority.

The objectives of the study may take the form of questions, when research is exploratory or a survey where specific facts are being sought. It may be possible to state objectives in the form of testable hypotheses where there is a basis for predicting results. It is more convincing if hypotheses are stated whenever possible. However, these need to be precise and relationships clearly specified. Further guidance on developing research aims and objectives can be found in Chapter 6.

Plan of investigation

This section could be called *plan of investigation, procedure or method* and is likely to be the section most carefully scrutinised by those reviewing the proposal. It is when procedures are spelled out that those reading the proposal gauge the applicant's capacity both to undertake and complete the proposed work.

The specific format of this section will depend on the methods adopted. Different emphases will be required depending on whether the study takes a survey, an experimental or qualitative approach. Irrespective of method there are several important matters to convey and these are best written in discrete sections.

Method/design

The design to be adopted and the precise methods and techniques to be used should be clear. Simple descriptions are available for particular types of experiment and for survey research and can be specified in advance. Equally it is straightforward to indicate whether the study is prospective or retrospective, cross-sectional or longitudinal. For exploratory studies, case studies or ethnographic research, the basic method should be made clear and this section will often require appropriate adaptation when the application forms issued are set out as if for clinical trials.

For experimental studies details will be required about which variables are controlled and how control is to be achieved. In some instances, there may be complete randomisation while in others subjects may be matched on known relevant variables, or included in a factorial design. It is important to show awareness of relevant variables and how control can be realistically managed. In health services research, control of all variables is virtually impossible. The challenge is to make the best use of available situations and be sophisticated in designs that offer the closest approximation to experimental proof.

When compromises have to be made to facilitate experimental design in the 'real world', the reasons for such compromises should be made clear. For example, if patients are to be allowed some degree of choice of treatment or randomisation is clustered by wards or general practices rather than individual patients, the reasons for doing so need to be made explicit.

Specification of design in observation studies and survey research should make clear that this is the intended method. Where particular qualitative methodologies have been chosen, for example, grounded theory, ethnography or phenomenology, it is important to explain why this is the case. The overall design should be detailed in advance of specification of the particular methods of data collection to be used, such as questionnaires, in-depth interviews, particular clinical tests or outcome measures. Further details on different research designs are provided in Section 3, Chapters 11–21.

Population and sample

The initial literature review will have indicated the nature of the population relevant to the study as well as giving a clue to the generalisability of the study findings. This section will include a clear statement of the population from which the study sample will be drawn, and details of the characteristics of the sample. When particular sampling techniques are used, for example, stratified or cluster sampling, as described in Chapter 12, this choice should be justified.

Evidence should be provided that the sample is available and can be recruited and that, where appropriate, a sampling frame exists. Clear criteria for inclusion and exclusion should be specified, or variables by which individual subjects will be matched.

Critical also are questions of sample size, which will be dealt with in greater detail in Chapter 12. Reviewers will be looking for indications that the sample size is appropriate to answer the research question. In the case of quantitative research, the sample needs to be big enough to detect differences or carry out other appropriate statistical manipulations so as to come up with a clear answer. It is generally expected that proposals for experimental designs include power analysis providing a statement of the expected and acceptable size of effects, at what degree of power, and the sample size required to detect them. The assistance of a statistician may be required in calculating the sample size.

It is equally important to specify the sampling intended in qualitative research studies. Case studies or individuals will be selected on some criteria and sometimes some or all of these can be specified in advance, for example, to include a gender, ethnic or occupational mix or other theoretically relevant variables. In some qualitative approaches, such as grounded theory, it may not be appropriate to specify the precise sample size in advance as this is dependent on ongoing theory development. However, it is important to explain how the sample will be generated during the course of the research and it can be helpful to the reader to give some indication of the limits of the anticipated sample size and how this will be determined.

Data collection

In this section measures and procedures to be used for data collection are described. These should reflect the variables included, show that the measures to be used represent acceptable operational definitions of them, and that they have appropriate measurement or psychometric characteristics. In many topics of relevance to nursing research, well-validated scales exist and it would be foolish to develop a new scale when this is unnecessary. Where proposed measurements have been used in other relevant studies it is helpful to indicate this. When methods of measurement do not already exist and new methods are proposed, these are best described in detail as an appendix to the proposal. In some cases reviewers wish to see copies of instrumentation, test items, questionnaires or interview guides. It makes sense to find out if this is required. However, for some studies, a substantial part of the work entails such methodological developments.

In addition to conventional data collection techniques like questionnaires and interviews, other methods may be involved such as anthropometric or clinical measures or assessment of observed behaviour. It may be appropriate to mention the apparatus to be used to obtain these data and whether any special conditions are required for their use. If the data to be collected or the methods used to collect them are likely to be sensitive or controversial, then plans indicating how anticipated problems would be dealt with should be included.

Pilot and development studies

Providing evidence that the study plan is based on findings of a pilot study increases the chances of impressing reviewers about the viability of the project. Indeed many proposals are submitted to enable pilot work to be carried out as a preliminary to a larger, definitive study. A pilot study will tell reviewers what steps will be taken to ensure that the proposed methods are workable, are acceptable to subjects and manageable. The pilot study is worth specifying in some detail. For example, to conduct a postal survey from first principles would involve going through several stages to arrive at a questionnaire before going on to a postal pilot study to gauge its acceptability and response rate. If an already validated instrument was to be used, then the amount of development and pilot work would be much less, but details of its acceptability to the population for the study may need to be ascertained. It is always worth investing time and effort to ensure that the development, feasibility or pilot work for a study is thorough, and stressing this in the proposal. Pilot work may be presented as the first phases of a project.

Analysis

It is essential to have considered analysis in the development of any study, even though doing the analysis is some way off. Most important is to show that the methods of analysis are consistent with the objectives, design of the study and data. Often this is easier to specify in advance for quantitative studies. It is more difficult to describe the analytic procedures used in qualitative studies especially if reviewers are unfamiliar with these techniques. Providing detail of the specific framework or approach for qualitative analysis to be used will demonstrate to the reviewer that the researcher has a good understanding of how the data will be analysed. In cases where complete specification is not possible, the stages of data analysis can be outlined indicating an appreciation of the kinds of methods likely to be used.

   If studies rely on multivariate or discriminant techniques or longitudinal analyses, this should be specified even if it has to be at a general level. It should be indicated that sufficient statistical expertise is available to inform and, if necessary, carry out statistical analysis. Knowing what techniques to apply to the analysis of data is more important than indicating that a statistical package such as SPSS for Windows is to be used. Similarly, stating that a qualitative data software package such as NUD*IST or NVivo is to be used is no substitute for detailing analytic methods. The reviewer needs to be convinced that you know which analysis is appropriate and have or can obtain the appropriate skills, hardware and software to achieve it.

Work plan

Details of the time scale and plan of work should be included to show the anticipated duration of each stage of the study. Providing a clear timetable with milestones to be achieved through the process of the study can demonstrate that the proposal is realistic and achievable. Sufficient lead-in time should be allowed to secure the necessary research governance and ethical approval. Major milestones, like having all data collection tools ready, targets for patient recruitment and completion of data collection and analysis should be included. When the study is complex and different activities are happening simultaneously, flow charts may be necessary to identify the anticipated progress of work. Often a diagram like a Gantt chart says more than words.

Generally, the time taken to complete each part of a study is underestimated, particularly data collection which depends on a prospective series. The tendency is to be over-optimistic. This can also apply to the time it takes to negotiate entry to study sites and gain research governance and ethical approval. Formal project planning activities should be undertaken to determine the timescale required in relation to critical events.

Project management

The reviewer of the proposal will want to be reassured that the researcher has the necessary expertise to undertake the study. In the case of a novice researcher they will be looking for appropriate support from an experienced researcher. If the study is complex, involving a large research team and possibly collecting data in different settings, it will be important to identify who carries overall responsibility for the project and how the different components will be co-ordinated.

Increasingly in health-related research there is an expectation that service users will have been involved in informing the design of the study. As Chapter 5 illustrates, this involvement will vary depending on the research question. Where service users have been consulted it is important to identify their contribution. It may also be appropriate to have a Project Steering Committee to act in an advisory capacity to the research team for the duration of the project. This can be a useful way of involving services users and in bringing in additional expertise to complement that of the researcher team.

Ethical considerations

Reading the methods section will have alerted the reviewer to any ethical problems. The proposal may be reviewed by a committee whose primary objective is to assess the scientific methods of a study. However, they will not be unaware of ethical issues and they are likely to assess whether 'the ends justify the means'. Some grant-awarding bodies require that a study has approval from an ethical committee (e.g. MREC/LREC) prior to any award being made. However MRECs will not review a proposal until it has been funded!

Whereas ethics committees may consider the science of the proposal, they will be giving most attention to the protection of participants from undue distress. As outlined in Chapter 10, when submitting a proposal for ethical approval, documentation about information for participants and how written consent will be obtained and the forms used to collect data should be submitted with the approval forms. Ethical matters may also be relevant to describing the protection of participants from any negative consequences of a study, and protection of staff can equally apply when they may be involved in handling noxious substances or administering procedures. How data will be stored and measures taken to protect the identities of participants or collaborating institutions should be included through adherence to the requirements of the Data Protection Act.

Products arising from the project

The end products of most research studies are a final report to the funding or commissioning body or a thesis and publications. However, research products may also be new research instruments or methods of data collection as well as teaching or clinical aids. If the study is likely to yield a product of commercial value, then ownership of the intellectual property rights and the patents to the product need to be made clear at the outset. This is especially so if an industrial company is involved. It may also be appropriate to include costs for product development in a proposal. Novice researchers may need to seek advice on intellectual property rights (IPR) from their employing organisation. Contracts of employment increasingly include a clause about who owns the intellectual property arising from the work of an employee. The funding body and the organisation in which data are to be collected may also have an interest in intellectual property.

Dissemination

Increasingly attention is required to the dissemination of the results of research. Reports and published papers are taken for granted but they are not the only way to present results. Videos and presentations may be equally relevant as a means of disseminating findings to particular audiences. It may be appropriate to make specific suggestions about how this is to be achieved, especially through executive summaries of findings targeted to specific audiences. Some grant-awarding bodies are more interested than others in dissemination over and above traditional publications. Research governance approval often includes the expectation that the researcher will feedback relevant findings to the organisation(s) in which the research is conducted.

Resources

It is important that the resources required to carry out the study are realistically appraised. Resources, whether human, material or financial, need to be specified.

Personnel

The person(s) who will direct the project, the principal investigator(s), should be clearly identified together with the amount of time they intend to devote to the project. It may be that this is a proposal for a full-time commitment or for only a few hours in a week. The relationships with academic and clinical collaborators and their responsibility and commitment to the project should be included. Where a complex study is involved, the right mix of expertise may be an important element. Such personnel may include a consultant or other clinical experts in the field, a statistician, health economist or social scientist. Each might be costed in for a few hours per week or month, or a flat fee as consultancy. It must be clear how they have contributed to the proposal.

It is especially important for inexperienced researchers to obtain the support of established research workers. In this respect it can be useful to show that active consultation has taken place in the development of a proposal. Indicate the kind and amount of assistance offered by those experienced in research or particular technical competence associated with data processing, analysis, costings and so on.

Other resources

Describing particular services or back-up facilities such as IT, library facilities and secretarial support can strengthen a proposal. Where established networks are integral to a project or co-operation has been obtained from particular agencies or institutions, some indication of this, such as letters of agreement, may be included as a helpful appendix. There are considerable benefits to the proposed study being hosted by an established research centre.

Budget

Even where no external funding is being sought, for example, if the costs of the research are notional and will be absorbed by the researcher's employer, or the research is undertaken as part of an educational programme, it is important to identify the costs of undertaking the research. Applications for research governance approval frequently require the researcher to make explicit any costs that will be incurred by the NHS, for example, if investigations additional to routine care need to be undertaken, or if staff will be required to provide or collect data.

Preparing a research budget requires as much skill as preparing other parts of the proposal. It is amazing, when a maximum amount of money is specified in calls for proposals, how many are costed at just that amount! Part of the skill in budgeting lies in locating other people who know the prices of commodities – staff salaries as well as equipment and other consumables. However knowing the details of data collection and processing makes costing much easier – how many hours it takes to collect data, how much travel time and mileage, how much data processing will be required. Preparing a budget means translating the timescale and plan of work into financial terms.

Novice writers have a tendency to skimp on the budget, earnestly believing that if a project costs less, then it improves the chance of being funded. Undercutting the budget simply reflects inexperience. Sharp-eyed critics will quickly notice where there has been undue trimming and what is feasible in the costs quoted. Equally where excesses are included, such as a new computer for a short project, or large travel budgets, they will be cut. Sometimes budgets can be a matter of negotiation if they are thought to be too high by virtue of over-elaborate sampling or extended timescales. However, to be caught short of cash and time can be disastrous and funding bodies do not take kindly to requests for extensions of time or increased budgets. Box 9.1 provides a checklist for preparing a budget.

Box 9.1   Checklist for preparing a budget.

- research staff salaries
- secretarial staff salaries
- data collection costs, for example purchase of equipment and other materials, printing, travelling expenses, stationery and postage
- data processing costs, for example coding questionnaire data, transcribing interview tapes
- book purchases/library costs such as inter-library loans
- conference attendance
- product development
- dissemination
- overheads

It is sometimes useful to distinguish between capital costs, to include the purchase of necessary equipment, and recurrent costs. It is useful to check whether your library will expect a fee for inter-library loans and special book purchases. Some organisations, especially universities, ask for overheads. Check whether this is so and the current rate. Hosting organisations also wish to check a budget statement before it is submitted and salaries, etc. usually have to be countersigned by someone with specific expertise in this matter. An appropriate budget is always a matter of careful specification rather than just pulling some notional figure out of the air.

Curriculum vitae

Attach appropriate *curricula vitae* for all principal investigators. The contents should be appropriate and include details of:

C ✓

- name
- age
- qualifications
- education
- work experience
- research experience
- recent relevant publications

One or two pages are usually sufficient to show whether the applicants have the appropriate experience and performance record to conduct the study.

Final review

Research proposals usually go through several drafts. Indeed, there would be a major cause for concern if they did not! There are a number of things to be achieved in reviewing proposals. Not least is to consider its physical presentation. Neatly spaced typescript with a major effort on legibility, lucidity and clarity of presentation are all important. While readers of a proposal will not be consciously evaluating it on how it is presented, nevertheless the relatively small amount of time it takes to ensure a pleasant layout that is easily followed will be time well-spent. Devices such as a bold typeface, italics, spacing, using diagrams, flow charts and tables are useful to attract the reader's eye. The latter are often more useful in presenting details than reams of text. Use a font size of at least 10 points and use Arial, Times or Helvetica typefaces.

It is also useful to ask others with experience of successfully submitting proposals to check over your efforts. Most people are pleased to assist, so long as there is evidence that you have made proper attempts to produce a good piece of work and adequate time is allowed.

Additional considerations

Guidelines for proposal development

Different review bodies considering a proposal will be looking at quite different things, and it is important to identify their primary concerns and give special consideration to them. Check if they have any particular requirements in the manner in which a proposal is presented. Some organisations have a checklist or a particular form on which proposals must be made. It is wise to adhere strictly to notes of guidance. Other organisations regard the form of the proposal as a measure of the worth of the researcher and offer no guidance on preparing a proposal.

Check whether a funding body has any special focus in terms of the subject matter, whether there is any specific geographical area or limits to funding. In Chapter 4, several sources of research funding were identified. Some funding bodies offer the opportunity to submit an outline proposal for approval before submitting a full proposal. This permits a degree of negotiation about the focus, content, methods and so on.

This book is intended primarily for people who are relatively new to research and this chapter may be used to assist some who have never before developed a proposal, or developed a successful one. Some funding bodies are keen to support new researchers but are not likely to want to risk large sums of money or invest in potentially unmanageable studies. It is wise, then, to begin in a relatively small way or to ask for only funding for the pilot work or first stage of the project. This safeguards both the funding body and the researcher should something go drastically wrong. Better still would be to have an experienced researcher as a co-applicant. It is always helpful to obtain copies of proposals that have been funded by the body to which you are applying. This does not imply slavish adherence to that particular format but it does give some indication of the type of proposal more likely to be welcomed and hence succeed in being funded.

Proposal review

It is also helpful to know how proposals are reviewed. Sometimes they are sent to external referees with particular expertise for comment, while others are dealt with completely 'in- house'. As well as scientific referees, there may also be 'customer' referees who are looking for the utility of the research in practical or policy terms, rather than the quality of the science. Knowledge of the membership of a review committee can be useful in anticipating areas to which special attention or orientation should be given. When a committee of mixed expertise reviews proposals, then all members should be able to understand the nature of the study. At times there could be a problem of orientation – when biological or physical scientists are asked to review a proposal with a social science orientation. In instances like this, it is important to avoid excessive jargon while maintaining appropriate specificity.

There is skill in achieving a balance between identifying every single possibility and spelling out every detail and providing sufficient detail to convince reviewers that the applicant has the ability to complete a worthwhile study. To some extent the degree of specificity is related to the state of knowledge in a particular field and to the extent to which the study is exploratory or explanatory. Writers of proposals have to rely on their judgement to some extent but, as a general principle, it is better to include more information than leave out something others may regard as important. However, the reviewing panel will be abreast of standard methods and these do not have to be detailed.

The length of the proposal can be of some concern. Sometimes maximum length and number of pages is specified. If lengthy details of specific steps are required, then these can be included as appendices so as to avoid crowding too much into the main text and so losing the crispness of the presentation. The purpose of appendices is to provide additional supportive information for reviewers who do not feel that the main text is sufficiently detailed but should not require to be read to obtain a clear impression of the study.

Conclusion

This chapter has discussed the need to write down a clear statement of proposed research in the form of a protocol to assist researchers clarify their own intentions and communicate these to funding bodies and committees granting ethical or research governance approval. Matters of making explicit a proposed time schedule and proper project management techniques can be fundamental to the successful execution of a project. However even more helpful is gaining the assistance of experienced researchers who have themselves submitted successful proposals to offer advice in the development phase of a study proposal. Gains to be made from others' experience in such matters are invaluable.

Finally, do not be dismayed if a first attempt is rejected. One can always learn from it. Unfortunately, not all grant-awarding bodies provide information detailing why a proposal is rejected and this is singularly unhelpful to the recipient of the rejection slip. However, increasingly, referees' comments are given to applicants. Proposal review bodies may refer the project, that is suggest that the researcher rework it with some specific types of guidance. In some cases it is almost as if referral is the rule and few proposals are accepted the first time round. There are several books, chapters in research texts and other publications devoted to offering advice about writing research proposals and some are listed below. These offer useful suggestions and go beyond this introductory chapter.

Further reading

Mores J (2004) Preparing and evaluating qualitative research proposals. In Seale C, Gobo G, Gubrium J, Silverman D (eds) *Qualitative Research Practice*. London, Sage pp493–503

Fraser J (1995) *Professional Proposal Writing*. London, Gower

Grant D (1998) How to get a grant funded. *British Medical Journal* 317: 1647–48

Hodgson C (1989) Tips on writing successful grant proposals. *Nurse Practitioner* 14:2 44–49

Locke LF, Spirduso WW, Silverman SJ (1999) *Proposals That Work: Guide for Planning Dissertations and Grant Proposals*, 4th edition. London, Sage

Ogden TE, Goldberg IA (2002) *Research Proposals: A Guide To Success*, 3rd edition. New York, Raven Press

Punch K (2000) *Developing Effective Research Proposals*. London, Sage

Ries JB, Leukefeld CG (1995) *Applying for Research Funding*. Thousand Oaks, Sage

Robson C (2002) *Real World Research*, 2nd edition. Oxford, Blackwell Publishing
Sandelowski M, Davis DH, Harris BG (1989) Artful research: writing the proposal for research in the naturalist paradigm. *Research in Nursing and Health* 12:2 77–84

Websites

rdfunding.org.uk/flowchart/Flowchart.html – provides an overview of all stages of the research process, how and where to start. Section 4 considers how to write a research proposal and has some useful links to other relevant websites
www.esrcsocietytoday.ac.uk/ – Economic and Social Research Council (ESRC) guidance on how to develop a robust proposal for external funding

10 Gaining Access to the Research Site

Amanda Hunn

Key points

- Approval from an NHS research ethics committee is required for all studies involving patients or their data, or using staff as participants.
- Approval from the NHS trust R&D department as part of the research governance approval process is required over and above any approval obtained from a research ethics committee.
- Researchers need to pay particular attention to issues around confidentiality and informed consent.
- Early contact with the trust R&D department is desirable, so you will need to allow adequate time for this and plan accordingly.

The need for regulation of research

Researchers today need to abide by a wealth of regulation and guidance. Most professional bodies have their own set of research ethics guidance, such as the Royal College of Nursing (RCN 2004), but these guidelines are not mandatory and can be conflicting. Researchers have followed the Declaration of Helsinki since 1964 with the most recent version agreed in 2002, but again this is not compulsory. The UK has had a research ethics system in place since the 1970s. However, since 2004 this has been regulated by law.

Historically researchers only required approval from a research ethics committee before starting their research. Recently, however, a series of scandals involving retention of children's organs without consent – and other sensitive issues – has caused concern in the world of clinical research. Formal enquiries held after each episode called for a system of research governance in the UK. In 2001 the government responded with the Research Governance Framework for Health and Social Care. This document, which is available from the Department of Health website (*www.dh.gov.uk/*) was revised in 2003.

The Research Governance Framework in the UK

The Research Governance Framework for Health and Social Care (Department of Health 2001; 2003) aims to set out the standards and promote good quality research, and reduce adverse events and poor performance. Research governance requires that approval from the NHS trust host site is gained, in addition to approval from the ethics committee. The Framework document lists responsibilities under five main headings:

- ethics
- science
- information
- health and safety
- finance and intellectual property

In addition the document sets out the responsibilities of researchers, sponsors, funders, hosts, and all NHS employees.

Social care research is also included in these regulations. At the time of writing, the system for reviewing social care research was not in place. If involved in a study that includes social care and/or social services it would be wise to check with the local research ethics committee administrator as to the latest requirements.

The system for ethical approval

While there has been a formal research ethics system operating in the UK for many years, it only became a legal system in 2004 with Medicines for Human Use (Clinical Trials) Regulations. The Act follows the EU Directive in Good Clinical Practice in Clinical Trials, which sought a single system across the whole of the EU. Under these regulations, it is a legal requirement to obtain a favourable ethical opinion for all clinical trials of medicinal products. The Act also requires a single system across the whole of the UK offering a single ethical opinion regardless of the number of sites involved, and controlled by a single authority known as the UK Ethics Committee Authority. This applies to all types of research, not just clinical trials. The implementation of the Act by the Central Office for Research Ethics Committees (COREC) has brought about a number of significant changes in the system.

There are currently four types of research ethics committee (REC):

- Type I RECs are recognised to review Phase 1 studies using healthy volunteers only. A Phase 1 study is an initial safety trial on a new medicine undertaken on healthy volunteers prior to a full clinical trial.
- Type II RECs are recognised to review clinical trials of medicinal products within a single health authority area
- Type III RECs are recognised to review research studies including clinical trials across more than one health authority. Researchers wishing to carry out such

studies must apply to either a Multicentre Research Ethics Committee (MREC) or a Type III Local Research Ethics Committee (LREC).
- The remaining RECs are authorised to review studies other than clinical trials of medicinal products, which take place within the boundaries of a single health authority.

Figure 10.1 shows how to establish which research ethics committee to apply to. Further information on which research ethics committees are recognised can be gained from the COREC website.

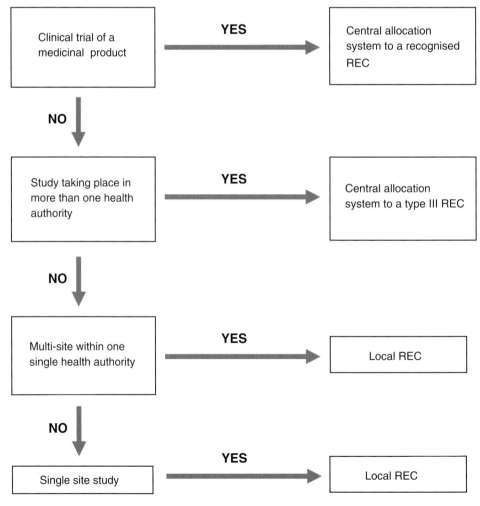

Figure 10.1 Identifying the appropriate research ethics committee.

Research ethics committee applications

Multi-site studies

Studies undertaken on a number of different sites only receive one ethical review. For a multi-site study that involves the delivery of an intervention at more than one site, an application is made to one main research ethics committee for a full ethical review. Applications for a site-specific assessment (SSA) will also need to be made at each of the remaining sites. A site is normally defined as an NHS trust, although in a GP led study, each GP practice is regarded as a site. In carrying out a site-specific assessment, the committees at the remaining sites will not be allowed to ethically review the study again. Instead they will only be able to assess the suitability of the local researcher, the local facilities, and other local issues.

Multi-site studies with no local investigator (NLI)

For a non-interventional study involving a sole researcher at a number of different sites, an application for ethics approval as a 'no local investigator' (NLI) can be made. An example of an NLI study would be a nurse wishing to carry out a postal survey across eight NHS trusts. The lead researcher would need to apply to a single research ethics committee approved for multi-site studies, but would not be required to apply for site-specific assessments at the remaining seven sites. However, the researcher would still be obliged to seek research governance approval from the R&D lead in each of the Trusts. Other examples of NLI studies are epidemiological research, and interview-based research, where the same individual or same small team of researchers from one site carry out all the interviews.

The remit of a research ethics committee

It is important to understand the remit of a research ethics committee. Ethical approval is required for studies that include:

- patients and users of the NHS
- relative/carers of NHS patients
- access to data, organs, and other bodily material past and present
- fetal material
- recently dead in NHS premises
- use or access to NHS premises
- Phase 1 studies of healthy volunteers, and
- NHS staff as subjects

Mote

The inclusion of NHS staff as subjects within the remit of research ethics committees is not a legal requirement and it is possible that the inclusion of staff may change in the future.

Building the approval process into research plans

Figure 10.2 shows the overall process when setting up a research study at a single site in the NHS. The key point to note here is that approval from the Trust R&D department as part of the research governance approval process is required over and above any approval obtained from a research ethics committee. Although many ethics committees are located on Trust premises, they are independent committees operating separately from the Trust and do not represent it. It is therefore possible that you could obtain a favourable opinion from a research ethics committee but still have your study rejected by a Trust and *vice versa*. Approval is required from both the ethics committee and the Trust before a study can commence.

The research governance process varies from trust to trust, but the vast majority will expect researchers to notify them in advance of applying for ethical approval. Once you have drafted a research proposal, you will need to approach the Research and Development (R&D) department of your local NHS Trust (and/or university if you are doing it under university auspices). If you have not been through this process before, you are advised to make contact in the earliest phase of planning the study in order to find out their requirements. The R&D department will want to look at the study with respect to a number of different issues. First, they will want to ensure that a scientific review of the study is completed. Research that has obtained external funding, for example, from a grant giving body such as a charity will probably have undergone scientific review already. However, unfunded research will require scientific review. The R&D department will arrange this. However, if the study is being carried out for educational purposes, i.e. as part of a degree, then the university may wish to carry out the scientific review.

Second, most R&D departments will want to do a risk analysis of the study in case they are required to provide indemnity. Research studies that carry an element of risk may be required to have indemnity in place in order to provide some form of compensation to participants in the event of something going wrong. NHS indemnity provides the research participants with compensation in the event of negligent harm. In contrast to this, most commercial pharmaceutical studies provide research participants with insurance, which would also provide cover in the event of non-negligent harm. The R&D department will help to arrange NHS indemnity should this be required.

The R&D department will want to examine the financial aspects of the study including the cost implications for the Trust, such as payment of overheads, staff costs and any other costs incurred by the Trust. If the researcher is not a Trust

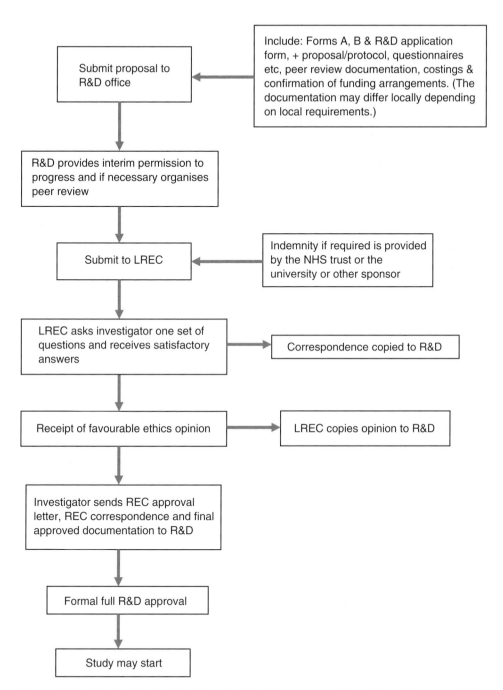

Figure 10.2   Single site studies: flowchart for the process of securing ethics committee approval and host organisational R&D approval.

employee they will need to arrange an honorary contract with the Trust. Finally the Trust may want to consider how the proposed research will fit in with their overall research strategy.

Most R&D departments want to work with researchers in a facilitative manner and many offer expert advice, guidance and support in terms of writing research proposals, statistical advice for calculating sample sizes and data analysis, and advice on how to fill in the COREC form. Time spent discussing the project with the R&D department at an early stage of the process may well save time later.

Once interim research governance approval to the research study has been granted, the researcher can then seek an ethical opinion from a research ethics committee. The committee may ask to see a copy of the scientific review and also evidence of indemnity if this is required.

The key to successfully working through all these stages is planning and allowing sufficient time for the approval process. The research ethics committee is required to reach a decision about a study within 60 calendar days, however, the time taken by the R&D department of a Trust for the research governance process varies considerably. Bear in mind it will nearly always be quicker to confine a study to a single site, rather than a multi-site study which will necessitate seeking research governance approval from several NHS Trusts. A researcher wishing to embark on this process should contact the R&D department of each trust at the beginning of the study in order to find out their local requirements and timescales. The process of gaining research governance in several Trusts can be complicated as there may be differing requirements and different forms to complete. Some trusts use the COREC form in addition to the NHS R&D form that is specifically for research governance. However, other Trusts have developed their own documentation.

Applying to the research ethics committee

The COREC application form is available electronically from the COREC website. Although lengthy, it provides useful prompts to the researcher in terms of the issues that need to be considered before a study can commence. The form is completed online. The study then needs to be booked onto an ethics committee agenda by telephoning the Central Allocation System (see the COREC website for the telephone number) or a local research ethics committee depending on the type of study (see Figure 10.1 for further information). When telephoning, you will be given a reference number, which needs to be inserted at the top of the form. The form can then be 'locked' electronically, printed off and the required authorised signatures obtained before sending off one single paper copy of the form to the ethics committee and submitting your electronic copy online. If you are applying for ethics committee approval as part of a student project, the academic supervisor must sign the form and a copy of the supervisor's CV needs to be submitted along with the form.

It is important that the date and version numbers are entered on all accompanying documentation that is submitted, for example, research proposal, participant information sheets, consent forms, invitation letters and questionnaires as appropriate.

The ethics committee administrator will give the date on which the application will be considered. Researchers are invited to attend this meeting. Attendance is not compulsory, but it is advisable if at all possible, since any initial misunderstandings can be resolved quickly which otherwise might result in lengthy correspondence. Attendance at a research ethics committee may seem to be a daunting prospect but you are not expected to present your study to the committee. Your presence is required only so that the members can ask you any questions that they may have. If you are attending the committee as a student it may be advisable for your academic supervisor to accompany you.

Box 10.1 illustrates some of the common concerns of research ethics committees. Although the main focus is on the ethics of the research, the committee is also concerned with the science of the study. A study will be rejected if the science is considered inadequate. With quantitative studies, they will expect to see a sample size calculation, either a power calculation for a trial with two or more arms, or confidence intervals for a survey so it may be advisable to consult with a statistician when developing the proposal.

Data protection and confidentiality issues that may arise from the study require careful consideration. Think about how participants will be identified and approached. For example, a study where patients are contacted directly by letter

Box 10.1 Issues of concern to research ethics committees.

- poor science/inadequate sample sizes
- poorly-worded patient information sheets or consent forms with inadequate information or written in technical language
- identification and initial approach to participants – an approach should be made by somebody who is already party to their information and should not breach confidentiality
- lack of time to consider joining the study – participants should be given wherever possible at least 24 hours to consider whether they wish to participate
- storage of data (transcripts, tapes, etc) and including electronic data – consideration needs to be given to secure storage of data and information (linking sheets that hold codes that enable data to be linked to individual participants need to be stored separately)
- potential identification of participants in qualitative research in the written report – consideration is required to sufficiently disguise participants in small-scale studies with unusual cases
- coercion of staff to be participants under line management control of the researcher – researchers often wish to conduct research amongst staff in their own workplace, sometimes staff that are managed by themselves – this raises concerns about coercion and honesty

from a university researcher, inviting them to take part in a survey of patients with prostate problems, would probably not get approval. Patients do not expect their confidential data to be passed to a third party without their permission. The first approach to the patient should always be from someone involved in his or her care.

Wherever possible allow potential participants sufficient time to read the patient information sheet and to consider whether or not they wish to take part in the study. Participants should normally be given enough time to take the patient information sheet away with them and to discuss it with their friends and family before committing themselves. Obviously this would not apply if the research were concerned with the delivery of an intervention in an emergency situation. However, most studies are not of this nature and it is usually possible to build sufficient time in to the process, for example, by sending out the patient information sheet by post first before meeting the participant.

Finally, if planning to undertake a qualitative study with a small sample size be prepared to explain to the committee how the data will be written up in such a way as to protect the identity of the participants. For example a qualitative study looking at how clinical staff cope with serious critical incidents with a sample size of just five based in one hospital, might pose problems for the researcher in terms of how to present the data without revealing the identity of the individuals even without the use of names.

Informal access negotiations

While there are formal hoops to be jumped through in order to gain approval for research, it is best if the individual researcher can also establish informal access in order to facilitate the process.

Gatekeepers

'Gatekeepers' are those people who control access to either participants or data. They may be external to the organisation such as ethics committee administrators or they may be internal such as the R&D lead (*see* below). In the vast majority of cases, these gatekeepers are willing to help facilitate research and will point the novice researcher in the right direction and support them with excellent advice. So it pays to make time to approach these individuals in the early stages of the project and to develop a rapport with them over time. Examples of gatekeepers are as follows:

- *R&D leads*. Most trust R&D leads are able to offer help and advice in terms of research design, choosing an appropriate methodology, sample size and data analysis. Many also assist researchers in completing the application form for the research ethics committee. Many trusts have a dedicated nursing professional with responsibility for nursing research. If applying for a research grant, the R&D department should be able to help you cost the different elements of your study including the overheads.

- *Caldicott Guardians* – Since 2001 each NHS Trust has appointed a Caldicott Guardian, usually a senior manager, who is responsible for the safekeeping of patient records, to ensure their rights are respected and to oversee how staff use personal information. Research requiring access to patient information may need the approval of the Caldicott Guardian. The first step is to identify whether the Trust has a policy on accessing patient records/data for research.

Consideration will need to be given to confidentiality issues, in particular, protecting the identity of participants and handling the storage of data. Plans for dealing with this aspect of the study will be of interest, not just to the ethics committee but also to the Trust and in particular the Caldicott Guardian. Showing that you have thought through and addressed these issues in your research proposal will inspire confidence and speed up the overall approval process. Points to bear in mind include:

How is the initial sample being identified and how will participants be approached? Does it involve anybody who would not normally have access to personal data?

Do you need to retain the identification of the participants once you have collected the data?

Could data be made confidential? i.e. the data would have a code number, which would link it back to the subject? The linking sheet would need to be stored separately under lock and key.

Could the data be made anonymous? All identifying details including linking codes would be removed so that it would not be possible to link the data back to an individual.

How and where will the data be stored – under lock and key – in an archive?

When will it be destroyed? Good practice is to destroy data after three to five years unless specifically agreed with the research participants that it will be kept for longer.

How will the sample details and data be protected on computer? Is the computer password-protected? How will tapes and transcripts be stored, will identifying labels be removed? Consider how to prevent the identity of individual participants being revealed, especially when labelling quotations if the sample size is very small.

Ethics committee administrators – each research ethics committee is run by an experienced administrator. Most administrators, given sufficient time, are happy to give advice on how to complete the COREC application form and on the issues that need to be considered when planning the study.

User involvement

Chapter 5 considers how users can be involved at different levels and stages in the research process. Users involvement can take many forms, they may be patients, carers, or members of the general public. It is deemed to be good practice to involve the participant group in the research as much as possible.

Locating and contacting research participants

Irrespective of the chosen methodology, studies involving people, be they patients, carers or staff, normally require a sampling frame (*see* Chapter 12). The source of the sampling frame will have implications for the type of approvals that need to be gained. Non-interventional studies which do not involve the use of an NHS sampling frame do not require a favourable opinion from an NHS research ethics committee, although university-based researchers may require approval from a university research ethics committee. So for example, if you wish to carry out a face-to-face interview with parents of children with eczema, it is possible to select the sample from a self-help group or by advertising in the local paper and NHS ethical review would not be required. Likewise it may be possible to get a list of health care staff from a university or a Royal College, in which case an ethics opinion from an NHS research ethics committee would not be required. Obviously studies that are interventional, involve a clinical trial of medicinal products, take place on NHS premises or with NHS patients or their data or tissue would still require a favourable opinion from a research ethics committee.

Whatever sampling frame is used, it is important that the initial contact with the research participant is made by somebody they know. For instance, if the participants are patients or carers and an NHS sampling frame is being used to select them, it is important that the first approach to gain their consent is made by a member of their clinical care team and not from somebody outside the organisation. Only after the participant has consented for their data to be passed to a third party can this take place.

Research ethics committees are often concerned that research participants are being 'induced' or pressurised to join a study. This may be in the form of monetary incentives or gifts. Obviously these should be kept to a minimum, but another example of inducement that often affects nursing research is the use of staff as participants. For example a nurse manager doing a higher degree might decide to undertake a qualitative interview study of nursing experiences of stress at work, and want to interview all the nursing staff that she manages on her ward. The ethics committee may well consider that staff in such a situation are under pressure to join the study, as they may not feel able to say no to their line manager. There is also a concern that where the participants know the researcher and where their individual responses will not be anonymous, they may not feel able to be honest and this will therefore weaken the findings. When planning to recruit participants from staff, try to select a sampling frame from a unit outside your immediate control, e.g. another general practice, ward or hospital.

Maintaining goodwill and co-operation

Access will need to be negotiated to the chosen sampling frame. This may involve writing letters to senior managers (including the Caldicott Guardian) in the organisation requesting access to potential research participants. It may be helpful to follow up this initial contact with a meeting. It is important to ensure that the relevant local practitioners are informed of the project. There is always a possibility that the study may conflict or overlap with the work of others and this should be avoided if possible. You may be dependent upon other people to search records and select the sample on your behalf. Likewise you may need people to consent participants on your behalf or distribute questionnaires for you. A good working relationship will need to be developed with these people if you are to maintain their input. It is sometimes helpful to put together a steering group of key stakeholders. This could include some of the key clinical leads and gatekeepers within the organisation as well as potential research participants. Individuals may feel more favourably inclined towards a project if they can influence its design and implementation.

Gaining informed consent from research participants

Informed consent should be sought from every research participant. At the initial contact with the potential research participant, the researcher would be expected to explain verbally the study in addition to giving them a copy of a participant information sheet (PIS) which they could take away with them to look at. The research participant should be given every opportunity to ask questions and discuss any anxieties they may have. In particular it should be made clear to them that if they decide not to participate in the research that this will not affect their treatment in any way. If the study is a clinical intervention it is necessary to explain what the 'standard' treatment would be and how the experimental treatment may differ from this.

The participant information sheet should explain the benefits and the risks of taking part and also what would happen if something went wrong. When explaining the benefits it is important not to oversell the study and make exaggerated claims that cannot be justified. It should be explained to the participant that they may withdraw from the study at any time. The contact details of someone independent of the researcher should be included in the event of a participant wishing to complain.

One of the main reasons for studies failing to gain a favourable ethical opinion is a poorly-written participant information sheet. It is essential that the information is presented clearly in a language that can be understood by a lay person without clinical knowledge. The researcher should aim for a low reading age, the equivalent of a tabloid newspaper, and avoid any jargon or acronyms.

A model patient information sheet and consent form are included in Boxes 10.2 and 10.3. The example used is based on an interview survey. Bear in mind that

Box 10.2 Example of participant information sheet.

Study reference number: **Date:**   **Version number:**

PATIENT INFORMATION SHEET
An interview survey of heart surgery patients after discharge

You are being invited to take part in a research study. Before you decide, it is important for you to understand why the research is being done and what it will involve. Please take time to read the following information carefully and discuss it with others if you wish. Ask us if there is anything that is not clear or if you would like more information. Take time to decide whether or not you wish to take part.

Thank you for reading this.

What is the purpose of the study?

The Well City Hospital is interested in finding out what happens to its patients after they have been discharged from hospital following heart surgery. We want to find out how you and your family cope when you are back home and what we could do to make this difficult time easier for you.

Why have I been chosen?

You have been chosen because we are planning to contact and interview a random sample of patients who have had heart surgery at our hospital over the last year. This is approximately 300 patients. You had surgery at this hospital earlier this year.

Do I have to take part?

It is up to you to decide whether or not to take part. If you do decide to take part you will be given this information sheet to keep and be asked to sign a consent form. If you decide to take part you are still free to withdraw at any time and without giving a reason. A decision to withdraw at any time, or a decision not to take part, will not affect the standard of care you receive.

What will happen to me if I take part?

If you decide to take part then you will need to return the reply slip to Mrs Smith the lead researcher. She will then contact you by phone to arrange a convenient time and place for the interview. The interviewer can visit you at home if that would be convenient for you. The interviewer will go through the patient information sheet with you and if you are happy to consent to taking part in this study she will ask you to sign two copies of the consent form. You will keep one copy and she will keep the other copy for our records. The interview is likely to last around one hour and will be tape-recorded. We will contact you again in 12 months' time to repeat the interview to see how much things have changed over that time.

What do I have to do?

You do not need to do anything apart from returning the reply slip to Mrs Smith using the reply paid envelope. Mrs Smith will then contact you to arrange a date for interview.

What are the possible disadvantages and risks of taking part?

There are very few disadvantages to taking part. As we said earlier the interview will be tape-recorded to help us with the analysis. If you are unhappy about this, then you should not return the reply slip. If you say something to the interviewer that indicates that you might need extra medical help, the researcher may have to pass this information to your doctor.

(Continues)

What are the possible benefits of taking part?
There is no intended clinical benefit to yourself from taking part in this study. We will use information to develop and improve our care and aftercare in the community, so this study may benefit future patients.

What happens when the research study stops?
The study should be finished in three years' time. This will not affect any treatment that you might be receiving.

What if something goes wrong?
If you are harmed by taking part in this research project, there are no special compensation arrangements. If you are harmed due to someone's negligence, then you may have grounds for a legal action but you may have to pay for it. Regardless of this, if you wish to complain, or have any concerns about any aspect of the way you have been approached or treated during the course of this study, the normal National Health Service complaints mechanisms should be available to you. This study does not involve any treatment so the risk of anything going wrong is very small.

Will my taking part in this study be kept confidential?
All information that is collected about you during the course of the research will be kept strictly confidential. Any information about you that leaves the hospital will have your name and address removed so that you cannot be recognised from it. We may need to link the information that you give us in the interview to some of the information in your notes but once this information has all been collected and linked we can destroy the code information linking the data to your name so that we will not be able to trace it back.

What will happen to the results of the research study?
When all the data are analysed the study will be written up for publication in a number of health service research journals. It will not be possible to identify you from these written reports. If you are interested in receiving a copy of the final report, please let the researcher know today and we will arrange for you to be sent a copy. Your data will stored in a secure place and will be destroyed after publication of the findings. We will also use the results of the study to review and change the services we provide.

Who is organising and funding the research?
This research study has been funded by the Made-Up Charities Research Fund. They have also agreed to fund the salary of a research assistant to organise the study and analyse the study findings. Your doctor is not being paid to include you in this study.

Can I claim travel expenses?
If you are interviewed in your own home, travel expenses will not be payable but if you would rather be interviewed at the hospital we will pay for travel expenses to and from the hospital.

Who has reviewed the study?
This study has been reviewed by the Science Review Committee of the Made-Up Charities Research Fund.

Contact for further information
If you would like more information about this study and what is involved then please contact Mrs Smith on telephone number 3579 at the Well City NHS Hospital Trust.

M₆ te

Box 10.3   Model consent form for research involving patients.

(form to be on headed paper)
Centre Number:
Study Number:
Patient Identification Number for this study:

CONSENT FORM

Title of project: An interview survey of heart surgery patients after discharge

Name of researcher: Mrs Smith

Please
initial box

1.   I confirm that I have read and understand the information
     sheet dated .... (version .....) for the above study and
     have had the opportunity to ask questions.

2.   I understand that my participation is voluntary and that I am
     free to withdraw at any time, without giving any reason,
     without my medical care or legal rights being affected.

3.   I understand that sections of any of my medical notes may be
     looked at by responsible individuals from [company name] or
     from regulatory authorities where it is relevant to my taking
     part in research. I give permission for these individuals to
     have access to my records.

I agree to take part in the above study.

_____   _____   _____
Name of patient   Date   Signature

_____   _____   _____
Name of person taking consent (if   Date   Signature
different from researcher)

_____   _____   _____
Researcher   Date   Signature

1 copy for patient; 1 for researcher; 1 to be kept with hospital notes

different methodologies require different information in the patient information
sheet. The more interventional the study, the more information will be necessary.
Further information on what to include is included on the COREC website (*www.
corec.org.uk*). The COREC guidance follows a question and answer format and
much of it can be applied generically to all types of research. A separate consent
form is normally not required for postal surveys – consent is assumed on the basis
of the person returning a completed questionnaire.

Guidance on research involving human tissue will be included in the new Human Tissue Act. It is likely that any surplus tissue taken from a living individual for the purposes of research will not require consent if it is to be anonymised. The MRC Guidelines on Human Tissue and Biological Samples (2001) for use in research provides helpful guidance on what information should be included in a patient information sheet and consent form.

Taking consent

With regard to clinical trials of medicinal products, the Declaration of Helsinki requires a physician to obtain consent. However guidance provided by International Conference for Harmonisation (ICH) Guideline for Good Clinical Practice (*www. ich.org*) allows the chief investigator to delegate this process, so for example, it could be delegated to a study nurse. With all other types of studies, consent would normally be gained by the investigator, regardless of their professional group.

Consenting vulnerable groups

A vulnerable individual may be considered to be one of the following groups:

* babies, infants, younger children, adolescents
* people with learning difficulties
* people with mental health problems
* people who are seriously ill with severe pain or distress
* the terminally ill
* the frail elderly
* people who are unconscious

In many instances one would seek to avoid including people from the groups above. However there may be occasions when the very focus of the research is a vulnerable group. There are specific requirements when consenting a vulnerable adult or child into a clinical trial of a medicinal product. The law governing clinical trials of medicinal products specifically allows for a legal representative to consent for a vulnerable adult. It also makes provision for emergency situations when a legal representative may not be available. Normally one would expect a potential research participant to have 24 hours or more to consider whether or not they wish to join a study. The only exception to this would be in an emergency situation where an intervention has to be delivered immediately. So, for example, a study looking at the best treatment for people with head injuries presenting in Accident & Emergency departments would have to be able to override the need for the legal representative in the form of the next of kin. If the intervention was a medicinal product the law would allow the researcher to nominate another person to be the 'legal representative' in order to consent on behalf of the unconscious patient.

For all other types of research, the law does not allow for one adult to consent for another, it only allows for the process of 'assent' (although this may change with the Mental Incapacity Act). When a researcher wishes to enrol a vulnerable adult into another type of study, e.g. an interview-based study, it is necessary to gain the assent of the vulnerable adult's family or carer. If the vulnerable person themselves should raise any objections to the study and does not wish to participate this should override any views of the relatives or carers. The same applies to research including children. While it is vital that the parents of the child are asked to give their consent, if the child does not wish to participate then the parents' wishes should not over-ride those of the child.

Conclusion

The process of applying for permission to carry out research is much more regulated than it has been in the past. Researchers should not underestimate the time involved and plan accordingly. While the process of applying for research ethics committee approval has been made more consistent, the process for applying for NHS Trust approval as part of research governance is relatively new, and is extremely variable. Researchers wishing to carry out multi-site research need to allow for extra time, and in some cases, additional resources, in order for all the necessary approvals to be given. This may have implications for the level of grant funding required and needs to be built into the costing of any study.

References

Medical Research Council (2001) *Human Tissue and Biological Samples for Use in Research: operational and ethical guidelines*. London, MRC
Royal College of Nursing (2004) *Research Ethics: RCN guidance for nurses*. London, RCN
Department of Health (2001) *Research Governance Framework for Health and Social Care*, 1st edition. London, Department of Health
Department of Health (2003) *Research Governance Framework for Health and Social Care*, 2nd edition. London, Department of Health

Websites

www.wma.net/e/policy/b3.htm – details of the Declaration of Helsinki 2002
www.corec.org.uk/ – Central Office for Research Ethics Committees (COREC): details for the central booking system and all research ethics committees, COREC's standard operating procedures and guidance on writing patient information sheets and consent forms
www.rdforum.nhs.uk/ – R&D Forum: latest information on research governance
www.dh.gov.uk – Department of Health information on NHS R&D

Section 3
Choosing the Right Approach

This section forms the heart of this book, as research approaches in nursing are many and diverse, and it is important to understand the range of approaches available before choosing a specific one to answer a particular question.

The section begins with a theoretical chapter tackling the two broad approaches available to the nurse researcher. Chapter 11 considers the philosophical under-pinning of the qualitative and quantitative paradigms in research, and emphasises the necessity to engage in the complex debates raised in the extensive literature on this subject. Both approaches, however, are valid for nursing research, and the perspective adopted should be guided by the nature of the question to be answered.

Chapter 12 stands alone as an essential prerequisite to any research design, be it qualitative or quantitative. Sampling procedures are well established for many methodologies, and this chapter discusses a variety of the most common sampling strategies used in nursing research. Sampling cannot be considered separately from the issue of research design, as it will determine the feasibility and resources required for a project.

Three chapters follow which introduce the major approaches used in qualitative research. Chapters 13–15 are preceded by a short introduction to qualitative research and a useful figure that compares the three approaches discussed in this book.

The focus of Section 3 then moves to quantitative approaches. Chapter 16 introduces experimental design, and Chapter 17 discusses surveys. Both these approaches have a long and well-established history in medical and social sciences, and both are also widely used in nursing research. These chapters discuss the strengths and weaknesses of the methodologies, and highlight examples from the nursing and medical literature where they have been used to good effect. Chapter 16 includes a critical discussion of the randomised controlled trial and its place as the 'gold standard' of medical research evidence. Chapter 17 includes a short section on epidemiology, a well-established research tradition that has perhaps been overlooked in nursing research.

Chapters 18, 19 and 20 each take a major research approach commonly used in nursing research and take the reader through the essential characteristics of the methodology. Action research, evaluation, and case studies are all well suited to particular aspects of nursing research, and many examples can be found in the nursing research literature. Each approach is described and applied in a range of health and social care settings. All three approaches can combine quantitative and qualitative approaches to data collection, and so highlight the advantages of adopting an eclectic stance in nursing research.

Chapter 21 concludes this section with another new subject for this edition of *The Research Process in Nursing*. Systematic reviews are now seen as a research method in their own right, taking a rigorous approach to the ever increasing range of research evidence available, and integrating findings of studies to assess implications for policy and practice wherever possible. This chapter reviews secondary research of all kinds, and highlights the importance of following an explicit method in distilling conclusions from a body of evidence.

11 The Quantitative–Qualitative Continuum

Annie Topping

Key points

- Qualitative and quantitative research have different characteristics and derive from different scientific traditions and forms of knowledge.
- Quantitative research methods assume that the world is stable and predictable, and phenomena can be measured empirically. The positivist tradition of quantitative research derives from the biomedical sciences.
- Qualitative research methods take an interpretivist perspective, emphasising meaning and the understanding of human actions and behaviour. The tradition of qualitative research derives from the social sciences.
- Both are appropriate approaches for nursing research; the choice of methodology depends on the nature of the research question. In some cases the two approaches can be blended in the same study.

Introduction

Not that long ago the unique characteristics and differences between qualitative and quantitative research would have been described in a way more akin to an intellectual battleground with researchers aligned to a particular camp. That position has undergone considerable revision across many disciplines and this is particularly marked in nursing. Today, there is a growing recognition that the use of a range of approaches strengthens, rather than divides, nursing enquiry. Researchers, irrespective of their preferred way of approaching problems or questions, are involved in an endeavour with a shared purpose.

Quality in research is concerned with using the most appropriate approach for investigating research problems and for researchers to adopt a systematic, rigorous and transparent approach for exploring, discovering, confirming and understanding. Underlying the practice of research and its findings are fundamental questions about the nature of knowledge, termed as epistemology, and what we understand as reality. Recognising that nursing as a research-active profession does not function in isolation, the assumptions, and contribution of the sciences, western medicine and the social sciences will be examined.

The characteristics of quantitative and qualitative research

First let us turn attention to the defining characteristics of the two approaches. Philosophically, quantitative research is underpinned by a *positivist* tradition that proposes scientific truths or laws exist. These truths emerge from what can be observed and measured and can be studied as objects. Methods that minimise, or are free from, bias are used to do this so that greater confidence can be given to any findings. This approach is often referred to as the *scientific* or *empirical method*. Qualitative research, in contrast, fits more neatly within an *interpretivist* tradition based on assumptions that in order to make sense of the world, human behaviour should be interpreted in interaction with others. So research that seeks to understand human behaviour and the social processes that we engage in must employ approaches and techniques that allow interpretation in natural settings.

This interpretative stance goes further, as qualitative methodologies also strive to emphasise that there is no single interpretation, truth or meaning but recognise that just as human beings are different, so are the societies and cultures in which they live their lives. Box 11.1 sets out the different qualities and characteristics reported by various authors to describe the two approaches. Although of some value, information is presented in stark contrast and you may not always be able to recognise all these characteristics in any single report of a quantitative or qualitative study.

Box 11.1   Characteristics of quantitative and qualitative research.

Quantitative research	Qualitative research
hard science	soft science
objective	subjective
political	value-free
reductionist	holistic
logico-deductive	dialectic, inductive, speculative
cause and effect relationships	meaning
tests theory	develops, advances and reinterprets theory
control	shared interpretation
instruments as data collection tools	listening and talking, observation as ways of gathering data
basic unit of analysis: numbers	basic unit of analysis: words
statistical analysis	interpretation
generalisation	uniqueness/transferability

Sources: Burns & Grove (1997); Corner (1993); Silverman (2000)

Influences and contributions to the development of nursing research

It might seem a little odd to discuss the influence of other disciplines in a textbook targeted to a nursing readership but it would be naïve not to recognise the shared history and mutual dependency. Biomedicine, like nursing as we know it today, has it roots in the nineteenth century and that period of industrialisation and accelerated societal change. Pre-industrial thinking about illness also underwent revision as a result of scientific breakthroughs and different ways of controlling disease. Previously held notions of illness as an imbalance, loss of harmony between the individual and the environment in which they live were increasingly challenged in favour of more rational, objectively-based, approaches. During the same time period, modern nursing began to emerge under the leadership of such figures as Florence Nightingale and Mrs Bedford Fenwick in response to the plight of soldiers injured in the Crimean War and the growing demand for a different type of workforce to support the organisation and delivery of what has become hospital medicine.

What is now described as *reductionism* emerged as a way for studying the causes and treatment of disease(s). This approach allows disease to become objectified, and the experience of ill-health to be reduced to the signs and symptoms that allow it to be better classified, diagnosed, and the response, if any, to treatment to be monitored. This view of illness as an object inevitably distances the doctor or nurse, encouraging detachment from the influencing effects of subjectivity. You can still see this approach in medical practice where routine assessment in the form of taking a patient's history to establish diagnosis might more correctly be described as an illness history.

Objectification and distancing is ingrained in the scientific tradition through separation of the subject of research from the investigator. This belief that removing the doctor or researcher from the context in which health care is delivered, or research is undertaken, provides a sense of security that neither doctor nor researcher impacts on illness or makes judgments about it. That picture of medicine and research performed by an objective yet fundamentally altruistic scientist fails to recognise that 'medical knowledge is never disinterested' (Annandale 1998:5).

Indeed scientific neutrality has itself received considerable attention from social scientists (Foucault 1973; Hammersley, 1989; Shipman 1992). More recently, nurse researchers have begun to suggest that nurses are far from disinterested and neutral in their interactions (Johnson & Webb 1995; Porter 1995).

The study of societies, the people within them, and the ways in which they organise themselves, is the focus of sociology, which at its most basic is an acceptance that people are different from objects. Objects do not have thought, do not have consciousness, they do not reason, think or reflect and therefore are qualitatively different from people. Importantly, objects, unlike people, do not have free will or choice. For that reason the ways in which a researcher might study and understand objects will by necessity be different from the approaches used to understand human society or indeed nursing. This argument, however, does become quite complex when applied to health care where people become patients. In so doing they can be viewed objectively as a dysfunctioning machine, and subjectively as an individual interacting with people and systems designed to support their illness. This complexity of the subjective person and objective body aligned philosophically as interpretivisim and positivism respectively reinforces the importance of both quantitative and qualitative approaches contributing to our understanding.

The positivist approach to investigate the social and natural world draws on empiricism and the scientific method. It is based on the assumption that social life, like natural sciences, can be studied as facts. That is not to say that ways in which individual, groups and societies organise themselves or their beliefs and practices are objects, but more that they can be examined as such. Interpretivism, on the other hand, asserts that the purpose of research is to examine meaning and therefore interpretation must remain central. Groundbreaking research undertaken in the 1950s and 1960s introduced this interpretative approach and still today informs thinking about medicine (Becker *et al.* 1961), mental illness and stigma (Goffman, 1964) and the dying (Glaser & Strauss, 1965).

Empiricism and the scientific method

Science, western modern medicine and quantitative approaches have their origins in the philosophical movements of the 16th and 17th centuries. A logical approach for developing knowledge emerged built upon the three principles of scepticism, determinism and empiricism. First, anything irrespective of its origin or authority is open to analysis and doubt and thus is susceptible to *scepticism*. Second, that regular laws and rules of causation determine all things – *determinism*. Lastly, *empiricism* asserts that enquiry or problem-solving such as research should be undertaken through observation and verification. The application of the scientific method was a major developmental shift in thinking from previously-held explanations and it encouraged a way of looking at nature 'free of mystery, superstition and religious obscurity' (Shipman 1992:19).

The scientific method became a formula for the production of knowledge and as Figure 11.1 illustrates is based on the two processes of *induction* and *deduction*.

It might be useful to consider how the scientific method has become an ordinary part of how we understand events around us and moreover how information is presented to us through the media. Try to recollect your first introduction to science. Probably early in your school career you learnt how to undertake a simple experiment that involved learning how to describe accurately, measure reliably and record diligently observations about what occurred in order to help you understand whatever you were investigating. From that first exposure to the scientific method, children are taught to describe the equipment used, how to undertake a test and record any deviations from the approved recipe, what they used

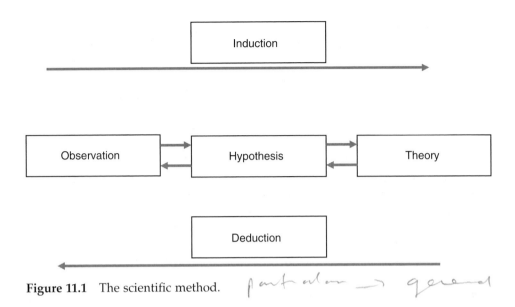

Figure 11.1 The scientific method.   *particular ⟶ general*

to measure any reaction or outcome, and to document the results. These skills form the basis of *observation, description* and *measurement* that underlie much of the conduct of science. In using this approach findings can be translated into *fact* explanations. These explanations are often expressed as *hypotheses* or *theories* that are themselves amenable to testing. This progression from observation to statement of a relationship between different observations (*hypotheses*) to *theory* and ultimately generalisation is termed *induction*. So theories derived through the process of induction, move from the particular to the general and could be seen as an organising system for what are essentially conjectures or tentative proposals based on observation (Polgar & Thomas 2000).

An essential feature of any scientific theory is the account of how the theory works, and its potential to predict. These predictions enable the researcher to *deduce* causal relationships, themselves expressed through theory but testable through controlled observation. The results of testing (*experimentation*) will produce data that can be translated into findings that may be consistent with the predictions expressed in the original hypothesis, thus verifying or providing support for the theory. Alternatively, they may fail to support the hypothesis and contradict the theory. Ultimately the volume of conflicting evidence may swell to such proportions until it causes the original theory to be discarded. Hence any scientific theory is not an absolute truth but only provisional and therefore can be modified, refined, disputed or invalidated (Popper 1972).

It might be helpful to illustrate the scientific method with an example. Imagine you are working on a surgical ward. You observe that patients admitted for elective surgery who do not receive pre-operative preparation about the impending events experience greater distress post-operatively than those who have received preparation. You also observe that the unprepared patients require more analgesia and appear to mobilise more slowly. You develop a theory that suggests a relationship between information and post-operative outcomes. In fact, two seminal studies undertaken by Hayward and Boore in the 1970s did just that (Hayward & Boore 1994). These studies demonstrated a relationship between information and the level of pain experienced by patients recovering from surgery. Applying the scientific method to Hayward's and Boore's studies leads us to ask whether the relationship between information and pain was established through theory and hypothesis testing (hypothetico-deductive reasoning) or from rigorous observation of patients who received pre-operative information. Probably the initial idea came from the latter but in order to demonstrate the relationship the former approach was used. As discussed in Chapter 2 initial ideas for research often come from observation but prior to investigation are checked by literature searching and analysis. In this way, existing understandings can be examined to prevent embarking prematurely on ill thought through research, and to assist in refining and honing original research ideas.

To extend this discussion, Wilson-Barnett (1988), drawing on many of the same theoretical ideas associated with the positive benefits of information, deduced that anxiety associated with radiological investigations could also be reduced by information giving. Her results supported in part the value of information in reducing anxiety, but also found that in some cases information could make some people more anxious. Although a deductive approach was used to undertake the work in the first instance the interpretation of the findings led to an inductively-driven revision and modification of the original theoretical assumptions. This reinforces the assertion that any knowledge is only provisional. Today we have far greater insight about the beneficial effects of information giving and best ways to provide that information to patients, their relatives and carers. Even so, some users of health services still have cause to complain about the poor quality of information received, despite the wealth of evidence confirming that the experience of health care is enhanced by effective education and information. This problem of translating what is known, the evidence base, into practice will be developed in much more detail in Chapters 31 and 32. Yet, something as fundamental as information giving still has many unanswered questions that deserve further investigation. For example: how to ensure information giving is appropriately targeted? Is information provided at the appropriate level? Do health care professionals have the skills or wherewithal to provide information effectively? What is it about health care organisations and the way(s) in which health professionals interact with users that prevents them from communicating effectively? These questions as research problems may require a number of different research approaches, as it is unlikely that one approach will provide all the answers.

In research that is largely deductive, the theory normally directs and drives the design and interpretation. In inductively-driven work, theory serves to provide a commitment to a particular way of looking at the world such as feminism or to justify a methodological approach (Sandelowski 1993). This is why you may be able to identify the theoretical framework that informed a research design in research reports. This explicit reference to the theoretical basis of the work can help the reader to navigate the interpretation offered. This can also provoke criticism when the theoretical framework itself appears to create a tension within the work, particularly if it appears incongruent with the research approach. For example, Patricia Benner's (1984) influential work *Novice to Expert*, which explored how nurses developed competence became the focus of some critical censure, albeit firmly countered by the author (Benner 1996), of the interpretation of the theoretical perspective adopted (Cash 1995). A further consideration concerns the role of theory in research. If data are collected in the absence of an organising framework or theory it could attract the criticism that the researcher is merely confirming their own biases (Grbich 1999). At this juncture it might be helpful to look at the two approaches in more detail.

Quantitative research

Quantitative research is a broad umbrella term for research that uses methods to collect evidence that can be transformed into numerical data and are based upon a *positivist* position. Often the numerical data produced in quantitative research can be statistically manipulated in order to confirm (or sometimes fail to confirm) the original hypotheses or research question. The findings can then be used to make predictions or indicate trends. Formal, objective and systematic processes are used to explain causal relationships between events or things (variables). Underpinning quantitative research is the principle that the world is stable and predictable and the quantitative researcher, by controlling external influences, can seek to minimise bias that might otherwise explain the findings. The ultimate aim is for the researcher and the consumer of the research to be assured that any results are *valid* and *reliable* (*see* Chapter 2). Classical experimental design is one such method but surveys, analysis of official statistics, and structured or non-participant observation are all quantitative methods (Silverman 2000). The use of quantitative research methods is illustrated in the study undertaken by Moore *et al.* (2002) where the research team set out to assess the effectiveness of nurse-led follow-up management of patients with lung cancer (Box 11.2). They defined, for the purposes of the study, the concept of effectiveness as those components that were most amenable to measurement. Outcomes such as quality of life, patients' satisfaction, general practitioners' (GPs) satisfaction, symptom-free survival and progression-free survival, use of resources and cost comparison were all used to generate numerical data. This produced a picture of the benefits of a nurse-led service contrasted with those achieved by conventional practice.

From this example you can see that for reality to be captured in quantitative research it has to be broken down, reduced, into those component parts that can be defined and are measurable. This provides greater assurance to the researcher and reader that the results are the product of consistent reproducible measurement that describes what the researcher sought to understand. The accuracy of any instruments developed to measure whatever is under investigation, and consistently reproduce results, is fundamental to undertaking quantitative research.

Box 11.2   Example of a quantitative research study.

Moore S, Corner J, Wells M, Salmon E, Normand C, Brada M, O'Brien M, Smith I (2002) Nurse-led follow up and conventional medical follow-up in management of patients with lung cancer: randomised trial. *British Medical Journal* 325: 1145–1147

This British study assessed the effectiveness of nurse led follow-up management of lung cancer patients. Mounting evidence casts doubt on the benefits of routine outpatient follow-up despite high levels of reported psychological morbidity in this client group. 203 patients three months following initial treatment were randomised to conventional outpatient follow-up or nurse led follow-up. The latter involved allocation to a clinical nurse specialist (CNS) for monthly telephone or clinic-based assessment. CNSs were also available via direct patient-initiated clinic attendance or telephone. The CNS intervention involved information-giving, support and co-ordinating care input from other agencies. Patient outcome measures were quality of life and patient satisfaction, survival, service use and cost. Results indicated patient acceptability and satisfaction was higher in the intervention group, some symptoms appeared better controlled and patients were more likely to die at home. The researchers concluded that nurse led follow-up was acceptable to patients and GPs and led to positive outcomes.

It also allows other researchers to replicate the study and therefore compare, confirm and question existing findings. The problem for the researcher is that dependency on measurement of what can be complex theoretical ideas or models is reliant on the clarity of the conceptualisation of the underlying concept, the technology available and the reliability of the researcher to use the instrument consistently. No matter how diligent a researcher is, or how well-designed a study, it could still only be reliable yet not be valid. In other words the research may measure something but not necessarily what was under investigation. That is why it is often more of a challenge in research to establish with any confidence that findings represent facts or truths about something than to construct an approach to measure it or some part of it.

Another feature of quantitative research is that it aspires to objectivity and therefore different approaches are used to keep the researched (participants) at a distance from the researcher. Detachment is used as a strategy for reducing bias and minimising any involvement that might contaminate the results or influence outcomes. There are numerous ways to increase detachment such as randomisation of participants, ensuring the researcher remains unaware (blind) of which subjects receive an intervention and which do not, referring to all subjects by a coded descriptors thus promoting anonymity, and by separating those delivering an intervention from those responsible for collecting data. In the study by Moore *et al.* (2002) a researcher rather than a clinical nurse specialist collected outcome data, thus removing any danger of bias by the nurses who were directly involved in delivering care.

Qualitative research

Defining qualitative research is often made more difficult by the absence of a common, unified set of techniques, philosophies or underpinning perspectives (Mason 1996). Qualitative research methods are used across a range of disciplines such as the social sciences, management and nursing and are beginning to be used more widely in the biomedical sciences.

Qualitative researchers use an array of terms, concepts and assumptions that may appear less familiar on initial encounter than scientific terms. These can be particularly confusing to the novice researcher who not only has to contend with the challenge to previously held notions of what is robust research, but also has to acquire what at times appears to be a new language. An analogy might be trying to cook from a recipe where all the ingredients and terms for techniques such as sieving, mixing, beating and combining were different, possibly unfamiliar. This would inevitably make you feel uncertain about what you had to use, how to use it and about what the final product might be like. Moreover the uncertainty if you persevere would require you to interpret to make sense of the recipe. This is not dissimilar from the processes involved in doing qualitative research. Ethnography, phenomenology, grounded theory, case study, are just some of the methodologies that are part of the cluster of approaches that can considered qualitative. Various attempts have been made to categorise what seems an incomprehensible array (Cresswell 1998; Denzin & Lincoln 1994). Some of these different methodological approaches will be examined in more detail in subsequent chapters, particularly Chapters 13–15. Box 11.3 presents a summary of a qualitative study by Roach (2004) using a particular methodological approach – grounded theory.

The subjectivity of using an approach where the researcher and the research are closely intertwined has its problems and reflexivity (critical self-reflection on the research process and interpretation of data) is an important part of the qualitative researcher's toolkit (Schwandt 1997). Reflexivity has some similarities and uses processes like those used in reflective practice. In qualitative research the acknowledgement of the influence, and hence the critical scrutiny, of the researcher is often subject to the same level of examination as the research itself (Carolan 2003). For this reason, emphasis is placed on recording in fieldnotes description of what was seen, said and done in the act of doing the research as well as interpretation of meaning in memos.

This emphasis on involvement and analytical detachment can seem paradoxical to the reader. The research approach encourages involvement, as the researcher frequently designs the study and collects, interprets and reports the data themselves. They can therefore influence and exert a bias on all stages of the research process. Yet the researcher(s), even though the report may be written in an engaging style more often than not using first person pronouns, employs a number of different devices to assure the reader that the study is trustworthy. For example: Koch *et al.* (2004) in a study examining how people with long-standing asthma

Box 11.3   Example of a qualitative research study.

Roach S (2004) Sexual behaviour of nursing home residents: staff perceptions and responses. *Journal of Advanced Nursing* 48: 371–379

This grounded theory study examined the perceptions of nursing home staff toward residents expressing affectionate or sexual behaviour. Data were collected from interviews with volunteers (n = 30), three nominal group interviews (n = 18) and interviews with key informants (n = 5) recruited from two centres in Australia and one in Sweden. Data were analysed using a constant comparative method that involved open, axial and selective coding. A core category emerged which was subsequently developed into the conceptual paradigm of *guarding discomfort*. This is offered as a framework to illustrate the ways in which expression of sexuality by residents was opposed or facilitated in nursing homes. The researcher concluded that nursing homes are not facilitative environments for residents to exercise their sexuality rights. Also, that attempts to do so infrequently result in discomfort in staff, and the combination of staff (dis)comfort and organisational ethos determine the residents' ability to express their sexuality.

manage the condition use the pronoun 'we' to signal to the reader the subjectivity of the approach, yet provide a transparent description of how the research was conducted, which of the research team undertook specific activities and how the findings were created and corroborated by the participants. They also suggest that readers can judge the authenticity of the findings by the inclusion of selected snippets of interview data in the report.

Data collection or generation is reliant upon using approaches that are sensitive to the social context in which the data are produced. So qualitative studies often lack standardisation or structure as too rigid or unsympathetic an approach might reduce the authenticity of the data. Semi- or unstructured interviewing and participant observation are commonly used methods in data collection and are often used in combination. Raw data may be recorded on to audiotape, videotape or in fieldnotes and then transcribed and transformed into words for analysis. Qualitative analysis inevitably involves breaking the data up and coding the different segments. Increasingly researchers use software packages to assist in managing data. Irrespective of whether the researcher uses paper based or electronic software for handling the data, the process involves a fracturing process that includes breaking down, coding, re-ordering and reconstituting in order to describe, explain or generate theory.

Critical accounts of research epistemology

Numerous commentators have offered critical accounts of the epistemology, methodologies and methods used in the name of research irrespective of perspective. Criticism should not necessarily be seen as negative, and debate could be considered an indicator of the health of a discipline and its practitioners. Much of the criticism centres on rigour of the approaches used to manufacture results and the questionable disinterest of research and researchers. Two of the arguments that cast doubt on the validity of many assumptions inherent in scientific enquiry are those offered by Popper (1972) and Kuhn (1972). Popper's argument is philosophical and examines the provisional nature of any knowledge or truth and maintains that researchers should seek to challenge hypotheses rather than set out to prove them. Kuhn offers a critical account of the culture of research communities and how they are self-maintaining and constraining. He terms this a paradigm that arguably limits the development of new ways for looking at problems.

It might be useful to apply these two critiques to nursing. In order to do this, it is helpful to think of nursing as a culture. One of the enduring narratives in the nursing literature is that associated with the concept of caring. Considerable effort has been exerted to define caring, understand it better through research and to theorise about the significance of caring to the experience of nursing. If, for the purposes of this discussion, caring is accepted as the paradigmatic framework of nursing, it serves as an explanation for the nature of nursing and by extension presents a way of interpreting what is done as nursing. In effect the way caring is theorised also prescribes the way(s) in which research will be undertaken to better understand it. It is not difficult, using a Kuhnian analysis, to distinguish a link between the volume of effort invested in understanding caring, its elevation as the primary contribution of nursing to care delivery and an explanation for the rapid assimilation of qualitative approaches into nursing research (Ramprogus 2002).

A different but associated criticism of research about nursing, undertaken by non-nurses, is that the work fails to make visible the work (caring) done by nurses. The result, it is said, makes the efforts of nurses and the unique contribution of nursing invisible with the consequence that the impact of 'caring for' done by nurses on health or patient outcomes goes unrecognised (Oakley, 1984). Applying a Popperian analysis, the research activity seeking to uncover caring should focus on critical appraisal of caring as the essential concept of nursing. In effect this would challenge the hypothesis or at least encourage critical analysis of any understandings that emerge. It has been suggested that too much effort is placed on securing a better fit or providing explanation for lack of fit (Johnson 1999), rather than seeking to question the assumptions surrounding the primacy of caring in nursing. Numerous arguments have been put forward to explain why particular methods used to demonstrate the concept are insufficiently sensitive, inappropriate to capture the nature of phenomenon, or when there is a lack of criticism of the underlying assumptions (Barker *et al.* 1995; Nelson & McGillon 2004). Kuhn would contend that it is only when there is enough substance to cast doubt, or a competing set of assumptions emerge, that a paradigm shift ultimately occurs. This is when a discipline changes its way of understanding problems. An example is how the understanding of infection transmission was overturned by germ theory, leading to the necessity for handwashing. This was despite the efforts of the Austrian obstetrician Semmelweiss (1818–1865) who encountered bitter resistance and incarceration in a mental hospital trying to disseminate his evidence relating to the positive benefits of handwashing.

Blending quantitative and qualitative approaches

A solution offered as an alternative to using one or other research approach is to blend qualitative and quantitative approaches through the use of mixed or combined methods (Becker 1996). The advantage this brings is the added value of using different yet complementary approaches, particularly if the relative weaknesses of one are offset by another (Corner 1991). The use of a number of methods within a research design is termed *triangulation*. The term has more traditionally been coined to refer to procedures used in surveying to pinpoint a particular geographic position by taking reference measurements from three or more points. In research it is used to describe a way to increase the types of information obtained from participants to produce a more holistic picture (Begley 1996).

There is, however, a difference between using a number of methods to provide convergent views yet still provide a coherent account, as in Moore *et al.* (2002) (Box 11.2); and an approach where a range of data collection strategies are used to provide a more complete but layered analysis. According to Denzin (1989) triangulation in research can take a number of forms – data, investigator, theory and method. Data triangulation involves using a number of different data sources that can shed light on a particular phenomenon, as in the study undertaken by Roach (2004) where she interviewed participants working in three different settings to enhance, and verify emerging understandings (Box 11.3). That said, Hammersley and Atkinson (1983) warn that using multiple data sources may not always confirm inferences but make differences more blatant and act as a further check to credibility. Theoretical triangulation encourages the use of competing theory to compare and contrast interpretations of data. By this means theory can be advanced and revised. Methodological triangulation can be within methods where compatible data collection methods such as participant observation, qualitative interviewing and fieldnotes can be used. Alternatively dissimilar data collection strategies from different research traditions may be used to illuminate the same phenomenon such as using a structured questionnaire with focus group interviews.

Criticisms of triangulation include concerns about philosophical incongruity between the position of objective truth (positivism) opposed to the interpretative traditions that make no claims to any single reality (Silverman, 1985; Johnson *et al.* 2001). Another criticism is that it can merely compound sources of error (Armitage & Hodgson 2004) inherent in the methods employed. Lastly, there is the issue of how the reader should judge quality, particularly if competing research traditions are used in the same study.

> **Box 11.4** Comparison of the criteria used to judge the trustworthiness of a study.
>
> | Quantitative research | Qualitative research Trustworthiness criteria (Lincoln & Guba 1985) |
> |---|---|
> | *Internal validity* – extent to which what is observed truly represents the variable under investigation | *Credibility* – fit between participant's views and researcher's representation of them |
> | *External validity* – extent that the results of a study can be generalised to other contexts and populations | *Transferability* – relates to the adequacy of the description to judge similarity to other situations so findings might be transferred |
> | *Reliability* – refers to the consistency and accuracy of the data collection approach or instrument | *Dependability* – relates to transparency of the research process and decision trail |
> | *Objectivity* – reliant upon physical reality, not amenable to individual interpretation | *Confirmability* – establishing that data, findings and interpretation are clearly linked |

Judging the quality of quantitative and qualitative research

Judgement inevitably introduces a comparison. In order to contrast something with something else the individual undertaking the comparison uses criteria to judge. In quantitative research these are normally the concepts of reliability and validity. Various commentators have questioned the appropriateness of using these concepts – which fit with a positivist world view – with research methodologies that do not sit comfortably with that way of thinking (Koch 1994; Koch & Harrington 1998; Mays & Pope 2000). Those voicing this position maintain that distinctive criteria are required to assess qualitative research. Lincoln and Guba (1985; 1989) offered one such set of criteria based on the concept of trustworthiness later refined as authenticity criteria (Box 11.4). An alternative position proposed is that researchers should adopt a more tentative position referred to as subtle realism (Mays & Pope 2000). This is a more conciliatory position and recognises that research is more concerned with representing what is perceived as reality rather than trying to accurately present truth.

yes.

Conclusion

This chapter has examined the key assumptions underpinning the research process. In doing so an attempt has been made to move attention away from the two approaches as divided by irreconcilable differences to what are different approaches with strengths and weaknesses, whether used separately or in combination. Subsequent chapters will emphasise that the purpose of research is to adopt the right tools for the task in hand. Just as a driver faced with a punctured tyre would select the appropriate equipment and most effective way to approach the task arguably the same principles apply to research problems. It would be naïve not to recognise that a researcher experienced in the use of a particular methodology or method, or holding a particular set of beliefs about the world, would be more inclined to explore research problems amenable to their preferred approach(es) – just as a chef will return to a tried and tested recipe. Research includes a broad constituency of competing perspectives, assumptions, methodologies and methods. All approaches can be criticised or found insufficient, and rightly so. Healthy constructive disrespect should be encouraged. Nevertheless this chapter has sought to emphasise that research problems or the pursuit of answers, however incomplete, should drive approaches not *vice versa*.

References

Annandale E (1998) *The Sociology of Health and Medicine*. Cambridge, Polity Press

Armitage G, Hodgson I (2004) Using ethnography (or qualitative methods) to investigate drug errors: a critique of a published study. *NT Research* 9: 379–387

Barker PJ, Reynolds W, Ward T (1995) The proper focus of nursing: a critique of the 'caring' ideology. *International Journal of Nursing Studies* 32: 386–397

Becker HS, Geer B, Hughes EC, Strauss AL (1961) *Boys in White: student culture in medical school*. Chicago: University of Chicago Press

Becker H (1996) The epistemology of qualitative research. In Jessor R, Colby A, Scheweder (eds) *Essays on Ethnography and Human Development*. Chicago, University of Chicago Press pp53–71

Begley CM (1996) Using triangulation in nursing research. *Journal of Advanced Nursing* 24: 122–128

Benner P (1984) *Novice to Expert*. Menlo Park, Addison-Wesley

Benner P (1996) A response by P Benner to Cash K: Benner and expertise in nursing: a critique. *International Journal of Nursing Studies* 33: 669–674

Burns N, Groves SK (1997) *The Practice of Nursing Research: conduct, critique and utilisation*, 3rd edition. Philadelphia, WB Saunders

Carolan M (2003) Reflexivity: a personal journey during data collection. *Nurse Researcher* 10:3 7–14

Cash K (1995) Benner and expertise in nursing: a critique. *International Journal of Nursing Studies* 32: 527–534

Corner J (1991) In search of more complete answers to research questions. Quantitative versus qualitative research methods: is there a way forward? *Journal of Advanced Nursing* 16: 718–727

Cresswell JW (1998) *Qualitative Inquiry and Research Design*. Thousand Oaks, Sage

Denzin NK (1989) *The Research Act: a theoretical introduction to sociological methods*, 3rd edition. New Jersey, Prentice Hall

Denzin NK, Lincoln YS (1994) *Handbook of Qualitative Research*. Thousand Oaks, Sage

Foucault M (1973) *The Birth of the Clinic*. London, Tavistock

Glaser BG, Strauss AL (1965) *Awareness of Dying*. New York, Aldine

Goffman A (1964) *Stigma: notes on the management of a spoiled identity*. Harmondsworth, Penguin

Grbich C (1999) *Qualitative Research in Health*. London, Sage

Hammersley M (1989) *The Dilemma of Qualitative Method*. London, Routledge

Hammersley M, Atkinson P (1983) *Ethnography Principles in Practice*. London, Tavistock

Hayward J, Boore JRP (1994) Research Classics from the Royal College of Nursing, Vol 1: *Information: a prescription against pain and prescription for recovery*. Harrow, Scutari

Johnson M (1999) Observations on positivism and pseudoscience in qualitative nursing research. *Journal of Advanced Nursing* 39: 67–73

Johnson M, Long AJ, White A (2001) Arguments for pluralism in qualitative health research. *Nurse Education Today* 22:1 85–93

Johnson M, Webb C (1995) Rediscovering unpopular patients: the concepts of social judgement. *Journal of Advanced Nursing* 21: 466–475

Koch T (1994) Establishing rigour in qualitative research: the decision trail. *Journal of Advanced Nursing* 19: 976–986

Koch T, Harrington (1998) Reconceptualizing rigour: the case for reflexivity. *Journal of Advanced Nursing* 28: 882–890

Koch T, Jenkin P, Kralik D (2004) Chronic illness self-management: locating the 'self'. *Journal of Advanced Nursing* 48: 484–492

Kuhn TS (1972) *The Structure of Scientific Revolutions*, 2nd edition, Chicago, University of Chicago

Lincoln YS, Guba EG (1985) *Naturalistic Inquiry*. Thousand Oaks, Sage

Lincoln YS, Guba EG (1989) *Fourth Generation Evaluation*. Thousand Oaks, Sage

Mason J (1996) *Qualitative Researching*. London, Sage

Mays N, Pope C (2000) Assessing quality in qualitative research. *British Medical Journal* 320: 50–52

Moore S, Corner J, Wells M, Salmon E, Normand C, Brada M, O'Brien M, Smith I (2002) Nurse led follow up and conventional medical follow up in management of patients with lung cancer: randomised trial *British Medical Journal* 325: 1145–1147

Nelson S, McGillon M (2004) Expertise or performance? Questioning the rhetoric of contemporary use of narrative use in nursing. *Journal of Advanced Nursing* 47: 631–638

Oakley A (1984) The importance of being a nurse. *Nursing Times* 80:59 24–27

Polgar S, Thomas SA (2000) *Introduction to Research in the Health Sciences*, 4th edition. Edinburgh, Churchill Livingstone

Popper K (1972) *Conjectures and Refutations*, 4th edition rev. London, Routledge & Kegan Paul

Porter S (1995) *Nursing's Relationship with Medicine*. Aldershot, Ashgate

Ramprogus V (2002) Eliciting nursing knowledge from practice: the dualism of nursing. *Nurse Researcher* 10:1 52–64

Roach S (2004) Sexual behaviour of nursing home residents: staff perceptions and responses. *Journal of Advanced Nursing* 48: 371–379

Sandolowski M (1993) Rigor or rigor mortis: The problem of rigor in qualitative research. *Advances in Nursing Science* 16:2 1–8

Schwandt TA (1997) *Qualitative Inquiry A Dictionary of Terms*. Thousand Oaks, Sage

Shipman M (1992) *The Limitations of Social Research*, 3rd edition. London, Longman

Silverman D (1985) *Qualitative Methodology and Sociology: describing the social world*. Aldershot, Gower

Silverman D (2000) *Doing Qualitative Research: a practical handbook.* London, Sage
Wilson-Barnett J (1988) Patient Teaching or Patient Counselling? *Journal of Advanced Nursing*
    13: 215–222

Websites

www.qualitative-research.net/fqs/fqs-eng.htm/ – *Forum: Qualitative Social Research* is an online
    peer-reviewed multilingual journal for qualitative research
www.nova.e/ssss/QR/web.html/ – *The Qualitative Report* is an online journal dedicated to
    qualitative research
www.data-archive.ac.uk/ – the UK Data Archive at the University of Essex houses the largest
    collection of accessible computer readable data in the social sciences and humanities

12 Sampling

Susan Procter and Teresa Allan

Key points

- Sampling techniques aim to produce the best science within the constraints of resources available.
- A variety of sampling strategies are used in both qualitative and quantitative research, depending on the context and the research design.
- Sample selection and sample size affect the validity of the research, and so should be done with maximum rigour.

Introduction

Sampling is a necessary aspect of all social research as by definition it is not possible, except in exceptional and limited circumstances, to carry out a census that collects data from the total population. Sampling reduces the costs of research projects and also reduces the time required to gather the data. As this chapter will demonstrate, research is a pragmatic activity and researchers are constantly trying to produce the best science within the constraints of time, resources and feasibility.

There is considerable overlap between the sampling techniques used in both qualitative and quantitative research, but also some important differences. This chapter will guide the reader through the sampling procedures that need to be considered when undertaking both quantitative and qualitative research.

Populations and samples

In all research it is important to distinguish between the target population, study population and the sampling frame used in the study. These are described below:

Target population

The target population is the total population that forms the focus for the study. In quantitative research it is the population to whom the study results will be generalised or applied. For instance, in the example given in Box 12.1 the target population would be all patients in the UK on oral anticoagulant treatment who correspond with the eligibility criteria for this study.

Qualitative research increases knowledge and understanding about the features of the target population under study. In Box 12.2 the target population is all medical patients experiencing repeat hospital admissions and/or delayed discharge.

Box 12.1   Example of a sample frame and simple random sample.

Fitzmaurice DA, Murray ET, Gee KM, Allan TF, Hobbs FDR (2002) A randomised controlled trial of patient self-management of oral anticoagulation treatment compared with primary care management. *Journal of Clinical Pathology* 55: 845–849

This study tested whether patients could manage to change their own dose of oral anticoagulation using a CoaguChek® international normalised ratio (INR) test and a simple dosing algorithm. The sampling frame consisted of all patients receiving warfarin from six general practices who satisfied study entry criteria. These patients were then invited to participate in the study; those who agreed were selected with simple random selection until the sample size was fulfilled. Eligible patients were randomised to 'self-management' (30 patients) or routine nurse-led clinics in primary care settings (26 patients). There was no significant difference in the main outcome measures of percentage time in an acceptable range of blood glucose levels (self-management 74% *vs* 77% control) and proportion of tests in the acceptable range (66% *vs* 72% controls).

Box 12.2   Example of a purposive sample.

Pearson P, Procter S, Wilcockson J, Allgar V (2004) The process of hospital discharge for medical patients: a model. *Journal of Advanced Nursing* 46: 496–505

In this study, patients anticipated to be at risk of unsuccessful hospital discharge were purposively sampled using criteria identified in an earlier phase of the study. All the health and social care professionals involved in the care of each patient before and after discharge were also sampled to ascertain the views of all those involved in the care of each patient as to their health care needs and ability to manage at home. The study demonstrates the strength of purposive sampling by focusing on only those patients which earlier research had demonstrated were likely to experience unsuccessful hospital discharge, and on the professionals caring for them. Therefore, most medical patients were excluded from the study as they did not fit the purpose of the study.

Study population

The study population is a subset of the target population from whom the sample is taken. Clearly in the examples given it would not be practical to recruit patients to the studies from across the UK. Instead, the researchers recruited patients who fitted the inclusion criteria for the study and were accessible locally.

Sampling frame

A sampling frame is a comprehensive itemised list of all people, patients, practices, hospitals or events, which comprise the study population, from which a sample will be taken. It includes the settings or individuals of interest to the researcher, and provides a transparent framework from which to derive a sample. When devising a sampling frame it is important to distinguish between the target population and the study population. The sampling frame is normally taken from the study population, which is assumed to broadly reflect the characteristics of the target population. If there are important differences between the two populations, these will limit the generalisability or transferability of the study findings and this should be noted as a study limitation. Once the sampling frame has been compiled it is possible to use it to derive a sample.

Types of sampling

There are two basic sampling schemes in research – probability, and non-probability sampling schemes. Quantitative research studies tend to use probability schemes as the errors or biases are more easily calculated and thus accounted for in the sampling procedures and analysis. This allows for generalisation to the study and target population more readily than non-probability schemes. Qualitative researchers predominantly use non-probability schemes as this allows for theoretical sampling.

Probability sampling

Probability sampling means that each unit in the target population has a known chance of selection. Usually it is an equal chance (as in the National Lottery) but sometimes it may be unequal, but known.

Probability sampling can only be used when an accurate and up-to-date sampling frame is available. Where the study population is known in advance (e.g. all patients receiving Warfarin in six GP practices as in Box 12.1) this provides a useful sampling frame for research. The strength of probability sampling arises from the fact that it generates a representative sample, which should ensure that the sample has the same characteristics as the study population, and where the study population is similar to the target population.

Non-probability sampling

Non-probability sampling is used when it is necessary to derive a sample from an unknown (hidden) population. It is frequently the case that the study population cannot be identified in advance or, more usually, that no up-to-date and complete list is available from which a sample can be derived. When it is not possible to obtain a comprehensive list of the study population, researchers must use non-probability sampling schemes. In quantitative research these are considered less rigorous because bias may inadvertently be introduced, making the sample not representative of the total population.

Nevertheless the alternative of not undertaking the research because a sampling frame is not available may impoverish our knowledge about important groups of people such as the homeless, family carers, single parents and other groups where a register does not exist. In-depth qualitative studies and descriptive surveys that identify the key characteristics and features of the sample population can be used to increase our knowledge and explanatory theories of this population and can be generalised to other populations which match the sample in ways identified as important by the researchers.

Non-probability sampling schemes are widely used in nursing research. In quantitative research they may be used in preliminary or exploratory studies, where random sampling is too costly, where an appropriate sampling frame is not available, or when it is the only way of getting the information required. In qualitative studies they are used to study the population of interest, and to ensure that the research samples rich sources of data that generate in-depth conceptual and theoretical understanding.

Sampling schemes in quantitative research

Simple random sampling

In simple random sampling each member on the sampling frame has a known and equal chance of being selected for the sample. To derive a sample of 390 from a list of 2,600, the list should be numbered systematically and a random number table or a software package such as Minitab or Statistical Package for the Social Sciences (SPSS) used to randomly generate the required number of 390. Simple random sampling can produce 'rogue' samples, especially if the sample size is small. In order to overcome this, either systematic or stratified random sampling can be used.

Systematic random sampling

Again a numbered list is used, but this time a sampling fraction is calculated. The sampling fraction depends on the sample size and how long the list is. If there are 400 on the list and 40 are required then this gives a sample fraction of 10% and selects 1 in 10. So the starting point on the list for selection (the start value) must be a number between 1 and 10, chosen randomly. Every tenth item on the list is chosen thereafter e.g. 6, 16, 26 etc, etc. Systematic random sampling leads to a more evenly spaced distribution of the sample from the list than simple random sampling (Bowling 1997). But even this can introduce bias if there is a cyclic pattern in the underlying list e.g. operations in hospitals that follow a weekly pattern would give the same type on the same day. Blocking schemes (Pocock 1983) can be used to overcome cyclical patterns. For instance over 7 weeks a different day each week is chosen at random before sampling takes place (using systematic random or random sampling) within each block.

Stratified random sampling

This is where the population is divided into well-defined sub-groups or strata, e.g. males/females, age groups, operation types, illness type, nurse grades. This means that people within a stratum are more similar to each other than across the different strata. There are two forms of stratified random sampling: *proportionate* and *disproportionate* sampling.

In *proportionate* sampling the same sampling fraction (e.g. 15%) is used to draw a sample from each group/stratum. This means that the different groups in the population (strata) are correctly represented in the sample, with larger groups contributing proportionately more people to the sample, as demonstrated in Table 12.1. This increases the precision of the estimates of error compared with simple random sampling and gives more confidence in the results.

In *disproportionate* sampling a variable sampling fraction is used to increase representation of particular groups that may have small numbers in the study or total population. For instance if an area had a very mixed ethnic population, the sample fraction might be increased in order to include people from a wider range of different ethnic backgrounds in the study. Similarly, some strata may be very small, giving rise to only a few members being selected if the standard sampling fraction is used. As Table 12.1 illustrates, a 15% sampling fraction of F grade staff nurses in a hospital yields a much higher number than a 15% sample of I grade nurses. However, because, in disproportionate sampling, the sample is no longer representative of the study or total population some variables will be over-represented. The analysis has to be adjusted to account for this over representation.

Table 12.1 Proportionate sampling from nurse grades.

Population stratum nurse grades	Number of people in the stratum	Number sampled from the stratum (15%)
F	1500	225
G	800	120
H	200	30
I	100	15
Total	2600	390

Cluster sampling

Here the entire population is divided into groups or clusters based on closeness of some kind (e.g. geographical), or similarity (e.g. type of hospital) or speciality (orthopaedic or cardiac) or particular wards (medical or surgical). First, a sample of the clusters is taken using simple, systematic or stratified random sampling. Then all members of each cluster selected are recruited, or members of each cluster are sampled using simple, systematic or stratified random sampling. Cluster sampling reduces the costs of research as it ensures that the population sampled is clustered together, so making access and communication easier. It also enables probability sampling to be used when a sampling frame of the population is not available. The clusters may be schools, hospitals, wards or departments for which a sampling frame is available. The sampling frame for each cluster can then be ascertained at a local level following recruitment into the sample as demonstrated in Box 12.3. The disadvantage is that sampling error is increased, and sample size has to increase accordingly.

Box 12.3   Example of cluster randomisation.

Chen HS, Horner SD, Percy MS (2002) Validation of the smoking self-efficacy survey for Taiwanese children. *Journal* of *Nursing Scholarship* 34:1 33–37

Two primary and one junior school were randomly selected from the 40 primary and 14 junior schools in the region of the study. Then two classes from each primary school and four from the junior school were randomly selected. All class members were invited to participate in the study.

Multi-stage sampling

This form of sampling uses more than two consecutive stages of random selection. It can combine simple random sampling, stratified random sampling and cluster sampling in some form.

Quota sampling

This is a non-probability method of sampling widely used in opinion polls. It is a form of convenience and judgement sampling where the data collector has to recruit a number (quota) of people fitting a particular category, e.g. white males over 50, but the selection of the sample is otherwise not specified. Often the size of the quota in the sample is proportional to the number of people in that category in the target population. Bias can be introduced, however, if data collectors consciously or unconsciously avoid certain types of people such as the homeless, or recruit in a particular area of a town. Quota sampling is not much used in health services research.

Calculating sample size in quantitative research

In quantitative research the size of the sample aimed for should be calculated at the design stage. In intervention and comparison studies, the sample size determines the *power* of the study to detect a statistically significant difference between groups.

The *significance* of a study relates to the probability of making a type I (α) error. A type I error means finding a real (i.e.) significant difference/effect between the two groups in the sample when one does not exist in the study or target population. In other words, saying the intervention works, or a real difference between groups exists, when it does not. A type II (β) error is the probability of finding there is no effect or difference between the two groups in the sample population when one does in fact exist in the study population.

If the significance level is set at 5% and a significant result achieved then it indicates with 95% confidence that a real difference exists. The confidence interval of 95% derives from the *probability* of obtaining the observed result due to chance alone.

Reducing the chance of making a type I error from 5% to say 1% and so reducing the chance of concluding that a difference exists, when it does not, requires an increase in sample size. In general terms, the greater the *power*, the larger the sample size has to be, which then has time and cost implications. Traditionally, most studies use either 90% or 80% power. So, for example, if a study has 80% power then there is an 80% probability of detecting a real difference, if it exists. However, this also means that there is a 20% chance of missing a real difference that actually exists.

Calculating sample size for intervention or comparison studies depends on an estimation of the expected differences between groups. In choosing the outcome variables that are going to be used for the calculation, it is helpful if there is some earlier information about the likely variability of the measures selected. Calculating sample size requires a measure of the *variability* of differences, usually the standard deviation or variance, to be expected in the total population. In clinical research the sort of clinical differences one is expecting from the intervention or between different groups that are under consideration, is required. For instance, in the study described in Box 12.1 the power of the study would relate to the ability to detect a real difference in the key outcome variables (time in range and proportion of tests in range) between patients using self-management and those receiving routine care. To calculate sample size, therefore, researchers have to identify in advance the likely size of the difference in measured outcomes that is clinically meaningful between the two groups and to provide a justification of the size difference selected.

In order to calculate sample size, it is necessary to identify the key outcome variables being measured, the tools used to measure those variables and the expected difference between groups. In order to estimate the expected difference between groups it is necessary to obtain as much information as possible from previous studies or from pilot studies about the distribution of the variables across the study and target populations. Armed with this information, researchers should seek the advice of a statistician.

Studies in which the sample size is considered too small to achieve the power required to obtain a significant outcome are often deemed unscientific and not worth undertaking because they will either produce flawed results (if significance testing is carried out) or fail to provide any new knowledge. In general if one wishes to generalise to the target population then sufficient power is a requirement for the validity of studies.

Small studies can, however, be used as pilots for larger studies in which a descriptive analysis of the findings (including percentages, means and standard deviations) of key variables across the study population may be useful for calculating the sample size required in subsequent studies. The power requirement may sometimes be waived in student research, although this is becoming less acceptable to ethics committees.

Sources of bias in quantitative sampling

In quantitative sampling there are two basic types of errors: random (sampling) and systematic (non-sampling). Bias is often introduced into a study through systematic errors.

Random errors create less bias as it is assumed that this type of error is evenly distributed across the sampling frame and therefore the sample, derived randomly, remains inaccurate but representative of the study population. Any errors will tend to average out across the sample and hence little or no bias is introduced. It is possible to control random errors by increasing the sample size and having an appropriate sampling technique.

Systematic errors are not reduced with increased sample size. If a study aims to recruit GPs from a particular list, for example, but certain sorts of GP practices are routinely excluded from that list (e.g. single handed practices), then these GPs cannot be selected and the error is not random. No matter how much the sample size is increased, the error will not be reduced. The key to reducing sample frame bias is to use as accurate a database (or list) as is possible.

In quantitative research the aim is to control as many sources of error as possible but it is a balance. In a large sample with systematic errors the analysis is not to be trusted. An unrepresentative sample makes it impossible to generalise to the study/target population. Sampling schemes, therefore, need to be as rigorous as possible, given the circumstances under which the researcher is working.

Sampling in qualitative research

Qualitative researchers are not so concerned with identifying the total population of people, events or settings in order to develop a sampling frame. They seek to identify key individuals, events or settings which provide a rich source of data. However, it is still important for qualitative researchers to pay attention to their sampling strategy. In assessing the rigour of qualitative research, Mays and Pope (2000) suggest the reviewer should ask the following questions:

> Did the sample include the full range of possible cases or settings so that conceptual rather than statistical generalisations could be made?

> If appropriate, were efforts made to obtain data that might contradict or modify the analysis by extending the sample (for example, to a different type of area or informant)?

In qualitative research the problem of diversity or variation is addressed through the development of a sampling strategy designed to ensure that a range of data are identified and collected as this increases the validity of the findings.

However, for some qualitative research the notion of selecting a sample is considered inappropriate and instead the research focuses on collecting data from a 'naturally occurring population' (Dreher 1994). Case study research may select a single case of an event or situation such as an individual experience of health care (for a good example of this see Allen *et al.* 2004), or study of a single ward, or hospital (Stake 1998). The populations studied, be they people, agencies or other units of study using naturalistic or case study research are recognised by qualitative researchers to be unique. However, they share sufficient commonalities with the population from which they are drawn to be recognisable as belonging to that population group (i.e. a classroom in a school could not be mistaken for a ward in a hospital). Consequently, the study is able to inform understanding of the wider population of which the case study or naturally occurring research is an example.

Convenience sampling

Qualitative researchers tend to study naturally occurring populations or events. They generally select an accessible population or setting in which they can develop a trustworthy relationship with the study participants rather than select a representative sample. Convenience may be a key feature in enabling this relationship to develop, for example, approaching nurses from a local hospital. In many ways all researchers use some form of convenience sample in the sense that the sample must be accessible to the researcher in some form.

Purposive sampling

A purposive sample is one where people from a prespecified group are purposely sought out and sampled. For instance, in the example given in Box 12.2 the researchers purposively sampled patients anticipated to be at risk of delayed discharge or readmission within six weeks. Purposive samples have an over representation of people or events of interest to the researcher. This means that they are not usually representative of the whole population under study. In the study depicted in Box 12.2 the researchers purposively sampled complex cases, or cases requiring complex discharge arrangements as these were considered to provide rich sources of data. Purposive sampling is used to justify the inclusion of rich sources of data that can be used to generate or test out the explanatory frameworks. Examples of purposive sampling given by Patton (1980) include sampling:

- extreme or deviant cases
- typical cases
- maximum variation in cases
- critical cases
- politically important or sensitive cases
- convenience sampling

Identifying the full range of possible cases or settings again requires the qualitative researcher to at least map out potential respondents or study sites from whatever information is available before deciding who, where or what to sample. Box 12.4 gives an illustration of how this can be achieved using matrix multidimensional sampling (Miles & Huberman 1994). Here a survey was used to obtain more detailed information and a matrix was drawn up with a range of different settings on one axis and the inclusion criteria on the other axis. Case study sites are chosen to provide a diversity of settings while covering as many of the inclusion criteria as possible. The process by which the sampling decisions are taken, perhaps distinguishes purposive sampling from convenience sampling in qualitative research.

Theoretical sampling

Further sampling in response to data analysis is sometimes referred to as theoretical sampling. Here the sampling strategy evolves iteratively in response to data analysis and in particular to the conceptual and theoretical aspects of the analysis rather than the characteristics of the population. For instance Canales and Bowers (2001) used purposive sampling to identify study participants but developed the

Box 12.4   Example of matrix multidimensional sampling.

Clarke CL, Wilcockson J (2001) Professional and organizational learning: analysing the relationship with the development of practice. *Journal of Advanced Nursing* 34: 264–272

Three case study sites were sampled by the use of a matrix for multidimensional analysis. To develop the matrix, questionnaires were sent to the total population of practitioners (n = 474) in one NHS region known to be undertaking practice developments at that time (as identified by the Practice and Service Development Initiative of the NHS Centre for Reviews and Dissemination). Criteria for selection as a case study site included: links with academic departments; identified model of practice development; evidence base used to inform practice development; level of central and local funding for practice developments; research and development strategy of the organisation; multidisciplinary involvement in practice developments. As such, the sites can be considered to be examples of good practice. All of the sites were within the NHS Region and included:

- a mental health/primary care health promotion initiative
- a nurse practitioner development in an A & E Department
- a whole trust practice development support mechanism.

interview schedule and therefore the data collected in response to their emerging theoretical analysis. Hupcey (2000), on the other hand, expanded her sample of participants in response to the emerging theoretical analysis.

As an indicator of rigour in qualitative research, Mays and Pope (2000) suggest that the researcher searches for contradictory or disconfirming sources of data or identifies exceptions to the patterns being described, in order to test out the findings from the study. These data sources can either be purposively identified at the start of the study and built into the sampling framework (purposive sampling) or identified during the course of the study in response to the analysis of the data (theoretical sampling). Either way a sampling frame that is used to map sampling decisions is a useful way to demonstrate rigour in qualitative research.

Snowball sampling

This strategy uses human networks to gather a sample or identify informants or situations where events might be observed e.g. homeless people often know others in the same situation; similarly people from ethnic minority populations may be able to identify others from their population who could inform the research. Snowball sampling (sometimes known as network mapping) can be used with professional staff and managers to identify colleagues who are for instance, championing or resisting a change in policy or practice. Snowball sampling can pose problems of definition, which requires the researcher to pay attention to how people define, or self-define themselves as group members. Faugier and Sargeant (1997) provide a good discussion of snowball sampling to access hard-to-reach populations.

Calculating sample size in qualitative research

Because sample size is not an intrinsic feature of the analysis in qualitative research there is very little guidance on the size of samples. In most cases the resources available and the feasibility of obtaining the sample combine to determine the size. The rigour of the approach used is determined by the rationale given for the sampling decisions taken by the researcher within the context of available opportunities for gaining access to events or naturally occurring populations.

Grounded theory uses the concept of *saturation* to determine sample size. Here data are collected and analysed until no new themes or perspectives are reported and it is assumed that all the component parts of the phenomenon under study have been captured. This approach creates difficulties in planning research as it is not possible to identify in advance how much data will be required to reach saturation and therefore how much resource is required to complete the study.

DePaulo (2000), in a paper designed to guide market research using qualitative methods, calculated the number of customer needs uncovered by various numbers of focus groups and in-depth interviews. Few additional needs were uncovered after 30 in-depth interviews; this was confirmed using quantitative methods. His work also indicates that if the researcher is not concerned with within group variation, only with typicality, then a sample of 10 should suffice. Similar estimates for sample size in qualitative research may be found in Morse (1994).

However, DePaulo (2000) is mainly concerned to produce a descriptive level of analysis that maximises the range of opinions or perceptions captured. He recommends that multiple analysts review the data to maximise findings. Qualitative researchers concerned to derive theoretical interpretations of data are not convinced by arguments for saturation or capturing maximum variation, viewing this as a search for descriptive completeness (Dreher 1994). Instead, they suggest that theory may be derived from a fragment of naturally occurring data if the researcher studies that data for what is not said or done and interprets absence and omissions in the data as well as inclusions.

Sampling strategies used in qualitative and quantitative research

Some types of sampling are used in both qualitative and quantitative research, although their use conforms to the principles of each type of sampling strategy as discussed above. These are discussed below.

Sampling for time, events and settings

Sampling for time, events and settings is difficult as these change over time, or vary from person to person or vary according to setting. Box 12.5 describes Meengs *et al.* (1994) quantitative observational study of handwashing in an emergency department. In this case information for a sample of 35 participants was gathered during three-hour periods over a number of days. Estimates of hand washing then have to be totalled or averaged over standardised periods.

Box 12.5 Example of sampling for time and events.

Meengs MR, Giles BK, Chisholm CD, Cordell WH, Nelson DR (1994) Handwashing frequency in an emergency department. *Journal of Emergency Nursing* 20: 183–188

This study examined the frequency and duration of handwashing in one emergency department and the effects of three variables: level of training, type of patient contact (clean, dirty, or gloved), and years of staff clinical experience. 11 faculty, 11 resident physicians, and 13 emergency nurses were observed. Participants were informed that their activities were being monitored but were unaware of the exact nature of the study. An observer recorded the number of patient contacts and activities for each participant during three-hour observation periods. Activities were categorised as either clean or dirty according to a scale devised by Fulkerson. The use of gloves was noted and handwashing technique and duration were recorded. A handwashing break in technique was defined as failure to wash hands after a patient contact and before proceeding to another patient or activity.

When undertaking this type of sampling it is important to make observations across time and space, as the pattern of event being observed, e.g. handwashing behaviour, may change both during the day and on different days and may vary according to how busy the department is, who is on duty and whether it is a weekday, evening, night or weekend shift.

Sampling in time and events and settings is an important feature of qualitative research, particularly observational research. It is often difficult to sample events as it is not possible to know exactly when or where they are going to occur. However, the selection of situations to observe is guided by the same sampling principles used elsewhere in qualitative research and tends, therefore, to focus on naturally occurring events during different time periods and in different settings. Qualitative sampling for time, events and settings can be purposive and/or theoretical. In undertaking purposive sampling of events the researcher would seek out settings where the event might naturally occur at a time when it might be expected (*see* Chapter 25 for a fuller account of this process).

Mixed sampling schemes

Quantitative researchers may use sampling schemes that are traditionally seen as qualitative methods. They can be used in either approach with only minor differences, mainly relating to sample size, in the way that they are used. For instance, if a convenience sample is used in quantitative research without random sampling it is not always possible to generalise to the wider population. However, if it can be demonstrated retrospectively that statistically the characteristics of the non-random sample match regional or national characteristics of a larger population for key variables such as gender, age groups, ethnicity etc. it may be possible to generalise to a wider population using non-probability convenience sampling.

Convenience sampling is a commonly-used approach to sampling, particularly in small-scale studies or student projects. For instance, a district nurse uses his/her caseload, a GP uses his/her patient list. However, if the patient caseload was used as a sampling frame and random sampling used to select a sample from this, then this would be a convenience sample but also a probability sample.

Judgement sampling

Judgement samples are used where the person in the sample is judged to have the right knowledge or information for entry. Some attempt is made to select this representative expert sample. Judgement samples can be derived purposively to access specific expertise, for example, a sample of clinical specialists recognised by their peers to be experts in that field may be selected. However, the sample is treated differently from a purposive sample. In judgement sampling deviant or non-conformist views are scrutinised to see if they reflect advanced expertise or poor judgement; in the latter case the view is rejected. Judgement samples are often used in Delphi surveys to derive a consensus where no other source of expert evidence is available.

Conclusion

This chapter has demonstrated that there is considerable overlap between the sampling techniques used in qualitative and quantitative research, but also some important differences. A limiting factor in undertaking quantitative research is the resources needed to undertake studies with a large enough sample to meet power requirements. Pilot work, however, is very valuable and does provide opportunities for students and less well-resourced researchers to undertake quantitative research. This chapter should have alerted readers to the idea that sampling in qualitative and quantitative research has many common factors, both are concerned to ensure rigour and this can be as difficult to achieve in qualitative research as it is in quantitative research. Expert advice from statisticians or experienced qualitative researchers should be sought before selecting a sample.

References

Allen D, Griffiths L, Lyne P (2004) Understanding complex trajectories in health and social care provision. *Sociology of Health and Illness* 26: 1008–1030

Bowling A (1997) *Research Methods in Health: investigating health and health services.* Buckingham, Open University Press

Canales MK, Bowers BJ (2001) Expanding conceptualizations of culturally competent care. *Journal of Advanced Nursing* 36: 102–111

Chen HS, Horner SD, Percy MS (2002) Validation of the smoking self-efficacy survey for Taiwanese Children. *Journal* of *Nursing Scholarship* 34:1 33–37

Clarke CL, Wilcockson J (2001) Professional and organizational learning: analysing the relationship with the development of practice. *Journal of Advanced Nursing* 34: 264–72

DePaulo P (2000) Sample size for qualitative research: the risk of missing something important. *Quirk's Marketing Research Review. www.quirks.com/articles*

Dreher M (1994) Qualitative research methods from the reviewer's perspective. In Morse JM (ed) *Critical Issues in Qualitative Research Methods.* Thousand Oaks, Sage pp281–299

Faugier J, Sargeant M (1997) Sampling hard to reach populations. *Journal of Advanced Nursing* 26: 790–797

Fitzmaurice DA, Murray ET, Gee KM, Allan TF, Hobbs FDR (2002) A randomised controlled trial of patient self management of oral anticoagulation treatment compared with primary care management. *Journal of Clinical Pathology* 55: 845–849

Hupcey JE (2000) Feeling safe: the psychosocial needs of ICU patients. *Journal of Nursing Scholarship* 32:4 361–367

Mays N, Pope C (2000) Assessing quality in qualitative research. *British Medical Journal* 320: 50–52

Meengs MR, Giles BK, Chisholm CD, Cordell WH, Nelson DR (1994) Handwashing frequency in an emergency department. *Journal of Emergency Nursing* 20: 183–188

Miles MB, Huberman AM (1994) *Qualitative Data Analysis: an expanded sourcebook*, 2nd edition. Thousand Oaks, Sage

Morse JM (1994) Designing funded qualitative research. In Denzin NK, Lincoln YS. *Handbook of Qualitative Research.* Thousand Oaks, Sage pp220–235

Muhajarine N, D'Arcy C (1999) Physical abuse during pregnancy: prevalence and risk factors. *Canadian Medical Association Journal* 160:7 1007–1010

Patton MQ (1980) *Qualitative Evaluation Methods.* Beverley Hills, Sage

Pearson P, Procter S, Wilcockson J, Allgar V (2004) The process of hospital discharge for medical patients: a model. *Journal of Advanced Nursing* 46: 496–505

Pocock SJ (1983) *Clinical Trials: a practical approach.* London, John Wiley

Stake RE (1998) Case studies. In Denzin NK, Lincoln YS (eds) *Strategies of Qualitative Inquiry.* Thousand Oaks, Sage pp86–109

Further reading

Armitage P, Berry G, Matthews JNS (2002) *Statistical Methods in Medical Research.* Oxford, Blackwell Science

Campbell MJ, Julious SA, Altman DG (1995) Estimating sample sizes for binary, ordered categorical, and continuous outcomes in two group comparisons. *British Medical Journal* 311: 1145–1148

Cohen J (1988) *Statistical Power Analysis for the Behavioural Sciences*, 2nd edition. Lawrence New Jersey, Erlbaum Associates

Introduction to qualitative research approaches (Chapters 13, 14 and 15)

Chapter 11 introduced the concept of *qualitative research* and outlined the underlying assumptions that shape research studies adopting this overall approach. Qualitative research fits within an interpretivist tradition based on the belief that human beings continuously interpret and make sense of their environment, and so research into their behaviour and social processes must take the meaning of events into account. Researchers undertaking qualitative studies employ approaches and techniques (for example in-depth interviewing or participant observation, narrative or thematic analysis) that allow insight into how people behave in natural settings, such as a ward.

There are, however, several different approaches to qualitative research. Whereas they all share the underlying assumptions outlined in Chapter 11, they differ in terms of their goals, research questions, techniques employed and the contribution they each make to knowledge development. The following three chapters examine three of the most popular qualitative approaches used in nursing research: grounded theory, ethnography, and phenomenology. The particular characteristics of each of these approaches are shown in Box S3.1. These chapters should be read alongside Chapter 27, which examines the analysis of data derived from qualitative research.

Box S3.1 Characteristics of ethnography, grounded theory and phenomenology.

Dimensions	Ethnography	Grounded theory	Phenomenology
Goal	Describe, interpret, and understand the characteristics of a particular social setting with all its cultural diversity and multiplicity of voices.	Develop a theory of how individuals and groups make meaning together and interact with each other; of how particular concepts and activities fit together and can explain what happens.	Describe, interpret and understand the meanings of experiences at both a general and unique level.
Research question	How are people positioned in a particular social context and how do they interact with each other, especially with significant others? What are the power relationships within the setting?	What theory can be formulated from real world events and experiences to explain this social phenomenon?	What is the structure of this particular experience? What is it like to be in or to experience a particular situation?
Data gathering	Through intensive fieldwork – participant observation and interviews – of key informants who are experts on the social setting and have rich knowledge of it. Also through visual data.	Open-ended beyond a general direction – breadth and depth at different phases; a variety of methods in which the questions may change at different stages depending on the data that are emerging and clues from the literature. Progressive focusing.	Focused on the depth of a particular experience; interviews, narratives – anything that is able to describe the qualities of experiences that were lived through.
Analysis	Coding and building patterns. Searching for the main building blocks of local culture and its themes.	Use the analysis to inspire a creative and plausible theory; constant comparison and organising the data into useful conceptual patterns by codes, categories. Construct and build credible models.	Thematic analysis, which clarifies the meanings by moving back and forth between whole meanings and part meanings.

Presentation of results	An ethnography – the story of people in their social and cultural context describing behaviour, activities, and social relations and the way they perceive their position in the setting under study and society.	A descriptive outline of the elements of the model and how they interact and fit together to form an explanatory theory that accounts for the range of the data collected. Often a diagram that represents these elements and relationships, followed by an exploration of the themes and concepts in relationship to both specific data examples as well as relevant literature.	Different levels depending on audience and purpose: a description of the essence (structure) of the experience, its 'bare bones'; followed by how each theme occurs in different and unique ways; sometimes, a more poetic and narrative account which communicates what the experience is like (its textures). Combinations of these.
Knowledge claim	Knowledge about people within a setting or situation and the way in which they relate to others and perceive themselves.	A plausible theory that can be applied and tested in other contexts. An explanatory model.	Transferable general qualities (essences) of what makes the experience what it is; description of unique contexts. Empathic understanding.
Historical background	Social and cultural anthropology.	Sociology and social psychology.	Philosophy, psychology.

Reprinted by permission from Sage Publications Ltd from Holloway I, Todres L. The status of method: flexibility, consistency and coherence. *Qualitative Research* 3: 345–357 © SAGE Publications, 2003

13 Grounded Theory

Immy Holloway and Les Todres

Key points

- Grounded theory is a systematic qualitative approach to data collection and analysis that is concerned with generating theory, although existing theories can be modified or extended through this process.
- Key features of grounded theory include theoretical sampling, coding and categorisation of data through a process of constant comparative analysis and the development of a core or central category.
- Researchers using a grounded theory approach need to develop theoretical sensitivity whereby they become attuned to important concepts that arise from the data. Reading the literature enhances theoretical sensitivity in that it creates awareness in the researcher of relevant and significant aspects of the data.
- The analytic process can be facilitated by the researcher writing fieldnotes and memos in which they initially record the development of ideas and provisional categories. Subsequently these ideas and categories become more theoretical.
- The data are analysed through coding and categorising.

Introduction

Grounded theory is a systematic approach within qualitative research originally developed by Glaser and Strauss (1967). It has its basis in sociology, particularly symbolic interactionism but the data collection and analysis procedures are also used in other disciplines such as psychology, health care or education. It became especially popular in nursing in the 1980s and 90s. Indeed, Schreiber and Stern (2001) suggest that it is the second most popular qualitative approach in nursing research.

Several informative books have been published on grounded theory, for instance *Theoretical Sensitivity* (Glaser 1978), *Qualitative Analysis for Social Scientists* (Strauss 1987), and *The Basics of Qualitative Research* (Strauss & Corbin 1990; 1998). Strauss died in 1996 but co-authored his last two books with Corbin, a nurse academic. Strauss and Corbin (1997) also edited a book demonstrating the use of grounded theory in practice. Glaser and Strauss used the approach in the health care field and helped students to apply it in particular in nursing and in education. One of the early books was the study by Benoliel (1973) on the interaction of nurses with dying patients. Others have described the techniques and procedures of grounded theory, for instance Charmaz (2000) and Hutchinson and Wilson (2001). An older but still useful text for nurses was edited by Chenitz and Swanson in 1986.

The purpose and main features of grounded theory

There are many similarities between grounded theory and other qualitative approaches. Grounded theory is initially at least, inductive. This means that researchers go from the specific, i.e. from the data, to the general, namely the theory. They gather data, analyse them and then build theory. This is the reverse process from that used more often in quantitative research. There is no hypothesis or theoretical framework prior to data collection in grounded theory; the data of the researcher have primacy. This means that researchers need to overcome preconceptions, be flexible and have an open mind. The most important kind of research questions are process, behaviour and meaning questions such as:

specific data | general Theory

What is going on in this setting?

How do people act and interact in this situation?

What is the meaning of people's experience?

How do things change over time?

What are the phases of the experience, treatment or condition?

However, grounded theory can be distinguished from other qualitative approaches. The main aim of grounded theory is the generation of theory from the data, although Strauss and Corbin (1998) suggest that existing theory may be modified or extended. Theory production differentiates grounded theory from other qualitative approaches. The theory is always grounded in the data and in reality; it focuses on process. It also demonstrates links and relationships between concepts and gives an overview and explanation of the phenomenon under study. It has to be applicable to a variety of similar settings and contexts.

The other distinct features of grounded theory are the interaction between data collection and analysis, and the procedure of theoretical sampling (*see* later sections of this chapter). While many other qualitative approaches end in description (albeit 'thick' or 'exhaustive' description), grounded theory goes further than generating a description by producing theory that has explanatory power. Nevertheless, it has many similarities to other qualitative research methods in that it is person-centred and focuses on the experience, behaviour and perspectives of participants. Grounded theory is most useful where little is known about a topic or a phenomenon, or where a new perspective is needed in a well-known or familiar setting or situation.

The use and relevance of grounded theory in nursing research

In nursing, the findings of grounded theory research will generally have implications for practice as they identify the meanings of participants' experiences, and
nurses can act on these (Wuest 1995). A few decades ago, nurse researchers used
traditional methods of inquiry to generate knowledge. They focused on hypothesis testing, using deductive rather than inductive approaches. Deductive reasoning means that the researcher goes from the general, for instance a general principle
or hypothesis, to specific instances that confirm or falsify this hypothesis.

More recently nurses have utilised qualitative forms of inquiry as the latter
produce rich and deep data. This has a number of advantages for nursing.

- Nurses will be able to understand patients' behaviour and emotions better
  than in the past, and this has implications for professional care and
  treatment.
- Nurses can study interactions between patients and health professionals, and
  this is important for professional action and interaction, and solutions to clinical problems might be found more quickly.
- Nurses learn to understand their own professional world better when studying the perspectives of their own and other professions as well as students'
  perspectives. Solutions to clinical problems might be more easily found.
- Through qualitative evaluation, programmes and processes can be
  improved.
- Nurses have learnt during their education to be structured and systematic in
  their approach to work; hence the structured and systematic approach of
  grounded theory has a particular appeal for them.
- Flexibility and openness is demanded of nurses in clinical practice and nurse
  educators. Nurses are able to apply these skills to grounded theory.

The theoretical basis of grounded theory: symbolic interactionism

Grounded theory has its roots in the movement of symbolic interactionism, a
theoretical perspective initially developed by George Herbert Mead in the 1920s
and 1930s. He saw the use of symbols in interaction as a major feature of human
life. Mead (1934) and Blumer (1971), one of his followers, claim that individuals
develop their own action in relation to others, in the sense that they take account
of each other's behaviour, interpret and respond to it. In the light of change
the meanings are re-interpreted. The emphasis is on the process of interaction
between people and the way they understand social roles. The self thus is a social

rather than a psychological phenomenon. Interactionists contribute to grounded theory the idea that human beings are active agents in their own experience through interpreting this experience and acting according to their interpretations.

Other people affect the development of a person's social self by their expectations and influence. When they start life, human beings develop through interacting with the important people in their lives, significant others. They learn to act according to others' expectations, thereby shaping their own behaviour through the process of socialisation. At a later stage, individuals as members of society analyse the symbols of others, such as language, gestures, mime and appearance, and interpret them. People share the attitudes and responses to particular situations with members of their group. The observation of these interacting roles and responses to each other is a source of data in grounded theory.

To understand action and interaction researchers look at the meanings human beings give to it. In grounded theory researchers explore these meanings and 'the definition of the situation' by those observing and living in it. Thomas (1928) claimed:

'if men (sic) define situations as real, they are real in their consequences' (Thomas 1928:584)

and suggested that individual definitions of reality and meanings they give to it shape perceptions and actions. Participant observation and interviewing help understand this process.

Human beings are creative individuals who plan, project and revise their thoughts and behaviour in relation to others within a particular context. Their conduct can only be understood in context. Grounded theory therefore stresses the importance of the context in which people function and share their social world with others.

Symbolic interactionism is sometimes criticised for neglecting society and its structure. This criticism is not wholly appropriate. It does see the individual in context, in relation with others and in their social situation, and 'conceptualisations are grounded in the empirical world' (Orona 1997:177).

Data collection and initial sampling

Nurse researchers use a variety of data sources for grounded theory research. These may be interviews, observation or documents such as patient diaries, letters or professional notes. Morse (2001), however, advises not to collect data by focus group interviews when carrying out grounded theory; she maintains that the 'snippets of data' obtained are not appropriate, as process cannot be easily uncovered in focus group interviews. In-depth or narrative interviews are more useful. Indeed, unstructured and semi-structured interviews are the favoured methods of data collection, although Strauss and Corbin (1998) stress the value of participant observation.

It must be emphasised that data collection and analysis proceed in parallel, and interact at each stage. Memos or fieldnotes are written throughout so that nothing of importance is forgotten. Researchers decide on the basis of the early collection and analysis what data to obtain next. Subsequently, concepts are followed up and the research becomes progressively focused on particular issues that are important for developing the theoretical ideas, for the participants, and for the researcher's agenda. It means that researchers formulate 'working propositions' which they can then test through further data collection and analysis. In this sense grounded theory, unlike other qualitative research approaches, has deductive elements as researchers develop ideas gained from working hypotheses. Indeed, Strauss (1987) sees the processes of induction, deduction and verification as essential in grounded theory. Grounded theory is mainly seen as starting with induction. Strauss and Corbin (1998) maintain however, that 'any interpretation is a form of deduction' (Strauss & Corbin 1998:136).

This has implications for sampling. The early sample might include a variety of participants, and concepts emerge from the very beginning in the inductive phase. Depending on the findings during the early stages of data collection and analysis, more people may be added to the sample. Others can be interviewed more than once to follow up later findings and to lead to saturation. This means that the number of participants at the beginning might differ from that at the end of the research. For instance, if a researcher finds during early stages that men feel differently from women about a particular issue or problem more men (or women) can be added to the sample.

Theoretical sampling

The preceding example is linked to the process of theoretical sampling. In this, grounded theory is distinctive from other approaches. Theoretical sampling is guided by concepts and constructs which have significance for the developing theory. At the beginning of the study initial sampling decisions are made regarding specific individuals or groups of people who have knowledge and information about the area of study. When initial data have been analysed particular concepts arise and are followed up by a choice of further participants, events and situations; this process can further illuminate the initial findings (*see* Box 13.1). The researcher can continue doing this, choosing a variety of settings or a particular age group to extend the conceptualisation. Certain concepts may be found initially, and during the analytic phase these will be tested out with a further search of these concepts. Theoretical sampling continues until the point of saturation. Although theoretical sampling has its roots in grounded theory it is used in other qualitative research approaches such as ethnography.

In theoretical sampling:

Box 13.1   Theoretical sampling.

A researcher carrying out a study using a grounded theory approach might interview patients about their pain experience, and find in the initial interviews that patients often mention 'lack of information'. The researcher would then follow this up in further interviews by asking questions about information – or types of information – which patients might have had.

'the emerging theory controls the research process throughout' (Alvesson & Sköldberg 2000:11)

The main differences between this and other types of sampling are time and continuance. Unlike other types of sampling, theoretical sampling is not planned from the outset but proceeds throughout the study. However, the fact that details of the sample and interview questions are not fully known beforehand may raise challenges during the process of ethical review.

Theoretical sensitivity

Grounded theory, and in particular theoretical sampling, demands theoretical sensitivity. Glaser (1978) first employed the term in order to help the researcher develop theory. Theoretical sensitivity means that the researcher becomes aware of important concepts or issues that arise from the data. Paying attention to detail and immersion in the data are essential in becoming sensitive. Not only do personal and professional experiences guide researchers, but reading the relevant literature throughout the process of research is also a useful tool in recognising important concepts. There are, however, dangers inherent in having theoretical sensitivity as it might mean reliance on prior assumptions or research developed by others. Hence the grounded theorist needs to take care not to be directed to certain issues.

In summary, sensitivity derives from personal and professional experience; it needs a continuous dialogue with the data and knowledge of the relevant literature.

Data analysis

Data analysis in grounded theory is iterative and interactive. Iteration means that researchers go backwards and forwards during the course of the research, returning to previous data and the issues contained in them. Constant comparison and theoretical sampling go on throughout the research and decisions are not made once and for all but are provisional.

Data analysis includes the following procedures:

- constant comparison
- coding the data
- reducing the codes and developing categories
- linking the categories and finding patterns
- discovering the core category
- discovering or building the theory

Constant comparison

Grounded theory is characterised by the *constant comparative method*. Constant comparison means that researchers take a series of iterative steps in which they compare incidents in, and sections of, the data. Glaser and Strauss (1967) explain that researchers not only compare qualitative data from interviews, documents and observations but also related information found in the literature. Differences and similarities across incidents in the data are explored. Ideas that develop within a category are compared with those that previously emerged in the same category. Through comparison, properties and dimensions (characteristics) of categories can be produced and patterns established which enhance the explanatory power of these categories and help in the development of theory.

Computer software may be used to assist in data analysis. Qualitative software packages, for example, NVivo or Atlas/ti, are intended for in-depth inductive analysis and allow for theory building models and diagrams. There are, however, limitations to the use of computers, particularly for novice researchers. Charmaz (2000) maintains that where researchers are deeply involved with the participants and need sensitivity, computer analysis might have a distancing effect. Computers, however, can be useful tools (*see* Chapter 27).

Coding and categorising

Initially the data will be coded line-by-line or sentence-by-sentence. Coding is the process by which the researcher identifies and names concepts. The first step is *open coding*. This involves breaking down and conceptualising the data and starts as soon as the researcher has collected the first group of data. It includes *in -vivo* coding, when the researcher examines phrases that the participants themselves have used. For instance, a patient might say 'nurses always spend time with patients.' 'Spending time with patients' is then an *in vivo* code. Box 13.2 provides an example of open coding.

The researcher generates a great number of open codes in the first stage of analysis and then has to collapse or reduce them. This process is called categorising. Categories tend to be more abstract than initial codes and group open codes together. Box 13.3 provides an example of a category developed from three open codes.

Categories are provisional in that new ideas can be integrated. Also their characteristics (properties and dimensions) should be uncovered as well as the conditions under which they occur and the consequences that they have. For instance

Box 13.2 Open coding.

Lines	Codes
1. I was frightened when I had my first test	1. Fear of the unknown
2. I felt I was thrown in at the deep end, but . . .	2. Thrown in at the deep end
3. . . . the nurse really reassured me I was ok	3. Feeling reassured

Box 13.3 Category development.

Initial code	Category
Being lonely	
Lack of attention	Feeling abandoned
Missing visits	

the analysts might explore the specific conditions and consequences around a category *Being in Control*. What are the conditions that determine whether patients see themselves as 'in control'? What are the consequences of 'being in control'? Strauss and Corbin (1998:224) give the properties and dimensions of *the pain experience* as an example; properties refer to intensity, location and duration.

Relating categories and linking them with their characteristics and 'subcategories' is important for the emerging theory. Relationships and links are connected with the 'when, where, why, how, and with what consequences an event occurs' (Strauss & Corbin 1998:22). Strauss and Corbin call this type of categorising *axial coding*. Box 13.4 provides an illustration of axial coding.

The next stage involves the search for patterns. At this stage data are combined. The constructs developed are major categories formulated by the researchers and rooted in their nursing or academic knowledge. These constructs contain emerging theoretical ideas and through developing them, researchers reassemble the data. There is no reason why researchers cannot occasionally use the categories that others have discovered. Constant comparison of new data, incidents, codes and categories is needed throughout, but especially at this stage.

The last phase of the analysis is *selective coding*. Selective coding involves integrating and refining the categories and identifying the story line. This means that the theory is starting to emerge; the categories are grouped around a central or core concept – or occasionally concepts – which have explanatory power.

Box 13.4   Axial coding.

Jacobsson A, Pihl E, Martensson J, Fridlund B (2004) Emotions, the meaning of food and heart failure: a grounded theory study. *Journal of Advanced Nursing* 46: 514–552

Jacobsson *et al.* (2004) carried out a study that developed a theoretical model of experiences of food among patients with heart failure. They reported that psychosocial and physiological meaning was associated with particular feelings and how patients' experience of food and eating changed during the development of the disease.

The account of the study shows how the researchers searched for patterns by sorting the information and linking categories with subcategories. Through this process they discovered cause and effect from the empirical data. They state:

Examples of axial coding were: 'I eat [strategy] because I have to [circumstance], not because it tastes good . . . or because I'm hungry [phenomenon] . . . but because otherwise I would die.'

Developing the core category

Through finding relationships between categories, the researcher discovers the core category from the data. Glaser (1978) and Strauss (1987) identify the characteristics for the core category:

- It is a central phenomenon in the research and should be linked to all other categories so that a pattern is established.
- It should occur frequently in the data.
- It emerges naturally without being forced out by the researcher.
- It should explain variations in the data.
- It is discovered towards the end of the analysis.

The core category is the basic social-psychological process involved in the research that occurs over time and explains changes in the participants' behaviour, feelings and thoughts. Box 13.5 provides an example of a core category.

Theoretical saturation

Saturation is a particular point in category development. It occurs when no new relevant concepts can be found that are important for the development of the emerging theory. Sampling goes on until categories, their properties and dimensions, as well as the links between the categories are well established. The theory will not be wholly adequate unless saturation has been established. When time is limited, researchers may not have sufficient data to reach saturation or may stop

Box 13.5   Core category.

Calvin AO (2004) Haemodialysis patients and end-of-life decisions: a theory of personal preservation. *Journal of Advanced Nursing* 46: 558–566

In using a grounded theory approach, Calvin (2004) studied decisions about end-of-life treatment of people with kidney failure who were undergoing haemodialysis. She found that participants focused on living rather than death. *Personal preservation* was uncovered as the core category of this research. This variable accounted for the behaviour of participants in relation to their decision-making. It connected both *being responsible* and *taking chances*. This category also linked other concepts and categories that emerged. The theory grounded in the data became *the theory of personal preservation*.

without fully analysing the data: this is known as premature closure (Glaser 1978).

New researchers do not always understand what saturation means. Sometimes it is thought that saturation has taken place when a concept is mentioned frequently and is described in similar ways by a number of people, or when the same ideas arise over and over again. This does not guarantee saturation. It is difficult to know when saturation has been established (Backman & Kyngäs 1999). It occurs at a different stage in each project and cannot be predicted at the outset.

The theory

Categories in grounded theory are more abstract than initial codes and assist in building theory. A theory must have 'grab' and 'fit'; it should be recognised by other people working in the field and grounded in the data. The 'theory of personal preservation' (Box 13.5) would resonate in the thinking of nurses as it is grounded in the real world of patients. Strauss and Corbin (1998) demand that:

- Theory shows systematic relationships between concepts and links between categories.
- Variation should be built into the theory, that is, it should hold true under a number of conditions and circumstances.
- The theory should demonstrate a social and/or psychological process.
- The theoretical findings should be significant and remain important over time.

Glaser and Strauss distinguish between two types of theory, substantive and formal. While substantive theory is derived from the study of a specific context, formal theory is more abstract and conceptual. For instance, a specific theory of negotiating between patients and nurses about pain relief would be substantive theory. A theory about the concept of negotiation in general that can be applied to many different settings and situations becomes formal theory. Most researchers, in particular novices, produce substantive theories that are specific and can be applied to the situation under study or similar settings.

Strauss and Corbin consider the applicability of theoretical ideas to other settings and situations. For instance the concept of 'transition' or 'status passage' may be applied to a variety of situations, such as 'becoming a mother' or 'seeking a diagnosis'. Indeed, Morse (1994) uses the term 'theory-based generalisation', meaning that a theory can be re-contextualised in a number of situations, and verified in a variety of settings.

Writing memos

In the early stages of a study important ideas may emerge and as the work progresses the researcher becomes increasingly aware of theoretical perspectives. These thoughts need to be recorded in a field diary and memos. Memos are: 'records of analysis, thoughts, interpretations, questions and directions for further data collection' (Strauss & Corbin 1998: 11).

They might be physical descriptions of the setting or theoretical ideas. The researcher should date them as well as supply detail.

Memos are meant to help in the development and formation of theory. Initially they are simple, but become progressively more theoretical. In theoretical memos researchers develop ideas and occasionally working propositions, compare findings and record their thoughts. Strauss (1987) provides examples of different types of memos that might be written. Diagrams may be used in memos to help the researcher capture ideas. They can guide the researcher to base abstract ideas in the reality of the data (Holloway & Wheeler 2002).

The use of literature in grounded theory

Grounded theory research is generally carried out where little is known about the phenomenon to be studied. Researchers need to identify a gap in knowledge that their research questions will address. They should read around the topic as this can generate questions and some initial concepts. However, if researchers are steeped in the literature from the very beginning, they might be directed to certain issues and constrained by their expectations developed from previous reading rather than developing their own ideas. Strauss and Corbin (1998) warn that researchers might become rigid and stifled through reading too much. Indeed, a full search of the literature would not be appropriate for grounded theory. Of course there is a need to review the literature on the research topic but researchers should enter the arena without major preconceptions.

Nurse researchers generally start their research with certain assumptions as they often have some knowledge of the field they wish to explore. Moreover, their professional experience and reading of the literature can enhance their research as it generates theoretical sensitivity to concepts and issues that are important for the developing theory. Researchers do need to be explicit however, and uncover their own preconceptions.

As a grounded theory study progresses, categories and theoretical concepts are developed. The literature relating to these concepts is reviewed and a dialogue takes place between the literature and the emerging ideas of the researcher. The researcher's data have priority over those of other studies in the same topic area. Concepts arising from the research can be compared with those emerging from other studies. In this sense Strauss and Corbin (1998) see the literature as a potential source of data. As categories are identified, researchers trawl the literature for confirmation or refutation of these categories. Grounded theorists examine what other researchers have found and whether there are any links to existing theories. In the dialogue with the literature, researchers should explore why other studies come up with similar or different findings and the reasons for any discrepancies. This interaction with the literature, and the debate about it, is integrated into the discussion section of the research report.

The choice between Glaserian and Straussian grounded theory

Glaser and Strauss started together on the path of developing grounded theory but subsequently diverged from each other. Glaser (1992) criticised Strauss and Corbin (1990) accusing them of distorting the procedures and meaning of the grounded theory approach. A full discussion of the differences between the two perspectives can be found in MacDonald (2001). Glaser and Strauss (and Corbin) differ mainly on the following points:

The research topic

Glaser suggests that researchers approach the topic without preconceptions and have a research interest rather than a research problem. While Strauss and Corbin advise researchers to identify a phenomenon to be studied at the beginning of the study, Glaser claims that this would arise naturally during the process of the research. This has implications for the initial literature review, which would be somewhat more detailed for Strauss and Corbin while Glaser believes that it might 'contaminate' the participants' data, although he too suggests that the literature should be integrated into the developing concepts. Annells (1997) suggests that

Strauss and Corbin see theory as a construct 'co-created by the researcher and the participants' while Glaser sees it as emerging from the data.

Coding and categorising

Coding is mentioned by both authors but seems to have slightly different meanings. Although Glaser does not like the term axial coding, his 'theoretical coding' seems very similar to axial coding.

Verification

One of the main factors that distinguish the ideas of Glaser and Strauss is the issue of verification. Strauss and Corbin suggest that working propositions are examined and provisionally tested against new data (as, indeed, the original text by Glaser and Strauss had suggested). Glaser believes that these hypotheses should not be verified or validated at this stage by the researcher, and new data should be integrated into the emerging theory.

The process of generating theory

While Strauss and Corbin advocate the building of theory through axial coding, Glaser suggests that the theory will eventually emerge naturally as long as the researcher continuously engages with the data, and they are analysed adequately and in depth. There are also differences of opinion regarding the generalisability of grounded theory. Strauss and Corbin consider that grounded theory is generalisable whereas Glaser considers this not to be the case.

Which approach?

Both approaches are viable forms of grounded theory research so researchers have to decide for themselves which one to adopt. The more prescriptive and formulaic approach of Strauss and Corbin (1990; 1998) may be easier for novices, while experienced researchers might find the Glaserian perspective more appropriate and flexible. Researchers may modify the approach to fit their own purposes; however, they should be thoroughly familiar with the original approach to justify their modification and deviation from it.

Problems and strengths of grounded theory

Grounded theory has been criticised for its neglect of social structure and culture, and the influence of these on human action and interaction. Indeed, Glaser and

Strauss (1967) advise researchers not to research topics linked to structure and culture. Symbolic interactionism as the basis of grounded theory is also more concerned with interaction, action and meaning rather than macro-issues such as societal factors.

Layder (1982), in particular, criticised the lack of emphasis on such concepts as power, gender and ethnicity. MacDonald (2001) develops these points in a critique of grounded theory and symbolic interactionism.

Researchers who use other qualitative approaches also stress process and human agency rather than society and structure. One might, however, argue that there is no rule stating that these approaches cannot be used in the discussion of macro-issues. After all, processes change; Layder wrote more than two decades ago, and early writings by Strauss and Glaser have been superseded by later texts. A large number of grounded theory studies have been carried out, some of which do centre on macro-issues such as gender and power, in particular work by feminists. Others, focusing on policy or health education and promotion cannot help considering structural, cultural and societal factors.

Nevertheless, it should be stressed that most qualitative approaches, including grounded theory, are used for the exploration of micro rather than macro issues. They are designed to focus on the meanings people give to their experience and behaviour.

Some problems with grounded theory are not connected with style or procedures but with the inexperience of researchers. Many novice researchers end up with a conceptual description rather than a theory. There is nothing wrong with dense, conceptual (sometimes called 'analytic') description but this alone cannot be called grounded theory.

Conclusion

Grounded theory is a systematic and processual approach to collecting and analysing data. Good grounded theory produces a theory that has explanatory power, or modification of a theory that already exists. Such theory generation is unique within qualitative research.

There are some major elements that are always present in this type of research:

- Data collection and analysis are in constant dialogue and interaction with each other.
- Constant comparison of data occurs throughout the research process.
- The researcher uses theoretical sampling by following up concepts.
- The data are analysed through coding and categorising.
- The researcher discovers the core category through links between other categories.

- The theory or the theoretical ideas that are generated should always have their basis in the data themselves.

References

Alvesson M, Sköldberg K (2000) *Reflexive Methodology: new vistas for qualitative research.* London, Sage

Annells M (1997) Grounded theory method, part 2: options for users of the method. *Nursing Inquiry* 4: 176–180

Backman K, Kyngäs HA (1999) Challenges of the grounded theory approach to a novice researcher. *Nursing and Health Sciences* 1: 147–153

Benoliel JQ (1973) *The Nurse and the Dying Patient.* New York, Macmillan

Blumer H (1971) Sociological implications of the thoughts of GH Mead. In Cosin BR *et al.* (eds) *School and Society.* Milton Keynes, Open University Press pp11–17

Calvin AO (2004) Haemodialysis patients and end-of-life decisions: a theory of personal preservation. *Journal of Advanced Nursing* 46: 558–566

Charmaz K (2000) Grounded theory: objectivist and constructivist methods. In Denzin NK, Lincoln YS (eds) *Handbook of Qualitative Research.* Thousand Oaks, Sage pp509–536

Chenitz WC, Swanson JM (eds) (1986) *From Practice to Grounded Theory: qualitative research in nursing.* Menlo Park, Addison-Wesley

Glaser BG (1978) *Theoretical Sensitivity.* Mill Valley, Sociology Press

Glaser BG (1992) *Basics of Grounded Theory Analysis.* Mill Valley, Sociology Press

Glaser BG, Strauss AL (1967) *The Discovery of Grounded Theory.* Chicago, Aldine

Holloway I, Wheeler S (2002) *Qualitative Research in Nursing*, 2nd edition. Oxford, Blackwell

Hutchinson SA, Wilson HS (2001) Grounded theory: the method. In Munhall PL (ed) *Nursing Research: a qualitative perspective*, 3rd edition. Sudbury MA, Jones and Bartlett pp209–243

Jacobsson A, Pihl E Martensson J, Fridlund B (2004) Emotions, the meaning of food and heart failure: a grounded theory study. *Journal of Advanced Nursing* 46: 514–522

Layder D (1982) Grounded theory: a constructive critique. *Journal for the Theory of Social Behaviour* 12: 102–123

MacDonald M (2001) Finding a critical perspective in grounded theory. In Schreiber RS, Stern PN (eds) *Using Grounded Theory in Nursing.* New York, Springer Publishing pp113–136

Mead (1934) *Mind, Self and Society.* Chicago, University of Chicago Press

Morse JM (1994) Designing funded qualitative research. In Denzin NK, Lincoln YS (eds) *Handbook of Qualitative Research.* Thousand Oaks, Sage pp220–235

Morse JM (2001) Situating grounded theory within qualitative inquiry. In Schreiber RS, Stern PN (eds) *Using Grounded Theory in Nursing.* New York, Springer pp1–15

Orona CJ (1997) Temporality and identity loss due to Alzheimer's disease. In Strauss AL, Corbin J (eds) *Grounded Theory in Practice.* Thousand Oaks, Sage pp171–196

Schreiber RS, Stern PN (2001) The 'how to' of grounded theory: avoiding the pitfalls. In Schreiber RS, Stern PN (eds) *Using Grounded Theory in Nursing.* New York, Springer pp55–83

Strauss AL (1987) *Qualitative Analysis for Social Scientists.* New York, Cambridge University Press

Strauss AL, Corbin J (1990) *Basics of Qualitative Research: grounded theory procedures and techniques.* Newbury Park, Sage

Strauss AL, Corbin J (1998) *Basics of Qualitative Research: techniques and procedures for developing grounded theory*, 2nd edition. Thousand Oaks, Sage

Strauss AL, Corbin J (eds) (1997) *Grounded Theory in Practice.* Thousand Oaks, Sage

Thomas WI (1928) *The Child in America.* New York, Alfred Knopf

Wuest J (1995) Feminist grounded theory: an exploration of the congruency and tensions between two traditions in knowledge discovery. *Qualitative Health Research* 5: 125–137

Further reading

Coyne IT (1997) Sampling in qualitative research: purposeful and theoretical sampling: merging or clear boundaries? *Journal of Advanced Nursing* 31: 374–630

Cutcliffe JR (2000) Methodological issues in grounded theory. *Journal of Advanced Nursing* 31: 1486–1484

Kelle U (ed) (1995) *Computer-Aided Qualitative Data Analysis: theory, method and practice.* London, Sage

Fielding NG, Lee RM (1998) *Computer Analysis of Qualitative Research*, 2nd edition. London, Sage

Glaser BG (1998) *Doing Grounded Theory: issues and discussion.* Mill Valley, Sociology Press

Glaser BG (2001) *The Grounded Theory Perspective: conceptualization contrasted with description.* Mill Valley, Sociology Press

Website

www.groundedtheory.com – Grounded Theory Institute

14 Ethnography

Immy Holloway and Les Todres

Key points

- Ethnography is concerned with the study of a culture or subculture. Large-scale macro-ethnographies examine a large culture with its institutions, communities and value systems. Small-scale micro-ethnographies investigate a single social setting such as a ward or small group of staff.
- Data collection involves immersion in the setting by means of participant observation and interviews with key informants.
- The researcher seeks to uncover the *emic* or insider view of the members of the particular culture being studied.
- 'Thick' description is used to provide a detailed account that makes explicit the patterns of cultural and social relationships and puts them into context.

Introduction

Ethnography is distinct from other qualitative research approaches in that it focuses on culture. It can be seen as a process that includes the methods and strategies of research – and a product, which is the written story as the outcome of the research. Researchers 'do' ethnography; they study a culture by observing cultural members' behaviours and ask questions about their actions, interactions, experience and feelings. They also write 'an ethnography', a narrative account in which they give a portrayal of the culture they study. Ethnography is both, 'doing science' and 'telling stories'.

Hammersley (1998) suggests that the term 'ethnography' is ambiguous, lacks clear definition and is sometimes used as synonymous with 'qualitative research'. This chapter adopts the original meaning of the term: an approach within anthropological traditions that can also be applied to our own society. The term 'ethnography' means 'writing culture' or 'writing people' and comes from the Greek language. Thus the major traits of ethnography have their basis in the first-hand experience of the researcher in the group or community that is being studied (Atkinson *et al.* 2001). Ethnographers may utilise both qualitative and quantitative procedures. In this chapter only qualitative strategies will be discussed as these are most commonly used (Tedlock 2000).

Ethnography is probably the oldest of the research approaches, as even in ancient times travellers to a country other than their own, studied and described foreign places and cultures and wrote about their experiences. It was particularly popular in the nineteenth and early twentieth centuries, when the approach became more systematic in the writing of anthropologists such as Malinowski (1922) and Boas (1928). They gave detailed descriptions of the cultures in which they immersed themselves for many years. Initially anthropologists explored only foreign cultures, often adopting a colonialist and ethnocentric stance. Today anthropologists are less ethnocentric, that is, they are less inclined to view other groups from their own (western) perspective.

The Chicago School of Sociology from 1917 to the early 1940s also influenced later ethnographic methods because its members examined marginal cultures such as ghettos, urban gangs and slums of the city. Researchers subsequently explored their own cultures researching that with which they were already familiar. These studies were carried out by members of many disciplines apart from anthropology, for example, by sociologists, educationists and also nurses. Janice Morse, the best-known nurse anthropologist and author of qualitative research texts, has discussed this approach in nursing for two decades (Morse 1994; Morse & Richards 2002).

Like most other qualitative approaches, ethnographic research is inductive. This means that it proceeds from the specific to the general, and that initially no preconceptions or hypotheses guide the researcher towards the outcomes of the inquiry. In ethnography, as in all forms of qualitative inquiry, the researcher is the main research tool.

Ethnography is distinct from other qualitative approaches in that it generates descriptions of a group in its cultural context, and focuses mainly, though not exclusively, on the routine activities and customs in the culture as well as on the location of the people within it.

The characteristics of ethnography

Roper and Shapira (2000) state that 'ethnography is a research process of learning *about* people by learning *from* them' (their italics) (Roper and Shapira 2000:1). The main features of ethnography are:

- immersion in a setting and a focus on culture
- the emic (insiders) dimension from the participants, in particular key informants
- 'thick', dense or analytic description

The focus on culture

Fetterman (1998) suggests that the interpretation of a culture (or subculture) is the main aim of most ethnography. Culture can be defined as the way of life of a group: the learnt patterns of behaviour that are socially constructed and transmitted. This includes a shared communication system in language, gestures and expressions: the messages that most cultural members understand and recognise. Individuals in a culture often share values and ideas acquired through learning from other members of the group.

Learning group values and behaviour is referred to as socialisation. For instance, members of the nursing profession have been socialised into the values and perspectives of their own group through their education and training. The perspectives of the group, the actions and interactions of group members, and the meaning they place on their behaviour, are legitimate areas of research for the ethnographer. Adopting an ethnographic approach to a familiar culture helps researchers to avoid assumptions about their own cultural group or take its working for granted.

Knowledge that the members of a culture share but do not articulate to each other is referred to as 'tacit knowledge'. Social behaviour and interpretations of the social world are based on this. Ethnographers uncover tacit knowledge and make it explicit. They also reveal some of the hidden meanings in the routines and rituals of a group and place.

Ethnographers have recently changed their perspective on culture from a monolithic understanding of culture where people share values, beliefs and perceptions to a focus on cultural diversity (Holloway & Todres 2003). They now demonstrate how cultural members are located within their setting and how they can only be understood within the specific context. For instance, although nurses and doctors in an Accident and Emergency (A&E) department might have certain perceptions in common (particularly about their patients) there are other elements where their beliefs and ways of working are in conflict with each other.

Emic and etic perspectives

The term *emic* perspective is often used in ethnographic research. Although the concept has a variety of interpretations, in its simplest form it means 'insider view'. The emic perspective is the perception of those who are members of a particular culture or group, or, in anthropological terms, the 'native' point of view. The linguist Pike coined this phrase, but it was used more extensively and with a different meaning by the anthropologist Harris (1976) and most ethnographers since. Members of a culture have special knowledge of this culture and can share this with the researcher. For instance, nurses in the A&E department know about the special problems facing members of the department, but they would also be able to narrate the dramatic events that might make this type of work exciting.

Insiders give meaning to their experiences and generate knowledge about the reasons for their actions. They know the rules and rituals of their group or subculture. The emic perspective is thus culture-specific. Outside observers would find it difficult to gain the same familiarity and intimacy with this setting that insiders do.

In contrast, ethnographers also speak of the *etic* perspective, that is the view of the outsider who may or may not be a member of the culture being studied. As an example an A&E nurse might wish to research the culture of A&E departments.

In this sense she or he is a 'native' of the group. Nurses are also researchers, and in this particular sense, they are outsiders, and they need to produce scientific knowledge about what they see and hear which means taking an etic view. Thus the emic perspective is the subjective view of insiders that has to be retold by the researchers in the account of the research. Indeed the A&E nurse researchers in the earlier example have to attempt to become 'naïve' observers or interviewers, taking the view of a 'cultural stranger' to the setting. The etic perspective is needed to transform the story into an ethnography with its roots in social science. Harris (1976) explains that etics are scientific transformations of the empirical data by the researchers who adopt an approach to the data that is more theoretical and abstract than that of the insiders.

Thick description

The concept of thick description has its origin in work of the philosopher Ryle and was taken on by the anthropologist Geertz (1973) who applied it to ethnography. He suggests that it is a detailed account that makes explicit the patterns of cultural and social relationships and puts them in context. It is a result of observations and interviews in the field. The notion of thick description is sometimes understood as a detailed description of a culture or group but this does not suffice. It must be theoretical and analytical in that researchers concern themselves with general patterns and traits of social life, and it gives the reader of the ethnographic text a sense of the emotional experience of the participants in the study. Thick description builds up a clear picture of the individuals and groups in the context of their culture and encompasses their meanings and intentions. On the other hand, thin description is superficial and factual and does not explore the underlying meanings of cultural members (Denzin, 1989). It does not lead to a good ethnography.

The use of ethnography in nursing

Many cultures and subcultures exist within nursing. One might think, for instance, of the culture of a hospital or the subculture of an orthopaedic ward. Ethnographic research is therefore helpful in:

- studying cultures, linked to nursing, with their rules and rituals and routine activities – this includes transcultural research, which examines different ethnic groups, their interactions, and meaning creation
- discovering the 'insider view' of patients and colleagues
- explaining phenomena related to nursing
- examining the conflicting perspectives of professionals within the organisational culture

Nurse researchers contextualise the perspectives, actions and emotions of their patients or colleagues and those of other health professionals through ethnographic methods. They become culture-sensitive and learn to identify the influences of the environment on the person. The aim of nurse researchers, however, is different from that of anthropologists. They do not merely generate knowledge, which is seen as the goal of ethnography (Hammersley & Atkinson 1995), but they also wish to change and improve professional practice through understanding the culture they study.

Leininger (1985) has coined the term 'ethnonursing' to refer to the use of ethnography in nursing. She describes this as an adaptation and extension of ethnography. Ethnonursing, she suggests, is concerned with studying groups and settings linked to nursing but also is specifically about nursing care, produces nursing knowledge and explains or demonstrates nursing phenomena.

Nurse ethnographers do not always investigate their own cultural members. In Britain, nurses care for patients from a variety of ethnic groups and need to be knowledgeable about different cultures. Indeed all nurses and patients belong to ethnic groups, and sometimes they come from different countries and have a variety of religions. Awareness of cultural differences is important because both nurses and patients are products of their group. DeSantis (1994) suggests that at least three cultures are involved in nurses' interactions with patients: the nurses' professional culture, the patients' culture and the context in which the interactions take place.

Nurse researchers usually proceed in the following way:

- they describe a problem in the group under study and, through this, they come to understand the causes of the problem and may prevent it
- they assist patients to identify and report their needs
- they give information to the readers of their accounts – their colleagues and other health professionals – to effect change in clinical and professional practice

When undertaking research with colleagues or students, nurse researchers proceed through similar phases. The ultimate goal of their research is to improve professional practice.

Savage (2000) draws certain parallels between ethnography (in particular participant observation) and clinical practice:

- the physical involvement with the setting is common to nursing and research
- the claims nurses and researchers make about knowledge through experience
- the theoretical assumptions they share as nurses and observers

Savage suggests that nurses and ethnographers should be concerned with the links between their own experience of the setting and that of their patients. Nurses and researchers also attempt to translate the understanding they gain of patients to others.

Descriptive and critical ethnography

There are two main approaches to ethnography: descriptive and critical ethnography. Thomas (1993) states the difference:

'Conventional ethnographers study culture for the purpose of describing it; critical ethnographers do so to change it' (Thomas 1993:4)

It should be noted however, that most nursing research that is carried out has implications for practice. While descriptive ethnography centres on the description of cultures or groups (Box 14.1), critical ethnography involves the study of macro-social factors such as power and control and examines commonsense assumptions and hidden agendas in this arena (Holloway & Wheeler 2002); it therefore has political elements (Box 14.2). Nurse researchers often use critical ethnography because women form the majority of these professions, and power relations are part of the complex factors influencing interaction between nurses and doctors or nurses and patients. Manias and Street (2001) speak of the need to reconstruct power relations in nursing because of the existence of inequalities and specific dominant ideologies.

Box 14.1   Example of descriptive ethnography.

Costello J (2001) Nursing older dying patients: findings from an ethnographic study of death and dying in elderly care wards. *Journal of Advanced Nursing* 3: 59–68

Costello (2001) utilised an ethnographic approach to explore the experiences of dying patients and nurses who cared for them in three wards for the elderly. The study focused on the management of care for dying patients and, in particular, communication issues. Participant observation in the ward areas was undertaken over a 15-month period, and semi-structured interviews were conducted with patients, nurses and doctors following the periods of observation. Interviews provided the opportunity to ask questions associated with the observations made. Detailed fieldnotes were recorded during observation periods and transcripts produced of the interviews. The findings showed that much of the care given centred on the physical needs of patients while emotional and spiritual care was neglected and nurses and doctors were reluctant to communicate about death and dying.

Box 14.2 Critical ethnography.

Manias E, Street A (2001) Rethinking ethnography: reconstructing nursing relationships. *Journal of Advanced Nursing* 33: 234–242

Manias and Street (2001) utilised a critical ethnographic approach to examine the world of critical care by researching the interaction of nurses with doctors and with their own nursing colleagues. Six registered nurses participated in the study. Through compiling a professional journal, one of the authors explored her professional interactions with doctors and other nurses in her role as a registered nurse in the critical care unit. Other data were collected by means of participant observation, individual and focus group interviews.

The researchers focused on exploring the power relationships inherent in communication processes such as the nursing handover, ward rounds and written policies and protocols. They found that uncritical uses of terms such as 'patriarchy' or 'oppression', for instance, did not do justice to describing the complex processes involved in interaction, and ignored already existing power relations. The paper also explores methodological issues associated with undertaken critical ethnography.

Whereas the same data collection and analysis procedures are used by ethnographers undertaking descriptive and critical ethnographies the latter are more intent on highlighting the power dimensions of interaction.

Selection of sample and setting in ethnographic studies

Ethnographers use purposive or criterion-based sampling; i.e. they adopt specific criteria to select their informants and setting such as patients undergoing orthopaedic surgery, children with diabetes, nursing students or a maternity unit. The criteria for sample selection must be explicit and systematic (Hammersley & Atkinson 1995) in order to ensure that participants are representative of the group under study. The participants in ethnographic research are usually called informants because they inform the researcher about issues in their world. Alternative terms include participant, cultural member or key actor. Key informants are those participants whose knowledge of the setting is intimate and long-standing. Patients are often the main informants in nursing ethnography. They tell of their experience and the meanings they attach to it, and of the expectations and health beliefs that form part of their perspectives (DeSantis 1994). Informants might be interviewed formally or participate by talking informally about the cultural beliefs and practices as well as ways of communicating. They become active collaborators in the research rather than passive respondents (hence the term 'informant'). Nurses can compare their own interpretations of the group with those of key informants through the process of member-checking, whereby they ask informants to check the script and interpretation (Lincoln & Guba 1985).

Data collection

Ethnographers have three major strategies for collecting data (Roper & Shapira 2000):

- They observe what is going on in the setting while participating in it.
- They ask informants from the cultural group they are studying about their behaviour, experiences and feelings.
- They study documents about and in the setting, in order to familiarise themselves with it.

Wolcott (1994) calls these data collecting methods 'experiencing' (participant observation), 'enquiring' (interviewing), and 'examining' (studying documents).

Occasionally researchers supplement interviews by taping oral histories from the cultural members whose world they study, or they examine photographs or pictures of the group and the setting.

Observing

Participant observation, the type of observation most commonly used, means that the researchers are immersed in the setting and become familiar with it. Prolonged observation produces more in-depth knowledge of a culture. Occasionally researchers need to withdraw from the setting in order to stand back and take stock. They also need to attempt to put aside their assumptions, come to the setting as 'cultural strangers' and keep an open mind in seeking to see the world through the eyes of the participants (Savage 2000). Ethnographers observe the setting and situation, the way people act and interact, the use of space and time, but they also observe critical incidents that may occur and the way rules are followed and rituals are carried out.

Spradley (1980:78), a well-known ethnographer, identifies the dimensions of the social settings that ethnographers study. These include:

Space	location of the research
Actor	the people who take part in the setting
Activity	the actions of people
Object	things located in the setting
Act	single actions of participants
Events	what is happening in the setting

Time   sequencing of activities and time frame
Goals   what people aim to do
Feeling   emotions that participants have

The observation setting can be open or closed. Open settings can be highly visible public spaces such as a reception area or a corridor whereas closed settings have to be more carefully negotiated and could be hospital wards or meeting rooms. In nursing settings, observation is normally overt where the researcher makes explicit their intention to observe the social setting. Covert observation, where participants do not know that they are being observed, is usually seen as unethical.

Observations are initially unstructured, although they become progressively more focused as important features emerge that might be of significance for the study. Observations inform the researcher's interviews with key informants. Incidents or issues that are puzzling or problematic are explored with participants.

The ethnographic interview

During and following observations researchers ask questions about the meaning of behaviour, language and events. This happens initially through informal conversations with participants. There are several consequences of these conversations: researchers familiarise themselves with the arena, bond with participants and acquire cultural knowledge from the informants.

In-depth interviews are commonly used to allow informants the opportunity to explore issues within the culture that they see as important. Although the researcher has an agenda, participants have control within certain boundaries. The researchers follow up the issues and ideas that the informant sees as significant without neglecting their own research agenda. The interviews may be formal or informal, in-depth, unstructured or semi-structured (*see* Chapter 22).

Spradley (1979) distinguishes between grand-tour and mini-tour questions. While the former questions are broad, the latter are more specific. An example of a grand-tour question might be: 'Can you describe your life as an orthopaedic nurse?' A mini-tour question might be: 'Tell me about the pain you had after your operation.' Researchers often start an interview with a broad question and the interview becomes more focused following up participants' answers (Box 14.3).

These questions are then followed up depending on the participants' answers. If something important emerges, gentle prompts can be used such as 'Can you tell me more about that, please?'

Ethnographers also listen to naturally occurring talk in the setting, for example, people communicating with each other on the ward, in meetings, or in the classroom. These conversations may be analysed in the same way as interviews. To make sure that data are not lost, interviewers generally tape-record participants' words, whereas detailed fieldnotes are made of conversations.

> **Box 14.3**   Examples of general and focused questions for ethnographic interviews.
>
> **General questions**
> Tell me about your experience of back pain?
>
> **Focused questions** (following the participant's ideas)
> What were your visits to the pain clinic like?
> What was the reaction of your family to this?
>
> **General questions**
> Can you describe your stay in hospital?
>
> **Focused questions**
> Tell me about the work of the nurses?
> You said that the nurses always have time for patients, please can you elaborate?

Fieldwork and fieldnotes

The field, fieldwork and fieldnotes are well-known concepts used in ethnography. The field is the physical environment in which the research is taking place (Schensul *et al.* 1999). It may be a ward, a hospital, or a specific community of people. The term fieldwork refers to the work undertaken in an ethnographic study such as collecting data from various sources. Fieldwork also includes the description and interpretation of cultural behaviour, the meaning people give to their actions, and the setting in which the study takes place. This is an ongoing process in the research.

Researchers keep a field journal or diary in which they jot down their thoughts about their experiences and make theoretical comments. These fieldnotes are used at a later stage to help remember important issues, questions or solutions to problems. They have their basis in the observations and interviews undertaken in the setting. Initially fieldnotes are only for the eyes of the ethnographer, but ultimately excerpts are used as data or extended descriptions in ethnographic writing. At first, fieldnotes tend to be simple but become more complex as the study progresses and may become notes about analysis and interpretation.

Spradley (1979) identifies different types of fieldnotes in terms of condensed and the extended accounts. Condensed accounts are short descriptions made in the field during data collection while expanded accounts extend the descriptions and fill in detail. Short fieldnotes are extended as soon as possible after a period of observation or interview if it was not possible to record the full detail during the data collection. Ethnographers also note their own biases, reactions and problems during fieldwork. They may use additional ways to record events and behaviour such as audiotapes, video film or photos, flowcharts and diagrams.

Macro- and micro-ethnographies

Spradley (1980) identifies macro- and micro-ethnographies, which can be viewed on a continuum of scale. At one end of this continuum are large-scale studies examining a complex society, one or more communities or social institutions (*macro-ethnography*); at the other are small-scale studies into a single social situation (*micro-ethnography*).

A macro-ethnography examines a large culture with its institutions, communities and value systems. In nursing this might be the wider culture of nursing. Such studies are rarely carried out by a single researcher. Both macro- and micro-ethnographies proceed in similar ways and produce an account of the culture being studied. The type of study depends on the focus of the investigation, the researcher's own interests or those who fund the research.

Novice nurse researchers often choose a micro-ethnography as it makes fewer demands on their time than macro-ethnography and seems more immediately relevant to the world of the nurse. Micro-ethnography focuses on small settings or groups such as a single ward or a group of specialist nurses. Box 14.4 provides an example of a micro-ethnography.

Box 14.4   Example of a micro-ethnography.

Cloherty M, Alexander J, Holloway I (2004) Supplementing breastfed babies in the UK to protect their mothers from tiredness and distress. *Midwifery* 20: 194–204

Cloherty *et al.* (2004) carried out a study on supplementary feeding of breastfed babies, using an ethnographic approach and lasting over nine months. The study involved participant observation of health professionals' and mothers' behaviour and the interaction between the two groups in a maternity unit of a hospital. Analysis of the observation data informed the interviews about breastfeeding and supplementation that took place with health professionals and new mothers.

Data analysis and interpretation

Analysis involves interaction with the data. The data are scanned and organised from the start of the research, and the focus on particular issues becomes clearer as the research progresses. Analysis and interpretation proceed in parallel. The analytic process is not linear but iterative; this means that researchers go back and forth, from the data collection and reading and thinking about them, to the analysis. They then return to collecting new data and analysing them. This process continues until the collection and analysis are complete.

The main steps in data analysis are presented in Chapter 27 and include:

- bringing order to the data and organising the material
- reading, re-reading and thinking about the data
- coding the data
- summarising and reducing the codes to larger categories
- searching for patterns and regularities in the data, sorting these and recognising themes
- uncovering variations in the data and revealing those cases that do not fit with the rest of the data, and accounting for them
- engaging with, and integrating, the related literature

When the audiotapes have been listened to and transcribed, and the observation notes ordered, the transcripts of interviews and observation notes are read several times. The researcher thinks about the data and their meaning. The next step is coding, the process of breaking down the data and giving each important section a descriptive label. For instance, the sentence from an informant: *I really was sick of all the grand words and could not understand anything that was going on*, might be labelled 'feeling frustrated', or 'lack of information', depending on the context. An observation note that reads: *The nurse comforted the critically ill patient*, could be labelled 'being there'. The names given to codes are determined by the individual researcher.

Once coding has been completed, codes with similar meaning or themes linked to the same area of analysis, are grouped together into larger and more abstract categories. For instance, the codes: *need for independence, wanting to be in control, reluctance to be helped, rejecting care from others* might be reduced to the category *the wish for self-determination* or *being empowered*. Thematically similar sets of categories are grouped together with links and relationships established between them. Broad patterns of thoughts and behaviour emerge at this stage, and major 'constructs' or themes are developed. The ethnographer needs to check that there is a fit between the data and the analytic categories and themes.

While ethnographers sometimes produce theories, they often generate typologies. This means developing a classification system that points to variations in the data. For example, an ethnographer might find two types of nurses in a particular ward, those who take control and make firm decisions, and others who generally ask their colleagues and doctors for advice and rarely make difficult decisions. The ethnographer might call these types *decision-makers* and *advice takers*. As in all typologies, these are types at the end of a continuum. At some point on the continuum these types overlap.

Interpretation of the data or 'going beyond the results' (Roper & Shapira 2000) means that researchers uncover the meaning of the patterns and themes that they developed. It allows them to answer the research question and to reveal elements of the cultural phenomena studied. Interpretation starts in early data collection and proceeds throughout, but data are often reinterpreted at a later stage. While interpreting the data, researchers make inferences and discuss the possible meanings of the data. Interpretation, although linked to the analysis, is more speculative, involving theorising and explaining. Interpretation links the findings of the project, derived from the analysis, to previously established theories through comparing other researchers' work with one's own. At this stage, the research literature related to the themes and patterns will be considered. It might confirm or 'disconfirm', that is, challenge the findings of the study. The researcher discusses this in a critical and analytical way. The processes of analysis and interpretation are stages in which a phenomenon is broken down, divided into its elements and 'reassembled in terms of definitions or explanations that make the phenomenon understandable to outsiders' (LeCompte & Schensul 1999:5). Thus researchers build a holistic portrait of a culture from a number of building blocks.

Relationships and problems in the setting

Ethnography is an appropriate approach when addressing questions about culture and subcultures or a particular group with common traits. However, problems do exist for nurses who wish to carry out ethnographic research. Ethnography needs prolonged engagement and immersion in the setting under study. Gaining admittance to the group, and establishing rapport takes time and commitment. Many nurse researchers who study groups other than their own are unable to undertake participant observation over a long period of time such as a year or more. Hence some nursing ethnographies are not as fully developed as they might be.

Insider researchers also experience problems. They must attempt to see familiar events with new eyes (DeWalt & DeWalt 2002). Nurses who carry out research in their own setting may be seen as health professionals and not as researchers, and this might prevent their colleagues, who are participants in the research, from making themselves explicit. They might have preconceptions and make assumptions about the setting under study and miss nuances or fail to observe important details. Patients too, might see them as carers who know them well and may be reluctant to disclose their thoughts for fear that this might prejudice their treatment. Nurse ethnographers might themselves experience conflict between their role as researcher and that of health professional (Bonner & Tolhurst 2002). On the other hand, it is easier to gain access and develop rapport with the research participants when an insider. Holloway and Wheeler (2002) identify a further problem. Nurses have a background in the natural sciences and learn to approach their clinical practice systematically. This means that they might find difficulty in dealing with ambiguity. Social inquiry is always provisional, and rarely unambiguous. It is better, however, to admit to uncertainty than to make unwarranted claims about the research. Findings can be re-interpreted at a later stage in the light of reflection or new evidence.

Fetterman (1998) warns that key informants might have assumptions about the culture or preconceptions about the researcher and may impose their own ideas about the culture on the study. This means that researchers need to compare the informants' accounts with the observed reality. There is also the risk that participants might only tell what they think researchers wish to hear. This danger is particularly strong in health care, as patients (and also nursing students) often want to please those who care for them or deal with them in a professional relationship. However, immersion in the culture by the researcher, and the prolonged relationship of researcher and informants helps to overcome this.

The ethnographic report

Wolcott (1994) claims that an ethnography consists of description, analysis and interpretation. Ethnographers describe what they observe and hear while studying cultural members in context; they identify the main features of the group and the setting and uncover relationships between separate and varied data through analysis; they also interpret the findings by asking for meaning and inferring such meaning from the data. It is important that the participants in the study recognise their own social reality and the traits of their culture and group.

Fetterman (1998) states that:

'ethnographic writing is a process of compression as the ethnographer moves from fieldnotes to written text' (Fetterman 1998:123).

The ethnography – the account of an ethnographic study – usually takes the form of a narrative and includes quotes from the interviews of participants and excerpts from fieldnotes that illustrate the descriptions and explanations. Thick description is one of the features of the report. An ethnography should be a clearly-written text that engages its readers.

Conclusion

Ethnography is the method of choice when the researcher wants to investigate a culture. The complete ethnography paints a detailed, yet holistic, portrait of the culture that has been studied. Ultimately a nursing ethnography contributes not only to nursing knowledge but also assists in applying that knowledge for the improvement of nursing practice.

Some of the main features of ethnography include:

- The data sources are mainly participant observation by immersion in the setting and interviews with key informants.
- The researcher uncovers the emic perspective.

- Thick description is used to make the study come alive.
- An ethnography is the description of a culture, a subculture or group.

References

Atkinson P, Coffey A, Delamont S, Lofland J, Lofland L (2001) Introduction to part one. In Atkinson P, Coffey A, Delamont S, Lofland J, Lofland L (eds) *Handbook of Ethnography*. London, Sage pp9–10

Boas F (1928) *Anthropology and Modern Life*. New York, Norton

Bonner A, Tolhurst G (2002) Insider-outsider perspectives of participant observation. *Nurse Researcher* 9:4 7–19

Cloherty M, Alexander J, Holloway I (2004) Supplementing breast-fed babies in the UK to protect their mothers from tiredness and distress. *Midwifery* 20: 194–204

Costello J (2001) Nursing older dying patients: findings from an ethnographic study of death and dying in elderly care wards. *Journal of Advanced Nursing* 35: 59–68

Denzin NK (1989) *Interpretive Interactionism*. Newbury Park, Sage

DeSantis L (1994) Making anthropology clinically relevant to nursing care. *Journal of Advanced Nursing* 20: 707–715

DeWalt KM, DeWalt BR (2002) *Participant Observation*. Walnut Creek, Altamira Press

Fetterman DM (1998) *Ethnography Step By Step*, 2nd edition. Thousand Oaks, Sage

Geertz C (1973) *The Interpretation of Cultures*. New York, Basic Books

Hammersley M (1998) *Reading Ethnographic Research*, 2nd edition. London, Longman

Hammersley M, Atkinson P (1995) *Ethnography: principles in practice*, 2nd edition. London, Tavistock

Harris M (1976) History and significance of the emic/etic distinction. *Annual Review of Anthropology* 5: 329–350

Holloway I, Wheeler S (2002) *Qualitative Research in Nursing*. Oxford, Blackwell

Holloway I, Todres L (2003) The status of method: flexibility, consistency and coherence. *Qualitative Research* 3: 345–357

LeCompte MD, Schensul JJ (1999) *Analyzing and Interpreting Ethnographic Data*. Walnut Creek, Altamira Press

Leininger M (ed) (1985) *Qualitative Research Methods in Nursing*. Philadelphia, WB Saunders

Lincoln YS, Guba EG (1985) *Naturalistic Inquiry*. Newbury Park, Sage

Malinowski B (1922) *Argonauts of the Western Pacific: an account of native enterprise and adventure in the archipelagoes of Melanesian New Guinea*. New York, Dutton

Manias E, Street A (2001) Rethinking ethnography: reconstructing nursing relationships. *Journal of Advanced Nursing* 33: 234–242

Morse JM (ed) (1994) *Critical Issues in Qualitative Research Methods*. Thousand Oaks, Sage

Morse JM, Richards KL (2002) *Read Me First for a Nurse's Guide to Qualitative Methods*. Thousand Oaks, Sage

Roper JM, Shapira J (2000) *Ethnography in Nursing Research*. Thousand Oaks, Sage

Savage J (2000) Participant observation: standing in the shoes of others. *Qualitative Health Research* 10: 324–339

Schensul SL, Schensul JJ, LeCompte MD (1999) *Essential Ethnographic Methods: observations, interviews and questionnaires*. Walnut Creek, Altamira Press

Spradley JP (1979) *The Ethnographic Interview*. Fort Worth, Harcourt Brace Jovanovich College

Spradley JP (1980) *Participant Observation*. Fort Worth, Harcourt Brace Jovanovich College

Tedlock B (2000) Ethnography and Ethnographic Representation. In Denzin NK, Lincoln YS. *Handbook of Qualitative Research*, 2nd edition. Thousand Oaks, Sage pp455–486

Thomas J (1993) *Doing Critical Ethnography*. Newbury Park, Sage

Wolcott HF (1994) *Transforming Qualitative Data: description, analysis, and interpretation*. Thousand Oaks, Sage

15 Phenomenological Research

Les Todres and Immy Holloway

Key points

- The phenomenological researcher uses descriptions and/or interpretations of everyday human experiences (the lifeworld) as sources of qualitative evidence.
- The purpose of phenomenology is to find insights that apply more generally beyond the cases studied.
- Descriptive phenomenology uses 'bracketing' of preconceptions and attempts to arrive at the 'essences' of experienced phenomena.
- Hermeneutic phenomenology uses interpretation and personal or theoretical 'sensitising' to highlight important themes. It seeks to enhance understanding in readers by presenting 'plots' or stories.

Introduction

Phenomenology as a discrete philosophical research tradition emerged in the early part of the twentieth century. Although Edmund Husserl (1859–1938) is credited as the central founder of this tradition (Spiegelberg 1994), he built on earlier philosophers who wished to describe human experience as the valid starting point of philosophy. This grabbed the attention of researchers who were looking for ways to study human experience on its own terms without reducing it to language that comes from other sciences such as chemistry or physiology. The promise of phenomenology was that human beings could be understood from 'inside' their subjective experience, which could not be adequately replaced by any external analysis or explanation. A view from within a person's perspective is needed for any comprehensive understanding of human behaviour. Phenomenologists thus emphasise the value of describing and interpreting human experience and seek to do this in credible and insightful ways.

This chapter will outline the main principles of phenomenology and illustrate some of the practical ways it is used in research. Some illustrations from published studies will be used to demonstrate particular principles or concepts. In some cases, only a brief excerpt of the study will be presented. In other cases, more detail and context will be given in order that readers may get a sense of the research study as a whole.

Purpose of phenomenological research

Phenomenological research begins with gathering examples of everyday experiences, describing them and reflecting on them. Husserl called these everyday experiences the 'lifeworld', while other phenomenologists have used the term 'lived experience'. So lived experiences such as 'having a baby' or 'the experience of back pain' are chosen as phenomena to be described and studied in depth. The purpose of focusing on such named experiential phenomena is: *to find insights that apply more generally beyond the cases that were studied in order to emphasise what we may have in common as human beings.* Husserl called such common themes 'essences', or they are also known as 'essential structures'.

One may find universal 'essences' in nature. For example, gravity can be described as the essence of all falling objects to earth. However, when it comes to human beings, one seldom finds common themes that are universal across all cultures and circumstances. Rather, one finds common themes that are typical within a context such as a particular culture or time in history. The other thing about 'essences' in relation to human experience is that the essential themes relate to other themes, like *in* a story. So when phenomenologists present their findings, they usually express this in such a way as to show how a number of common themes are related. This is referred to as 'the essential structure' of the phenomenon. The example in Box 15.1 provides insight into how an essential structure is like a story: it has a general plot that brings the essential themes together in an understandable way.

Another important concept in phenomenological research is the idea of 'bracketing' in which phenomenological researchers attempt to suspend (or bracket) their preconceptions so that they can approach the phenomenon to be studied with 'fresh eyes'. Husserl called this suspension of preconceptions 'the phenomenological reduction' where a certain open-mindedness is achieved. In such 'openness', something new can be discovered that is not tainted by previous theory or taken-for-granted assumptions. In practical terms, this involves a certain self-discipline similar to true listening in which one lets the information and data 'speak' more fully before imposing one's own understanding or interpretation.

Here is an example of 'bracketing' as an ongoing discipline during the research:

> Imagine an interview situation where something is said which reminds the interviewer of something he or she has read about. He or she then needs to be careful not to influence the interview in the direction of what has been read. Also, when analysing the interview, the researcher needs to be careful not to impose the ideas from his or her reading onto the analysis. This can be done later in a discussion

Box 15.1   Example of a section of an essential structure: women's experience
of self-harm through self-cutting.

Robinson FA (1998) Dissociative women's experiences of self-cutting. In Valle R (ed)
Phenomenological Inquiry in Psychology: existential and transpersonal dimensions. New
York, Plenum Press, pp218–219

'Emotional states prior to cutting include feelings of being trapped, inner emotional chaos and
noise, intolerable emotional pain, intense anger, and feelings of separation from significant
others. Cutters are wanting a release of tension, a relief from their enduring pain, and a quiet-
ing of the chaos and the noise. They reach a place where it feels as if they will explode or
die or where they are feeling out of control and desparate. It feels as if physical pain could
take away their emotional pain.
   Alters emerge who seem responsible for the cutting . . .
   Cutters shift into an altered mental state. They find a pleasurable place where they are
feeling in total control of their life. The pain subsides.
   The sight and feel of flowing blood has much symbolism for cutters. It represents life, the
possibility of death, relase of things trapped in the body, and survival . . .
   Cutters experience much fear and shame after cutting. Their good feelings and relief are
always temporary. They feel sad knowing cutting brings their greatest comfort and meets
their love and nurturing needs . . .'

section, but descriptive phenomenology seeks to stay very close to the data when
formulating meaningful themes.

Use of phenomenology in nursing

Phenomenological studies have become an increasingly important qualitative
approach in nursing. Topics have included the lived experience of postpartum
depression (Beck 1992), the lived experience of persons with chronic illness
(Gullickson 1993), being in pain (Bradley-Springer 1995), on surviving breast
cancer and mastectomy (Shin 1999), and the phenomenology of comfort (Morse
et al. 1994). By way of illustration, Box 15.2 summarises a phenomenological study
examining the lived experience of patients in a critical care setting.

   A strong indication that phenomenological attention to lifeworld descriptions
is entering mainstream health care is evidenced by the United Kingdom's National
Health Service modernisation agency, which is adopting a methodology of 'discovery interviews'. Here, detailed guidance is given to health care practitioners
of how to elicit experiential descriptions from service users in order that those
services may be improved (Wilcock *et al.* 2003). This approach, whereby users are

Box 15.2   The experience of a patient in an intensive care unit.

Todres L, Fulbrook P, Albarran J (2000) On the receiving end: a hermeneutic-phenomenological analysis of a patient's struggle to cope while going through intensive care. *Nursing in Critical Care* 5:6 284

Consider a patient in an intensive care unit. What kind of endurance does this require? What are the experiential tasks and stages that such a patient may be negotiating? What do nurses need to understand about the totality of this experience that could help them in their caring tasks? In such a phenomenological study, Todres *et al.* (2000) were able to provide insight into, for example, a challenging form of endurance at one of the stages of the intensive care experience: how, in relation to intubation, the body wants to resist what feels alien and unnatural, while the person understands at the same time that such 'intrusion' is not only *help* but *lifesaving help*. In articulating this structure, one may see how this could be a plausible transferable theme for other patients as well. Different patients may respond to this meaningful structure differently, but the structure helps us to understand these variations in terms of the central issue at stake, that is, having to accept bodily-repulsed intrusion as *help*. They were also able to articulate other stages of the experience such as entering a 'twilight world', the frustration of not being understood, ambivalent feelings during the weaning process, and the importance of having someone to advocate on one's behalf, amongst other themes.

It may be helpful for nurses to understand, for example, the transitions that a patient may be experiencing when being weaned from the ventilator after some time. Here is one of the essential structures that was formulated on the basis of an interview:

'Adapting to breathing again on her own marked a transition from the twilight world where she drifted between life and death, between technological and human support, between caring and not caring, between fight and flight. Anne's hand was now not just looking for human contact and reassurance, but beginning to become again what it used to be: a power towards personal competence and self-support. Issues in the social world again became relevant and particularly focused on the beginnings of power struggles between herself and others. Though she was still unpractised in negotiating interpersonal power, and even confused and ambivalent about this, she recognised that her growing self-assertion was a good thing. In 'being weaned' one re-enters again the world where saying yes and no is granted more meaning: clarifying the ambiguity of where dependence is still needed and where a degree of independence is possible, is both a personal and interpersonal task. Both patient and caregiver need to recognise and adjust to this transition. Its inconvenience and ambiguity needs to be welcomed. It is a *welcome back* like the protest and cry of a baby first gasping for breath. As such, protest is the beginning of choice and personal competence.' (Todres *et al.* 2000:284)

asked to describe significant experiences of care, is proving to be much richer than surveys that are based on preconceived questions.

This kind of knowledge of 'what it may be like' is particularly helpful in aiding nurses to imagine what the patient is going through. Such understanding can provide a kind of empathy that is an important foundation for making ethical judgements about care. As an adjunct to technical proficiency, this kind of knowledge may be action-oriented in the way, for example, a nurse having considered the above reflection about being weaned from an intubator, now begins to welcome a patient's protest, and is flexible in attuning her/himself to the patient's ambivalent struggles regarding dependence and independence. Such kinds and levels of knowledge may also be important in designing nursing education where a grasp of the 'world of the patient' may help to underpin the development of more uniquely tailored, person-centred practice. Such lifeworld-led education may increasingly expand the horizons of evidence-based education to include qualitative evidence about the world from the patient's point of view.

Main features

Phenomenological research as used by nurses is generally divided into two types: *descriptive* phenomenology and *interpretive or hermeneutic* phenomenology. Descriptive phenomenology stays close to Husserl and has been translated into an empirical research approach by Amedeo Giorgi, his colleagues and students (Giorgi 1970; 1997). Interpretive or hermeneutic phenomenology stays close to Heidegger, Gadamer and Ricoeur, and their philosophical insights are used in various ways to underpin qualitative research. Hermeneutic phenomenologists do not believe that researchers can be very successful in suspending their preconceptions. Rather, they should use their preconceptions positively, making them more explicit so that readers of the research can understand the strengths and limitations of the interpretations that the researcher makes. So, for example, a hermeneutic phenomenologist may use 'feminism' as an interpretive framework and demonstrate how this perspective may throw some new light on the phenomenon studied. Hermeneutic phenomenologists are also very cautious about finding common essences as they wish to emphasise uniqueness and diversity.

In the authors' view the distinctions between descriptive and hermeneutic phenomenology have been overemphasised. Both these types of phenomenology share the following features: starting from 'lifeworld' descriptions, the use of 'bracketing' or 'sensitising' as a reflective analytic method and arriving at 'essences' or 'fusion of horizons' to characterise the experienced phenomena.

Starting from 'lifeworld' descriptions

Both descriptive and hermeneutic phenomenologists use the term 'lifeworld' instead of using the traditional term, 'data'. This is because they are not gathering separate pieces of information but rather interrelated themes or stories. Individual experiences are the starting point for enquiry. This approach moves from the specific to the general. In other words it uses specific examples of concrete, every day experiences (lifeworld experiences) as a starting point for further analysis and reflection. With insight and reflection, more general insights across cases can then be formulated. So the phenomenological researcher studies 'experiential happenings', and one often finds that fresh insights are 'in the details'. The findings of a good phenomenological study can resonate at a feeling level and richly describe experiences that human beings can either identify with, or alternatively, understand something more about the differences from their own experience.

The use of 'bracketing' or 'sensitising' as a reflective analytic method

Descriptive phenomenology uses the term 'bracketing' while hermeneutic phenomenology is more likely to use the term 'sensitising'. Descriptive phenomenologists do not wish to start out with a hypothesis or preconceived idea or theory, which they then try to prove or disprove. Rather they wish to be open-minded about what they may discover and therefore try to suspend preconceptions and theories as much as possible. This attitude has been called the 'phenomenological reduction', whereby fresh meanings can be seen and expressed in language.

Both descriptive and hermeneutic phenomenologists would agree that the possibility of 'seeing something' freshly, differently or from a new perspective, is a crucial dimension of phenomenology's discovery-oriented approach. But hermeneutic phenomenological researchers may use existing preconceptions as a way of 'sensitising' themselves to what is missing or different. For example, Shin (1999) reflected on her own experiences as a nurse and as a woman living in South Korea, as part of the process of carrying out a hermeneutic phenomenological study of a number of women who had survived breast cancer and mastectomy in that country. Her own cultural background 'sensitised' her to certain meanings that helped to bring out valuable aspects of the experience of being a woman in a transitional period in South Korea, and these insights had an important bearing on the study.

The findings of phenomenological research: essences or 'fusion of horizons'

Descriptive phenomenology uses the term 'essence' or 'essential structure' while hermeneutic phenomenology is more likely to use the term 'fusion of horizons'. Learning about, and communicating the meaning and significance of an experienced phenomenon is a qualitative and literary effort. Husserl, in representing the descriptive emphasis, was interested in finding qualitative features that define what a phenomenon is most generally. For example, one defining feature of many different examples of anger may be the quality of wanting to change another person or something in the world. When formulating 'essences' from a number of cases of an experience, one notices and tries to put into words what is common, but also, what varies or is different between cases studied. So, the findings of phenomenological research should make sense of both the unique details, as well as the commonalities between the experiences studied. This has been referred to as the 'essential structure' of the phenomenon and is expressed in a narrative way that points out how everything fits together. Hermeneutic phenomenologists are also interested in communicating the meaning and significance of experience but express this differently. Meaning is 'pointed out' in multiple ways and relies on personal insight as well as helpful theories that may be relevant. It is less concerned than descriptive phenomenology to come to a specific conclusion, and may evoke deeper understandings in a similar manner as that of a good film-maker or novelist, who 'paints a picture' from various angles.

This kind of writing requires an artistic capability. Even though the different phases and parts of this writing may not be conclusive, they are aimed at forming a coherent picture so that they can offer the reader a place of 'meeting' and understanding about the topic. Gadamer, a hermeneutic phenomenologist, used the term 'fusion of horizons' to mean how different people's understandings could come together, thus achieving broad shared insights that, nevertheless, tolerate some freedom in how readers interpret the significance of findings for their own lives or situations. By this, he was pointing out that the validity of phenomenological findings are not based on their ability to correspond perfectly to all cases, but rather that they have sufficient coherence to be meaningfully applied in similar situations.

Whether the researcher adopts a descriptive emphasis or a hermeneutic emphasis, we would argue that a coherent phenomenological study would include all three features discussed above. Del Barrio *et al.* (2004) provide an account of how these features were applied in a study of patients' experiences of an intensive care unit following a liver transplant (Box 15.3) We now turn to the more practical details of fieldwork and analytical procedures. We can only be indicative here as the practice of these principles varies.

Fieldwork

It has been suggested that researchers adopting a phenomenological approach should read very little relevant literature about the research topic before starting in order not to be influenced by preconceptions. However, the research questions do need to be informed by what has already been done, and what the gaps are. 'Bracketing' is not about pretending that prior knowledge does not exist, but about looking freshly at the area of study, and questioning the assumptions that may be in the literature. So, for example, in a study on therapeutic self-insight, one of the authors was aware of the literature and research that referred to therapeutic self-

Box 15.3   Liver transplant patients: their experience in the intensive care unit.

Del Barrio M, Lacunza M, Armendariz AC, Margall A, Asiain C (2004) Liver transplant patients: their experience in the intensive care unit. A phenomenological study. *Journal of Clinical Nursing* 13: 967–976

Del Barrio and colleagues undertook a descriptive phenomenological study to explore patients' experiences of an intensive care unit following a liver transplant. In-depth interviews were undertaken with 10 patients. The interview began with a very general question: 'Tell me about your experience of your stay in the intensive care unit'. Beyond this, the interview was unstructured, and non-leading questions were asked to encourage participants to express their ideas in their own words. The researchers sought to bracket previous knowledge about the phenomena encountered so that it would not influence the interviews. The transcribed interviews were analysed using Giorgi's method for thematising meanings. Transferable themes between cases were finally expressed in an extensive narrative that highlighted both the common themes as well as some of the unique and different ways in which patients responded. Some of the general themes included:

- the hope they experienced by meeting other patients who had benefited from transplantation
- changes in body image
- pleasurable changes to their preconceptions that the intensive care unit would be a stress-ful, highly technological place

The general description was followed up by a more in-depth description of each of the themes, drawing on quotations from selected patients to elucidate the themes. The value and relevance of these insights for clinical practice were discussed at the end of the article. For example, the findings suggested how patients who were experiencing great discomfort after the operation would benefit from frequent positive reassurance that the body had already shown signs of improved functioning.

insight using different theories and terms such as 're-organising psychic energy', 'cognitive re-structuring', or 'transcending developmental fixations' (Todres 2002). This made the author more interested in describing what was occurring without these theoretical ideas, by going back to people's specific experiences and letting the concepts come 'from there'.

The kind of data that need to be gathered in phenomenological studies are from people who can give examples of experiences they have personally lived through. It is thus not enough that they just have general opinions or views about the topic. They must be able and willing to give descriptions of their own personal experiences. So it is often useful as a starting point to ask: 'Have you had something like this kind of experience?' Sometimes this is obvious and may not need to be asked, such as in approaching fathers about their experience of becoming a father for the first time. At other times it is less obvious, such as in a study of the experience of phantom limb pain. This kind of sampling has been called purposive sampling, in that selection of informants is made on the basis of a particular purpose. In the case of phenomenological research, such purpose is that the research participants included in the study can provide good personal accounts of the experience to be studied. It is also important to gather as much relevant context about the person and the experience as possible. This contextual information helps the researcher to not only make sense of the experience, but also to help specify the nature of the examples on which the reflections are built.

Phenomenological research can generate valuable transferable insights based on an in-depth analysis of only one case study, but value may be increased by studying a number of cases. Phenomenological research, in the authors' experience, has achieved the most profound insights with in-depth reflections on about six to twelve cases as 'windows' to, and illustrations of, a phenomenon. There is a danger to choosing a sample that is too large. A number of journal reviewers have commented that, in such cases, depth and thoughtfulness in the analysis is sacrificed. One then wonders why an alternative research design was not chosen that is better able to capture the quantitative incidence of themes.

In phenomenological research, cases of relevant experiences have been gathered from written descriptions, autobiographical texts, journals and from dialogues. Most phenomenological studies are, however, interview based. This may be because an in-depth interview is able to focus on the complexity of the experience, as well as provide a clear focus for exploration.

A phenomenological interview that gathers lifeworld descriptions of experiences is similar to, but different from other types of non-structured, open-ended interviews. It begins with a request that an interviewee describe a relevant experience as fully as possible. This request is generally similar for all respondents. Instructions are sometimes given which may help the respondent to focus on the details of the experience. One can study lived experience in retrospect because it still has meaning for the person even though the event may have taken place a while ago.

An account of an experience usually begins with some of the factual details but also includes what they meant to the person, the feelings and attitudes. However, the richness of the account is often better when it is closer to the experience in time. The interviewer then helps the interviewee to 'tell the story' as fully and concretely as possible, eliciting examples of the experience and what it was like for the respondent. The logic of the interview is: 'Have you had this kind of experience, and if so, how did it occur for you and what was it like for you?' The interview is open-ended, but the interviewer at times may become more focused on attempting to clarify in greater depth the nature of the phenomenon being studied. This often requires a sensitivity and timing so that the interviewee feels understood and comfortable about the interaction. Box 15.4 provides an example of an interview designed to obtain a lifeworld description.

Box 15.4   Using interviews to obtain 'lifeworld descriptions'.

Imagine that we wish to better understand what happens when a patient is given a diagnosis she or he was not expecting. Using a phenomenological approach that focuses on their life-world, we would ask patients who have had this experience to describe as fully as possible the story of the happening, the events in sequence, the interactions, the 'before' and 'after', their thoughts, feelings and actions – all that goes into the meaning of the experience for them. The value of such lifeworld description is that it provides sources of information that may have been unanticipated by both the respondent and researcher. It does not depend on the ability of the respondent to come up with already formulated views or articulate generalisations.

Analytical procedures

After gathering lifeworld descriptions of personal experiences, each account becomes a 'text' that is ready for the analysis of meanings, and for the formulation of these meanings into a coherent story of interrelated themes and insights. The analysis is different from procedures in other qualitative research such as coding or qualitative content analysis. The articulation and clarification of the meanings in the text, both explicit and implicit, requires a 'reading' or strategy that entails a back and forth movement between particular expressions and details within the text and a sense of the meaning of the text as a whole. It is only the whole of the text and its context that can make sense of the details within the text. On the other hand, the details contribute to, and refine, the process of formulating and synthe-sising meanings into a coherent overall structure as a whole. The danger of com-puter aided analysis packages is that they can divert attention in a way that over-emphasises a concern with 'parts', and this can obscure an understanding of the text as a whole.

There has been some controversy about how much to use a systematic method of analysis in phenomenology. Giorgi and his colleagues (Giorgi 1985; Giorgi & Giorgi 2004) have recommended and demonstrated a systematic procedure which includes:

- reading to get a narrative sense of the text as a whole
- dividing the text into 'meaning units' that discriminate changes in meaning
- expressing the meanings in more transferable and general ways (Box 15.5)
- formulating a narrative structure that highlights the common themes across experiences and cases
- illustrating the common themes in greater detail by elaborating further, and also by using quotations from research respondents' original descriptions – this phase also indicates some of the different and unique ways that different people 'lived out' a particular common theme

Box 15.5   Example of expressing 'meaning units' in more transferable and general ways: responding to a loved-one's memory loss through Alzheimer's disease.

Interviewee's narrative (one meaning unit divided from the rest of the text)	Transferable, more general meaning
In retrospect the earliest indication that there was a problem with Betty's memory loss was that we purchased our new car. Betty had extreme difficulty in the use of fifth gear. Indeed teaching her how to drive the new car was slow and tedious. It should be noted that at this time, Betty was very cognitive and was enjoying secretarial duties.	The earliest indication of him becoming aware of Betty's memory loss was her difficulty in learning an operational task that was, in his view, not in keeping with her usual competent functioning.

Other phenomenologists such as Van Manen (1994) take a less systematic approach and are more concerned with the insightful art of writing that is grounded in lifeworld experiences. Van Manen follows some of the thoughts of Gadamer who feels that no method can ensure insight. Insight emerges through the way the researchers interpret the experiences in the act of writing. Narrative writing is used as a method in itself for reflecting further in order to integrate the different strands of meanings that may be implicit in people's descriptions. Van Manen provides some guidance for writing which includes: involving the readers by writing in a compelling way, building a plot-line with sub-plots, providing enough details and concrete examples to illustrate the themes, and offering new insights that come out of the analysis. Box 15.6 illustrates this with an example of a her-meneutic phenomenological study exploring the use of touch by health professionals caring for older people.

As in other forms of qualitative research, the findings of phenomenological research are finally considered in dialogue with the literature and current research in order to offer critique, possible applications, and further directions for research.

Strengths and limitations

The central strength of a phenomenological approach is that it provides both philosophical and methodological support in attempting to capture and express the meaning of significant human experiences in a rigorous manner. When done well, this gives others deeper insight into what an experience or lived situation is

Box 15.6 The value of using touch in the care of older patients.

Edvardsson JD, Sandman P, Rasmussen BH (2003) Meanings of giving touch in the care of older patients: becoming a valuable person and professional. *Journal of Clinical Nursing* 12: 601–609

These researchers conducted a hermeneutic-phenomenological study influenced by the French philosopher Paul Ricoeur. The phenomenon studied was health care workers' experience of using touch when interacting with older patients. The study explored the experiences of 12 health care workers who had been trained in 'tactile massage' and 'tactile stimulation'. These methods involve the slow and soft stroking of the skin of patients in specific ways. In open-ended interviews, research informants were asked to describe their experience of giving touch to older patients. In order to increase the vividness of their descriptions, informants were asked to imagine themselves in a situation where they would be giving touch to someone, and to elaborate further on the thoughts and emotions connected with the situation. Each interview was transcribed to form a 'text' for interpretation.

The analysis of the texts involved a variation on the idea that the researchers go back and forth between their sense of the meaning of the text as a whole and an attention to the detailed meanings in the parts of the text. The findings showed that these forms of touch helped health care workers to feel more confident that they were able to intervene in a direct way in the suffering of older patients. The respondents also felt that it transformed their relationships with these patients in ways that emphasised their common humanity. The clinical significance of this study is in empowering health care workers with an understanding of, and rationale for, the benefits of using these types of touch with older patients.

like. Such forms of knowledge humanise our understanding, and this may be crucially important as one basis for ethical practice. The narrative product of such studies seeks to express insights in such a way that it may evoke a sense of recognition and understanding in readers. This kind of narrative knowledge is also interpersonal knowledge in that it describes people-in-situations in holistic and interactive ways, guarding against viewing humans as objects like other objects. This may be why the humanistic school of psychology has adopted phenomenology as one of its core methodological approaches. It is also resonant with some feminist contributions to psychology (Gilligan 1982) and sociology (Oakley 2000).

The central limitations of a phenomenological approach in our view are threefold:

- The use of observation is problematic in phenomenological research. Because phenomenology wants to get the inner perspectives of people from their own point of view, it is reluctant to judge behaviour from an external perspective. Critics of phenomenology have noted that descriptions of the world from an 'insider' perspective may be inadequate as an account of human behaviour. Such critics would say that it is not people themselves that can best explain their behaviour, as their behaviour may be caused by forces that are more appropriately analysed in other ways with reference to social, political or chemical analyses.

- Descriptions of lifeworlds depend on full and rich verbal accounts by people who are articulate. This raises challenges for phenomenological methodology, for example, when studying children. There are some ways forward in this regard, such as using photographs or drawings as prompts for people to talk about a particular topic.

- It can be élitist in that there is an artistic-literary capability required of the researcher when reflecting and writing. The 'method' does not guarantee the quality of the narrative coherence achieved in the writing of the final stages of the research product. This can be said to some degree of all research, but phenomenology is on the literary side of the scientific-literary continuum.

Conclusion

Phenomenology is a discrete qualitative research approach that is embedded in the philosophical traditions of the early part of the twentieth century. Phenomenologists emphasise the value of describing and interpreting human experience and seek to do this in credible and insightful ways that apply more generally beyond the particular cases studied. The phenomenological researcher uses descriptions and/or interpretations of everyday human experiences (the lifeworld) as sources of data. When undertaking descriptive phenomenology the researcher seeks to bracket any preconceptions and attempts to arrive at the essences of experienced phenomena. By contrast, hermeneutic phenomenology uses interpretation and personal or theoretical sensitising to highlight important themes. It seeks to enhance understanding in readers by presenting plots or stories in a narratively coherent way.

References

Beck CT (1992) The lived experience of postnatal depression: a phenomenological study. *Nursing Research* 41: 166–170

Bradley-Springer L (1995) Being in pain: a nurse's experience. *Journal of Phenomenological Psychology* 26:2 58–70

Del Barrio M, Lacunza M, Armendariz AC, Margall A, Asiain C (2004) Liver transplant patients: their experience in the intensive care unit: a phenomenological study. *Journal of Clinical Nursing* 13: 967–976

Edvardsson JD, Sandman P, Rasmussen BH (2003) Meanings of giving touch in the care of older patients: becoming a valuable person and professional. *Journal of Clinical Nursing* 12: 601–609

Gilligan C (1982) *In a Different Voice: psychological theory and women's development*. Cambridge, Mass, Harvard University Press

Giorgi A (1970) *Psychology as a Human Science: a phenomenologically based approach*. New York, Harper and Row

Giorgi A (1985) *Phenomenology and Psychological Research*. Pittsburgh, Duquesne University Press

Giorgi A (1997) The theory, practice and evaluation of the phenomenological method as a qualitative research procedure. *Journal of Phenomenological Psychology* 28: 235–260

Giorgi A, Giorgi B (2004) The descriptive phenomenological psychological method. In Camic PM, Rhodes JE, Yardley L (eds) *Qualitative Research in Psychology: expanding perspectives in methodology and design*. Washington DC, American Psychological Association pp243–274

Gullickson C (1993) 'My death as nearing its future': A Heideggerian hermeneutic analysis of the lived experience of persons with chronic illness. *Journal of Advanced Nursing* 18: 1386–1392

Morse J, Bottorff JL, Hutchinson S (1994) The phenomenology of comfort. *Journal of Advanced Nursing* 20: 189–195

Oakley A (2000) *Experiments in Knowing: gender and method in the social sciences*. London, Blackwell

Robinson FA (1998) Dissociative women's experiences of self-cutting. In Valle R (ed) *Phenomenological Inquiry in Psychology: existential and transpersonal dimensions*. New York, Plenum Press pp209–225

Shin KR (1999) On surviving breast cancer and mastectomy. In Madjar I, Walton JA (eds) *Nursing and the Experience of Illness: phenomenology in practice*. London, Routledge pp77–97

Spiegelberg H (1994) *The Phenomenological Movement: a historical introduction*, 3rd edition revised. Dordrecht, Kluwer Academic Publisher

Todres L (2002) Humanising forces: phenomenology in science; psychotherapy in technological culture. *Indo-Pacific Journal of Phenomenology* 3: 1–16

Todres L, Fulbrook P, Albarran J (2000) On the receiving end: a hermeneutic-phenomenological analysis of a patient's struggle to cope while going through intensive care. *Nursing in Critical Care* 5:6 277–287

Van Manen M (1994) *Researching Lived Experience: human science for an action-sensitive pedagogy*. London, Ontario, Althouse Press

Wilcock PM, Brown GCS, Bateson J, Carver J, Machin S (2003) Using patient stories to inspire quality improvement within the modernisation agency collaborative programmes. *Journal of Clinical Nursing* 12: 1–9

Further reading

Holloway I, Wheeler S (2002) *Qualitative Research in Nursing*. Oxford, Blackwell

Rapport F (2005) Hermeneutic phenomenology: the science of interpretation of texts. In Holloway I (ed) *Qualitative Research in Healthcare*. Maidenhead, Open University Press pp125–246

Todres L (2005) Clarifying the Lifeworld: descriptive phenomenology. In Holloway I (ed) *Qualitative Research in Healthcare*. Maidenhead, Open University Press pp104–124

Websites

http://phenomenology.utk.edu/ – Center for Applied Phenomenological Research, University of Tennessee

www.phenomenologyonline.com/ – public access to articles, monographs, and other materials discussing and exemplifying phenomenological research

16 Experimental Research

Andrea Nelson, Jo Dumville and David Torgerson

Key points

- Experimental research makes a useful contribution to nursing research as it is a powerful design able to distinguish between cause and effect.
- There are many different types of experimental design used in health care research.
- The randomised controlled trial is particularly valued for its ability to test rigorously the effectiveness of treatments and interventions – it is known as the 'gold standard'.
- Experimental research seeks to minimise all possible sources of bias and confounding.
- Strengths and weaknesses of the experimental design for different research questions and contexts must be acknowledged.

Background

Well-designed and executed experimental research can contribute to theoretical understanding and to nursing practice. There are several different types of health care interventions, including screening, drugs, information giving, education, and different ways of delivering care (e.g. walk-in clinics) that are amenable to experimental research as a way of testing their effectiveness. Since the thalidomide disaster, drugs must be evaluated in large randomised controlled trials (RCTs) before they are licensed for use. However, other types of interventions are not routinely evaluated in this way, with some commentators arguing that RCTs are of limited use in evaluating nursing interventions.

Experimental versus observational studies

True experimental studies are more powerful than observational studies in determining the cause of an observed outcome. Using an observational design, an association may be found between two variables, but it is difficult to be certain about the direction in which the causal effect is operating. For example, women who give up breastfeeding soon after birth use dummies more often than women who maintain breastfeeding. An RCT of discouraging dummy use found no effect on breastfeeding rates (Kramer *et al.* 2001). In fact, the association between dummy use was observed because women who were going to give up breastfeeding (for whatever reason) tended to use dummies more. Cessation of breastfeeding led to increased dummy use, not the other way around!

It may be tempting to address questions about the effects of interventions by surveying a large number of people. This approach can also be misleading as the intervention a person receives may be related to another factor. For example, in a study of the impact of support group meetings for people with angina on their quality of life, it may happen that those people who attended the support group report a higher quality of life, but this could be because the most active patients, with the least serious disease, attend the group. Concluding that support groups lead to a higher quality of life, *on the basis of this evidence alone*, would be inappropriate.

Results from observational studies of interventions should usually be used to generate further questions for study, rather than to give the definitive answer. Treatments with plausible modes of action, and some limited support through anecdotal evidence may in fact be ineffective or harmful when tested in a robust manner. This means that robust evaluation of interventions sometimes gives 'surprising' results (Box 16.1).

Box 16.1   'Surprising' results of treatments.

Question	Impact of intervention	Reference
Will driver training in older people prevent crashes?	There were no significant differences in the crash rate between people who had received training and those who did not after two years, either as number of collisions, or risk of crash per 100 person years of driving.	Owsley *et al.* (2004)
Does a midwife-led debriefing session after operative childbirth reduce rates of postpartum depression?	Rates of postpartum depression at six months were similar. Debriefing led to poorer health-related quality of life scores on 7 of 8 SF-36* scales (only the values for role functioning (emotional) were statistically significant) There was no difference in satisfaction with care.	Small *et al.* (2000)

36-item short form health survey

Characteristics of experimental design

In an observational study the researcher describes a number of variables. Conversely, in an experimental study the researcher manipulates some aspect of the phenomenon under study and observes what happens.

An experiment is carried out in order to test a hypothesis or research question. An example might be:

'Does patient-controlled analgesia (PCA) reduce post-operative pain?'

Formally, hypotheses are usually expressed as a statement rather than a question, for example:

'PCA is effective at reducing pain scores in the 48 hours post-operatively for patients undergoing major surgery.'

As discussed in Chapter 6, it is important to specify the components of the hypothesis precisely.

It is common to express the hypothesis as a null hypothesis (H_o), a statement that there is no relationship between the variables under investigation, for example:

'PCA is not effective at reducing pain scores in the 48 hours post-operatively for patients undergoing major surgery.'

Statistical testing is commonly set up with the assumption that the null hypothesis is true until there is enough evidence to reject it (*see* Chapter 29 for further information on null hypotheses). More recently there has been a resurgence of interest in statistical methods that do not assume that the null hypothesis holds, e.g. Bayesian analysis. These methods are complex and beyond the scope of this book.

In the PCA example the independent variable is the type of analgesia, and the pain score is the dependent variable. Increasingly the terms participant or population, intervention(s), and outcomes rather than independent and dependent variables are used when reporting the results of experiments. The relationship between these terms can be seen in Box 16.2. As with all study designs, when carrying out experimental research the characteristics of the study population, the type of interventions used, and the outcome(s) of interest, must all be well defined prior to the start of the study.

Box 16.2 Terms used to describe elements of an experiment.

Population	Independent variable	Dependent variable
Population e.g. people undergoing surgery	Intervention e.g. analgesia administered via a patient-controlled device	Outcome e.g. pain levels

Pre-post-test design

There are a number of forms of experiment used in health care. The simplest type of experiment uses a pre-post-test design (sometimes called a before-and-after study). Figure 16.1 shows a representation of this design.

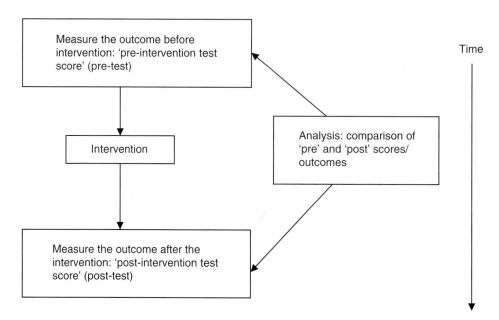

Figure 16.1 Diagrammatic representation of a simple experiment: pre-post-test study.

This design reports a change in an outcome following a change in an intervention. It does not, however, allow us to confidently state that the change occurred *due to* a change in the intervention; i.e. it does not allow us to ascribe cause and effect. There are three key reasons that a change in the outcome might not be due to the intervention being studied; temporal effects, testing effects and regression to the mean.

Temporal effects

A change in an outcome over time might be due to variations in the outcome being measured rather than the intervention. In our example, a reduction in pain scores after use of the PCA device might be due to the reduction in pain levels that would be observed anyway in the first few days after surgery.

Testing effects

These may affect the robustness of pre-post-test designs, particularly in studies of educational interventions, as the initial testing may affect the outcomes (Box 16.3) (Jones & Nelson 1997).

Box 16.3   Example of the possible testing effect on outcome.

Jones JE, Nelson EA (1997) Evaluation of an education package in leg ulcer management. *Journal of Wound Care* 6:7 342–343

A before-and-after study to assess the impact of an educational intervention on the knowledge of nurses managing venous ulcers.

Community nurses involved in leg ulcer care attended two study days. At the first day they attended lectures and workshops and were given an open learning pack and a video on compression bandaging. Between the first and second days they had a supported visit from a local expert in leg ulcer care to address any issues in practice. At the second day there were more lectures and workshops. Knowledge on leg ulcer aetiology and management was tested by means of a self-administered questionnaire at the start of the first study day, repeated at the end of the second study day. The numbers of correct responses were compared. The number of correct responses increased, but this may not have been due to the study day content, as the questionnaire itself may have helped nurses identify gaps in knowledge and prompted further study.

Regression to the mean

Regression to the mean describes a phenomenon that occurs when a variable is measured in a group of people more than once. In our example the researchers recorded pain scores from a number of people, introduced PCA and recorded pain scores for a second time. In the baseline pain scores, one would see a few people had very high pain scores, a few had low pain scores, and the majority of people had pain scores that clustered around the average (mean). If the pain scores are measured again, the people with low pain scores will tend to 'regress' upwards towards the mean, and the people with very high pain scores will tend to 'regress' down towards the mean due to measurement error. This phenomenon means that if an intervention is tested on people with a high pain level, then as a group, their pain scores will decrease, whether or not the intervention is actually effective (Bland & Altman 1994).

One approach to addressing the limitations of the pre-test/post-test design is to monitor the outcomes over long periods before and after the introduction of the intervention. An alternative is to form a group who are not given the intervention being studied but are still followed. The former is called an interrupted time series, the latter, a controlled trial.

Interrupted time series

The stability of the outcome can be assessed both before and after use of the intervention by measuring it several times prior to and after the intervention's introduction. This design might be used when it is impossible to allocate people to different groups, e.g. if there are ethical barriers to randomisation, or if it is not possible to control the release of the intervention, for example, advice from governments on the use of interventions (Sheldon *et al.* 2004).

Controlled trials

In a controlled trial a group (the control group) is formed to act as a comparison to assess whether changes in outcomes are unrelated to the intervention under study. Outcomes from the intervention group are then compared with outcomes from the control group (people not given the intervention). The design is similar to that shown in Figure 16.1 but has at least two groups so that you can be confident that any changes in outcome were not due to temporal effects (*see* Figure 16.2).

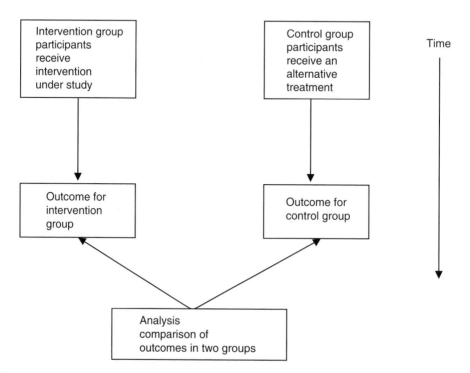

Figure 16.2 Diagrammatic representation of a controlled trial.

If the two groups have different outcomes it might be concluded that the differences were due to the experimental treatment being given to the first group (i.e. ascribing cause and effect). However, this is only the case *if the groups were similar at the outset*. If, for example, people self-selected their treatment group, or if clinicians chose which group a patient entered, then the groups are likely to be systematically different at the outset due to this selection bias, and therefore likely to have different outcomes regardless of the intervention received.

There are a number of ways of allocating people to groups so they are similar. 'Matching' patients with important characteristics is one approach, e.g. age, gender, medical history, etc. This approach, however, can only 'match' for those variables already known to be important. There are possibly many unknown factors that predict outcomes (such as genetic make-up), hence 'matched' groups might still be quite different in some important aspects. In order to address this problem, the most powerful way of allocating people to groups is to allocate them 'randomly'. People are allocated to the groups in a purely random manner, with no way of predicting which group the next person will be allocated to. A controlled trial in which the participants are allocated to the intervention groups at random is a randomised controlled trial (RCT) (Figure 16.3).

The randomised controlled trial

In addition to assessing the direction of causal effects and removing temporal effects, the key strength of the RCT is that it reduces the possibility of selection bias.

Randomisation

To ensure that such selection bias does not take place, the process of random allocation should be concealed from the person(s) recruiting participants into the study if possible. The methods of randomisation deemed to minimise selection bias have two components: randomly generated number sequences; and allocation either via remote telephone randomisation or sealed, sequentially numbered, opaque, envelopes. These are described as blinded or masked allocation methods. Failure to adequately mask allocation has led, in some studies, to inflated estimates of effectiveness of interventions (Schulz & Grimes 2002).

Comparator-control intervention

The control group in an RCT consists of people from the same population, who are treated identically to the treatment group except they receive a different intervention to that being tested. The choice of a comparison treatment may be 'standard care', or it may be a placebo or even nothing at all, depending on the clinical question and state of knowledge. A placebo treatment is one that is

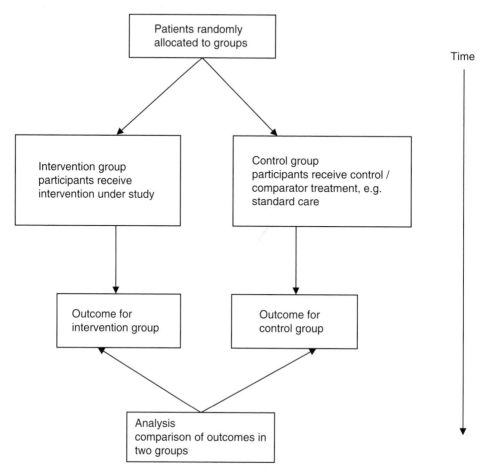

Figure 16.3 Diagrammatic representation of a randomised controlled trial.

identical to the active treatment in every respect, except that it does not contain the proposed therapeutic benefit of the active intervention. Placebo controls are easier to develop and use in pharmaceutical trials (e.g. a sugar pill) compared to many nursing trials, but the lack of a placebo does not preclude the design of RCTs with other, more meaningful, comparison interventions. Box 16.4 illustrates the different types of comparison that can be used.

In an early evaluation of an intervention, where researchers are asking the question 'can this work?' they commonly choose a placebo control (these are sometimes called efficacy studies). If an intervention shows some promise, then researchers may ask the question 'does this intervention make a difference in normal usage?' then the choice of comparator would commonly be 'standard care', and these are sometimes called effectiveness studies. If there is an accepted standard of care, then this should be used as the comparison, as failure to use this means the trial cannot be used to determine if a change in policy from current

Box 16.4 Examples of control groups.

Population	Intervention	Outcome	Control 1	Control 2	Comment
Young people with asthma	New low-allergy bedding	Reducing asthma attacks (number and severity)	Standard treatment – old bedding	Placebo – new 'non-allergenic' bedding	If one uses old bedding, then any reduction in asthma attacks may be due to the fact that newer bedding has fewer allergens. If new 'non-allergenic bedding' is used, and participants are not told which group they are in, then the control bedding is a placebo.
People with diabetic foot ulcers	Growth factor	Healing foot ulcer	Standard care – e.g. semi-occlusive dressings	Placebo – the gel 'vehicle' without the growth factor	If one uses a standard care comparator, then any improvement in healing with the growth factor gel may be due to the gel or growth factor or both.

practice to the new system would be beneficial. For example, an RCT of compression bandages compared a multilayered system with non-compressive technologies for venous ulcers (O'Brien *et al.* 2003). As we already know that compression is better than no compression, then this trial reaffirms what was already known and provides no information on the relative benefits of the multilayered system over any other compression system.

Randomised controlled trials and the reduction of bias

RCTs are designed to reduce an important source of bias – selection bias. However, there are other forms of bias that may lead to systematic error in the results of an RCT, and well-designed and executed RCTs will seek to minimise these.

Performance bias/confounding

In an RCT, if people are treated in different ways other than the treatment of interest, for example, one group gets an 'active' treatment plus extra attention such as more visits or diagnostic tests, then that group may fare better because of the effect of the extra 'care' rather than the treatment being evaluated. Where interventions are complex, in that they have more than one component that could contribute to the interventions' effectiveness, researchers should ensure they have an understanding of the various elements that make up the intervention. For example, in a study comparing cognitive behavioural therapy (CBT) with drugs for depression in primary care, it needs to be recognised that the CBT group would also receive, potentially, increased frequency and duration of contact with health professionals. Both may contribute to improvement in depression as well as the CBT. An RCT might take account of this by having a control group in which people received extra attention and contact but not CBT.

Attrition bias

Attrition bias refers to differences between the comparison groups due to the loss of participants from the study. These can be described as withdrawals, dropouts, or protocol deviations, and the way in which they are handled has potential for biasing the results of an RCT. This is because the reasons for 'withdrawing' from a trial can be related to the intervention or outcomes.

Having a significant minority of people without any final outcome data can threaten the validity of the results of an RCT as it is not known whether the missing people on the treatments fared well or badly. People who were 'lost to follow-up' should not be ignored in the results and analysis, as this would undermine what was achieved by using randomisation.

Figure 16.4 explains this. Two treatments, A and B, are being evaluated in a trial of 100 people (50 in each group), and in each group 10% of people are lost to

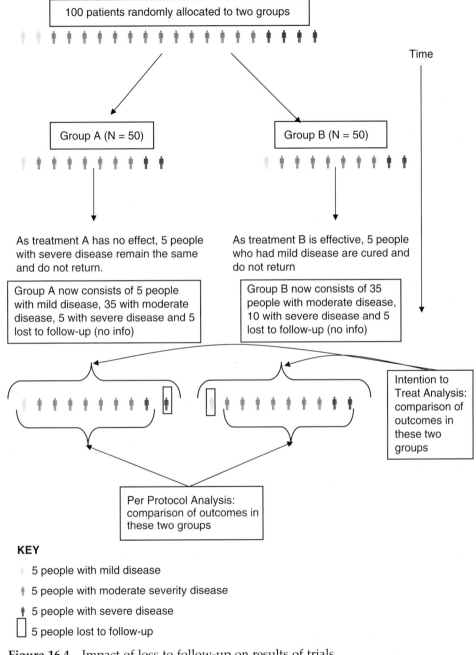

Figure 16.4   Impact of loss to follow-up on results of trials.

follow-up. The remaining two groups, of 45 people each, may differ in a systematic way. If one assumes that treatment A was ineffective, then it may be that five people lost to follow-up in that group had not improved and were demoralised, so did not return for follow-up. By contrast, let us assume that treatment B was mildly effective and the five people lost to follow-up did not return because they had experienced a complete cure. The 45 people remaining in group A would consist of people with mild to moderate disease (the more severe cases dropped out), whereas the people remaining in group B would be people with moderate to severe disease (the least severe cases having been cured). Making a comparison between the two groups on the basis of the 90 people remaining would not maintain the comparable groups obtained through randomisation, and could mislead.

An analysis in which all randomised participants are included, regardless of whether they received the intervention or not, or had any follow-up data is called an 'intention to treat' analysis. Analysing data only from those people who received the intervention and attended follow-up is called a 'per protocol' analysis.

In order to prevent RCTs being threatened by loss to follow-up, they should be designed and conducted to maximise follow-up. In some studies, e.g. cancer RCTs it may be possible to determine eventual outcomes by 'flagging' patients in national registers.

Measurement bias

Outcome data should be collected in the same way, and with the same rigour, for all the study groups. To facilitate this, where possible, participants, health professionals and outcome assessors may remain unaware of the intervention being received. Such blinding (also called masking) aims to prevent knowledge of the participant's treatment group consciously or unconsciously influencing the measurements made in the study (Box 16.5). Blinding can be especially important if the outcome measure has a subjective aspect to it. Various people may be 'blinded' to the allocation, for example, the person randomising the patients, the patient, the person delivering care, the outcome assessor, and the statistician analysing the results. 'Single-blind' studies usually mean that the patient is unaware of the group to which they have been allocated. In 'double-blind' studies both the patient and their clinician are unaware of treatment allocation. It is always possible to mask allocation and the person conducting the analysis. It is usually possible to mask the person performing the outcome assessment; while it is sometimes possible to mask the patient and their clinician.

Hawthorne effect

Franke and Kaul (1978) described the effect of being observed and studied on workers in the Hawthorne factory. A series of experiments were designed to assess if environmental changes, e.g. lighting, improved productivity. It was found that at each change in environment, productivity rose. Strangely, productivity even

> **Box 16.5**   An example of measurement bias.
>
> Reynolds T, Russell L, Deeth M, Jones H, Birchall L (2004) A randomised controlled trial comparing Drawtex with standard dressings for exuding wounds. *Journal of Wound Care* 13:2 71–74.
>
> In an RCT in wound care, a new dressing was compared with standard care. Both patients and nurses were aware of the allocation. The outcomes were assessed in two ways: by asking the nurse treating the patient if the wound was improving, deteriorating or static, and by taking photographs of the wound to be assessed by someone unaware of the dressing being used. When nurses knew which group the patients belonged to they rated the new dressing as being better than standard care. This apparent benefit associated with the new dressing disappeared when the wounds were assessed by blinded assessors looking at the photographs.

rose when there was no actual change in environment, as the participants (factory workers) knew they were being studied and the effect of being studied changed their behaviour. The Hawthorne effect emphasises the need for control groups in experimental research.

Other experimental designs

Cluster RCTs

In the trials described above, individuals were randomised to two or more interventions. An alternative is for natural groups of people (clusters) to be randomised, for example, hospital wards, or geographical areas. By allocating a cluster of people to an intervention, it is possible to be more confident that there will be no contamination between groups. For example, if testing the impact of advanced training for nurses to recognise and treat depression in primary care, one could not expect nurses with this additional training not to assess or treat a patient if the trial was designed with individual patient randomisation. It would be more appropriate to allocate whole practices to 'advanced nurse training' or not and compare the outcomes across the clusters. The reporting and analysis of cluster RCTs must take into account that people in clusters have shared characteristics and therefore cannot all be regarded as independent from each other.

Factorial RCTs

The majority of RCTs seek to test out the effect of changing just one element of treatment at a time. Factorial trials, by contrast, evaluate the effect of multiple interventions at the same time. These RCTs, therefore, may reflect clinical practice where multiple treatments are introduced, e.g. wound management, lifestyle changes. For example, with a factorial trial the effects of two wound dressings and two compression bandages for venous leg ulcers can be compared at the same time.

In a '2 by 2' factorial RCT there are two comparisons of two interventions being made: e.g. two bandages and two dressings. Half the people would get dressing 1, and half would get dressing 2; half would get bandage 1 and half would get bandage 2. Figure 16.5 shows a diagram of a factorial trial making this comparison for venous leg ulcers (Callam *et al.* 1992a; b).

In order to evaluate the two dressings, the healing rates in the columns are compared, and to evaluate the two bandages, the healing rates in the rows are compared. As people were randomly allocated to the dressings and to the bandages, the two dressings groups are assumed to be balanced for bandages, in the same way that age, sex, ulcer size, etc., are balanced across trial groups by randomisation.

One strength of a factorial trial is that it allows researchers to undertake more than one trial at a time, reducing the cost and increasing efficiency. The sample size needed is not usually increased beyond that of a simple, parallel group trial,

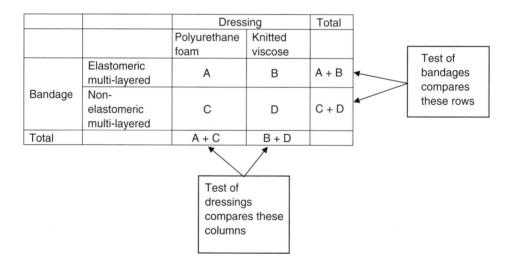

Cell A: 33 patients receive elastomeric multi-layered bandage with polyurethane foam dressing

Cell B: 32 patients receive elastomeric multi-layered bandage and knitted viscose dressing

Cell C: 33 patients receive non-elastomeric multi-layered bandage with polyurethane foam dressing

Cell D: 34 patients receive non-elastomeric multi-layered bandage and knitted viscose dressing

Figure 16.5   A '2 by 2' factorial trial.

so two trials can be completed in the same time, and at almost the same cost as a single treatment trial (as long as there is no interaction between treatments). The other advantage of the factorial trial is that it allows determination of whether the interventions being evaluated have a synergistic (additive) or an antagonistic (working against each other) effect.

Crossover trial

One of the reasons control groups are used is to determine whether any change in outcome is part of the pattern of the disease process, or whether it is due to the intervention. However, if studying the impact of an intervention in a very stable health condition, i.e. one in which there is unlikely to be rapid resolution or deterioration, it is possible to perform *some* evaluations with patients acting as their own control. Essentially, the effect of a treatment is evaluated over a period and then the participant is given an alternative treatment (the crossover). The outcomes at the end of each period are compared for each patient to see whether there is any systematic difference in outcomes. In order to check that any change in outcome is due to the intervention being evaluated rather than temporal changes in outcomes, it usual to randomise participants to either start on treatment A and crossover to B, or start on B and crossover to A (*see* Figure 16.6). This also allows determination of whether there is an 'order effect' whereby treatment B performs differently if preceded by treatment A than if B is given first.

Treatments should not have a prolonged effect, as otherwise their effects may not be seen until the second period of the crossover and therefore the effectiveness would be wrongly attributed to the second treatment used. The analysis of these trials also requires care, as the crossover design needs to be accounted for. Behavioural or educational interventions should not be evaluated in this way, as it is not possible to 'take away' the knowledge or behaviour from the first period.

Single case experimental design (n of 1 trial)

In the face of incomplete evidence to guide a decision about selecting a treatment for a chronic condition, or if a patient does not get relief from those treatments recommended in guidelines, there is a systematic alternative approach to 'trying things out'. In a 'n of 1' trial (where 'n' means number of participants), the clinician and patient work together to evaluate which of the treatments result in consistent benefit. As in the cross-over trial, the condition of interest should be a relatively stable one, e.g. arthritis, so that attributing the effect of the treatment to any improvement or deterioration is a robust conclusion, and not undermined by any natural change in the underlying severity of the condition over time. For example, in an 'n of 1' trial of two treatments for osteoarthritic knee pain, the clinician would draw up a randomly selected schedule of options being investigated, e.g. a magnetic or heat wrap. The patient would keep a pain and stiffness diary,

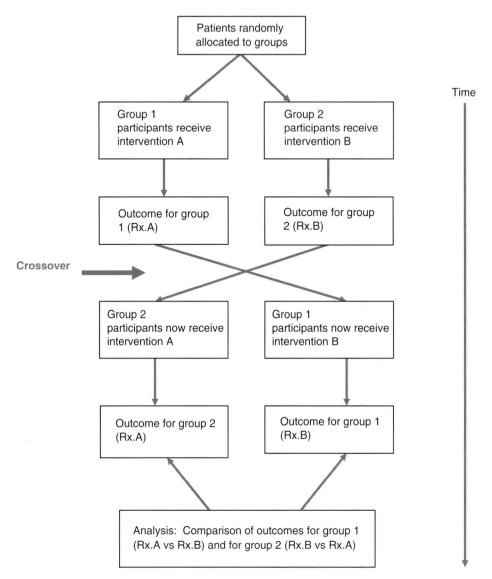

Figure 16.6 A crossover trial.

and agree to use one of the treatments for a specified time, before swapping to the alternative, and then back again, possibly a few times.

Evaluating the two treatments over a number of swap-overs allows the researcher to be more confident that any difference in pain or stiffness is due to the treatment rather than temporary changes in arthritis. If a drug is being evaluated in this way, the clinician may even arrange with a pharmacist to supply the preparation in a masked container so that the patient is 'blinded' to the effective treatment. The clinician and patient review the outcomes for the different treatments using the patient's diary, at the end of the trial, and decide on future management. Given the limited number of conditions for which this is relevant, and the need for relatively intensive input from the clinician, and the patient, this design is not common.

Reporting and reading RCTs

Given the important role RCTs have in informing clinicians of the effects of interventions, and the number of potential threats to their validity, it is important that researchers report exactly what they did in a trial. This allows readers to decide whether the study results are robust. A statement on the reporting of trials (CONSORT) (*http://www.consort-statement.org/*) describes what researchers should report, and journals are increasingly asking researchers to use the CONSORT framework to structure their articles on RCTs for publication (Begg *et al.* 1996).

There are a number of critical appraisal checklists and tools available to help the reader determine whether RCTs are valid and reliable, e.g. CASP (*www.phru.nhs.uk/casp/casp.htm*).

Important considerations in using randomised controlled trials

Securing ethical approval

In order to have ethical approval an RCT must conform to the procedures discussed in Chapters 3 and 10. Participants must usually give their informed consent to be involved in the RCT. However, it is possible, and indeed necessary, to conduct trials in people unable to give consent, for example, in emergency care, but approaches for obtaining consent are governed by individual country arrangements in the UK, following the EU Clinical Trials Directive.

Equipoise

Clinicians recruiting to an RCT must be in collective equipoise, that is, they must believe that the question of whether treatment A or B is better needs to be answered. If there is a clear preference for one intervention over another, then it is not appropriate to conduct an RCT in that area, as researchers would be asking clinicians to administer a treatment that they believed was less beneficial than an alternative.

There is a window of opportunity for RCTs, therefore, in evaluating interventions which clinicians think might be beneficial, before they become convinced that it is better than standard care, when RCTs will not be possible.

Complexity and cost

RCTs can be expensive to carry out. Adherence to the legislation that underpins trials (such as the EU Clinical Trials Directive and data protection), the need for ethical and research governance approval all increase the time it takes to set up a trial. RCTs also require the infrastructure to support randomisation and data collection and management. Trials may be cost-effective, however, if they demonstrate that a treatment is no more effective that standard care, or is better at a very high cost, and therefore inappropriate for many cases. Health economists study the cost-effectiveness of treatments within RCTs, comparing the cost of a treatment with its benefit to participants, to ensure that limited health care resources are used most efficiently. They can also assess the likely benefit of trials to determine which should be prioritised so that greater value for money can be obtained. An example of such an RCT is used throughout Chapters 28 and 29, and is summarised in Box 28.1.

Strengths and limitations of randomised controlled trials

Strengths

An RCT is the best way to determine, with certainty, whether an intervention works. It controls for those variables we know might influence outcome, like concordance, age, and disease severity, but crucially, for those factors which affect prognosis, but which are not measurable or are as yet unknown. Results from well-conducted RCTs are the most reliable research source for informing medical practice about the clinical effectiveness of treatments and interventions, and as such are regarded as the 'gold standard' for answering questions of effectiveness in evidence-based practice.

Limitations

Poorly designed and conducted RCTs can mislead, as often the sizes of effect we are observing in health care are small, and the potential problems with designing and doing trials well can introduce biases and errors that swamp the treatment effect between groups.

Learning curve for technologies

Designing, implementing and completing an RCT can take a long time – if an intervention is changing, the trial evidence may prove to be irrelevant unless particular types of trial are conducted, e.g. tracking trials.

It is important to consider when an RCT was conducted if there is likely to be a 'learning curve'. If a trial is done when few people know how to deliver the intervention effectively, then the trial may conclude no benefit when in fact there might be benefit if a trial was done in the middle or top of the learning curve, when more people were using it appropriately, for example, skills like compression therapy or endoscopy.

Explaining the results of trials

Experiments only answer the question of whether something works, not why it does so. For example, a few RCTs of hip-protector pads to prevent fractured hips on falling, have found that they do not work, and that many people did not wear them. The reasons why the participants did not wear them, or why, in those who did fall, the hip protectors did not reduce fracture rates are not explored. Qualitative studies are increasingly nested within RCTs to help explain the findings.

Poor choice of control groups

If a study has stated it intends to evaluate the effectiveness of a new treatment but compares it against a treatment not in current use, e.g. a sub-therapeutic dose of the standard care regimen, then it is likely to conclude that the new therapy was effective even if it offers no benefit over current best practice.

Surrogate/interim outcomes

Some RCTs may report outcomes that are easier or quicker to assess rather than the actual outcome of interest for patients and clinicians. For example, in an RCT investigating rehabilitation after myocardial infarction, to determine the effect on life expectancy, a long-term follow up would be needed. In order to avoid having to follow-up participants for decades, researchers might report a surrogate outcome instead, e.g. cardiac perfusion, or treadmill walking distance. They may assume that improvements in the physiological outcomes will mirror longer life expectancy. Such use of surrogate outcomes relies on their association with the more relevant, patient-oriented outcomes, such as incidence of disease or survival. Surrogate outcomes commonly mislead, and if they are used, there should be clear evidence of their ability to predict long-term outcomes.

Conclusion

Given the ever increasing pressure on health care systems to make efficient use of the limited resources available, the question of 'what works' needs to be answered by high-quality studies with minimal potential to mislead, and thereby waste resources. For evidence of effectiveness, RCTs are often described as 'the gold standard' as they seek to minimise confounding and selection bias, which may make the results of other comparative studies unreliable. There are a number of biases that may threaten the results of studies, including RCTs, therefore decision makers need to be able to understand how these may threaten the validity of studies, and to identify and appraise such studies to inform their decision-making.

References

Begg C, Cho M, Eastwood S, Horton R, Moher D, Olkin I, Pitkin R, Rennie D, Schulz KF, Simel D, Stroup DF (1996) Improving the quality of reporting of randomized controlled trials. *Journal of the American Medical Association* 276: 637–639

Bland JM, Altman DG (1994) Regression towards the mean. *British Medical Journal* 308: 1499

Callam MJ, Harper DR, Dale JJ, Brown D, Gibson B, Prescott RJ, Ruckley CV (1992a) Lothian and Forth Valley leg ulcer healing trial. Part 1: Elastic versus non-elastic bandaging in the treatment of chronic leg ulceration. *Phlebology* 7:4 136–141

Callam MJ, Harper DR, Dale JJ, Brown D, Gibson B, Prescott RJ, Ruckley CV (1992b) Lothian and Forth Valley leg ulcer healing trial. Part 2: Knitted viscose dressing versus a hydrocellular dressing in the treatment of chronic leg ulceration. *Phlebology* 7:4 142–145

Franke RH, Kaul JD (1978) The Hawthorne experiments: First statistical interpretation. *American Sociological Review* 43: 623–643

Jones JE, Nelson EA (1997) Evaluation of an education package in leg ulcer management. *Journal of Wound Care* 6: 342–343

Kramer MS, Barr RG, Dagenis S, Yang H, Jones P, Ciofanis L, Jane F (2001) Pacifier use, early weaning, and cry/fuss behaviour. *Journal of the American Medical Association* 286: 322–326

O'Brien JF, Grace PA, Perry IJ, Hannigan A, Clarke Moloney M, Burke PE (2003) Randomized clinical trial and economic analysis of four-layer compression bandaging for venous ulcers. *British Journal of Surgery* 90: 794–798

Owsley C, McGwin G, Phillips JM, McNeal SF, Stalvey BT (2004) Impact of an educational program on the safety of high-risk, visually impaired, older drivers. *American Journal of Preventive Medicine* 26: 222–229

Reynolds T, Russell L, Deeth M, Jones H, Birchall L (2004) A randomised controlled trial comparing Drawtex with standard dressings for exuding wounds. *Journal of Wound Care* 13:2 71–74

Schulz KF, Grimes DA (2002) Allocation concealment in randomised trials: defending against deciphering. *The Lancet* 359: 614–618

Sheldon T, Cullum N, Dawson D, Lankshear A, Lowson K, Watt I, West P, Wright D, Wright J (2004) What's the evidence that NICE guidance has been implemented? Results from a national evaluation using time series analysis, audit of patients' notes, and interviews. *British Medical Journal* 329: 999

Small R, Lumley J, Donohue L, Potter A, Waldsenström (2000) Randomised controlled trial of midwife led debriefing to reduce maternal depression after operative childbirth. *British Medical Journal* 321: 1043–1047

Websites

www.jameslindlibrary.org – history of trials in medicine and why we need them

www.phru.nhs.uk/casp/casp.htm – Critical Appraisal Skills Programme (CASP), resources to help appraise clinical studies such as trials

www.cochrane.org/index0.htm – Cochrane Library, databases of systematic reviews and trial reports (freely available via internet to people in England, Wales, Scotland, Northern Ireland and Southern Ireland)

17 Surveys

Hugh McKenna, Felicity Hasson and Sinead Keeney

Key points

- Descriptive surveys aim to describe what exists, whereas correlational and comparative surveys investigate and compare the relationship between variables.
- Surveys can capture the time dimension by being retrospective (past behaviour) and prospective (future propensities).
- Longitudinal surveys are conducted to monitor changes across a period of time.
- Data collection methods used in surveys include questionnaires, interviews, observation and analysis of secondary data.
- Epidemiology is a form of survey research that is concerned with how and why diseases and risk factors occur in populations.
- Epidemiological research has a long tradition in medicine, but is less commonly applied to nursing.

Historical development of survey research in health

It is impossible to determine when the first survey was conducted. Several accounts are given in the Bible, beginning with a census taken after Moses ascended Mount Sinai (Weisberg *et al.* 1996). Later the Romans carried out censuses to prepare for taxation. The social surveys that were at the heart of the early twentieth century survey movement were also total censuses of the cities studied, merging census data with special surveys of topics, such as housing conditions. In England, nineteenth century surveys were conducted by independent individuals and government agencies in attempts to study social conditions and the nature of poverty. For instance, in 1902 Charles Booth conducted his monumental inquiry into the *'Labour and life of the people of London'* (1889–1902). In 1912, Bowley undertook a study of working-class conditions. This was published as *'Livelihood and Poverty'* (Bowley & Burnett-Hurst 1915). Bowley's great methodological contribution was his use of statistical sampling, which came to act as a decisive stimulus to social surveys (Moser & Kalton 1971).

At the end of World War I, a new approach was adopted that was different to censuses; rather psychophysical laboratories were used in which a small number of consumers were brought for standardised product testing (Rossi *et al.* 1983). Market research psychologists introduced the techniques of questioning people on their preferences to a range of issues. The middle 1930s saw an expansion in the use of survey methods in public opinion polling. This was pioneered by George Gallup in America.

At the beginning of the twenty-first century, the survey is an established method of social inquiry. Since the time of Booth and Bowley, great changes have occurred in the amount of survey activity and in the interest by the public to this research approach. There have been considerable changes in methods of collecting and storing survey data due specifically to technological developments.

Descriptive surveys

The most common objective of survey research is to describe. In descriptive surveys, statistics are collected about a large group: for example, the proportion of men and women who view a television programme or who participated in a health-screening programme. They can be designed to measure events, behaviour, and attitudes in a given population or sample of interest. So a descriptive survey is used to obtain information on the current status of phenomena so as to describe, *'what exists'* with respect to variables or conditions (Sim & Wright 2000).

For example, a Gallup Poll conducted during a political election campaign has the purpose of describing the voting intentions of the electorate. Descriptive surveys are based on the assumption that the answer to the research question may exist in the present so the objective is to collect this information in a systematic way. They are indispensable in the early stages of studying a phenomenon (Dublin 1978), because from such phenomena concepts are formed which are the building blocks of theory.

Descriptive surveys are also carried out to describe populations, to study associations between variables and to establish trends and possible links between variables. While this is valuable, they cannot provide robust evidence about the direction of cause and effect relationships. Box 17.1 provides an example of such a survey.

Descriptive surveys have several advantages but perhaps the main one is that they are relatively easy to undertake as they only involve one contact with the study population. However, there is the potential problem that the respondents give the answers that they believe the researcher wants to hear, rather than their true views. Another disadvantage is that they cannot measure change, so if things change rapidly, the survey information may easily become outdated. To measure change it is necessary to have at least two observations, that is, at least two cross-sectional studies, at two points in time, on the same population. Furthermore, the results of surveys can be wrong. One of the most famous examples of this was the survey polls that predicted a landslide victory of Thomas E. Dewey over Harry S. Truman in the 1948 presidential elections. Truman won with a two million majority.

Box 17.1 Example of a descriptive survey.

Walczak JR, McGuire DB, Haisfield ME, Beezley A (1994) A survey of research-related activities and perceived barriers to research utilisation among professional oncology nurses. *Oncology Nursing Forum* 21: 710–715

The purpose of this study was to identify current research-related activities among oncology nurses, their knowledge of research utilisation, and perceived barriers to using research in practice. In this descriptive, cross-sectional survey a self-report questionnaire was used to collect data. A convenience sample of 82 registered nurses who were employed in a cancer centre returned the questionnaire. Findings revealed that although nurses appeared to be aware of the importance of using research and value it, they identified barriers to using research findings in practice and did not participate routinely in research-related activities. The findings provided baseline information for a departmental research utilisation program and suggested strategies and activities that could be incorporated into the program.

Correlational and comparative surveys

These types of survey are devoted to investigating and comparing the relationship between variables. For example, a questionnaire may be administered to a large number of patients to find out whether there is a difference in the self-reported levels of post-operative stress between those who received information and those who did not. In each case the question is whether there is a relationship between variable X and variable Y. In correlational studies, a researcher can collect demographic details such as age, occupation, gender and educational background and seek to establish links between these and other characteristics of participants such as their beliefs and behaviours (Parahoo 1997). The purpose is often to develop hypotheses and in turn contribute to theory development. It does so from theory-based expectations on how and why variables should be related. Hypotheses could be basic (i.e. relationships exist) or directional (i.e. the relationship is positive or negative). Such surveys only tell us that there is a relationship between the two variables; they do not tell us whether one variable 'caused' the other. Correlational studies have little control over the respondents' environment and thus have difficulty ruling out alternative explanations for causation.

In comparative surveys, data are collected that allow comparisons to be made according to demographic features such as age, gender or class. Therefore, the main purpose of such studies is to compare variables across people, places or time. If changes are surveyed over time we may need to compare data collected as a baseline with those collected some time later. If we want to know the effects of behaviour such as smoking or drinking, we can compare those who indulge in these practices with those who do not. Such studies can be quantitative, qualitative or both.

Comparative surveys encounter a number of potential limitations including problems in ensuring comparable measures and samples. For example, over 65 countries participate in the World Values Survey *(www.worldvaluessurvey.org)*. This involves comparing results across countries. Different sample designs in different countries, different methods of administering surveys, different acceptance of survey research and different levels of interviewer training and technique can cause problems. This can result in design-based measurement errors arising in which the same methods of data collection and the same questions are used in very different cultural contexts.

Prospective and retrospective survey designs

While surveys can capture a snapshot of the attitudes, beliefs and behaviours of individuals and groups in the present they can also be applied retrospectively and prospectively.

A retrospective design is one in which researchers study a current phenomenon by seeking information from the past. Researchers have to work backwards and search for variables or factors to help shed light on issues. Such a design aims to describe or explain a phenomenon by examining factors with which it was associated. For example, patients' notes hold a considerable amount of information on the treatment and progress of their illness as well as demographic details. These can be used retrospectively to explain phenomena. Most cross-sectional studies are retrospective. This is a relatively inexpensive research method as large numbers of people can be surveyed quickly and data are easily coded (Bowling 1997).

One of the main drawbacks of retrospective designs is that the researcher relies on existing data that were, most probably, not collected for research purposes and therefore lack the required rigour. Furthermore, many archives that could be of interest to future researchers are being lost. For example, with the closure of many psychiatric hospitals, patients' notes and other materials are being destroyed. Also, descriptions of past behaviour may be highly subjective, records may be incomplete and/or rely on respondents' memories. For instance, respondents may be asked questions about past diet and other lifestyle factors and the potential for selectivity in recollection and recall bias is great. Despite these shortcomings, retrospective studies have been useful in, for example, studying the perspectives of older women regarding their experiences of living with ovarian cancer (Fitch *et al.* 2001).

The prospective survey is one that takes place over the forward passage of time with more than one period of data collection. Such studies attempt to establish the outcome of an event or explore what is likely to happen. For example, nurses may want to know the effects of new practices on patients' behaviour. Researchers using this design can have control over what they want to include in their study and how data are collected. Another example could be noting if and how the lifestyles of newly diagnosed cancer patients change over time. The researcher may compare this group of respondents with another group who do not have the illness (control group). With this design, data are collected at one or multiple points in the future. Such studies require careful definitions of the groups under study and careful selection of variables for measurement.

Prospective surveys can be expensive, take a long time, need a great amount of administration (e.g. update and trace addresses) and can suffer from high sample attrition through natural loss, geographical mobility or refusals over time. Respondents can also become conditioned to the study and learn the responses that they believe are expected of them. In addition, there can be reactive effects of the research arrangements – the 'Hawthorne effect' as people change simply as a result of being studied (Roethlisberger & Dickson 1939). Chapter 16 has a fuller discussion of this effect in experimental research. There needs to be a clear rationale to support the timing of repeated survey points, retaining the respondents' interests and participation and employ sensitive instruments with relevant items that will detect change.

Longitudinal surveys and cohort studies

Longitudinal surveys are normally conducted over a long period of time. Data collection takes place at regular intervals throughout the life of the study. The purpose of this is to monitor changes over time. Such surveys are sometimes referred to as panel studies. The British Household Panel Survey (Box 17.2) is a large-scale example of a longitudinal survey. The purpose of this survey is to monitor householders over a long period of time to analyse their responses to changes in the social and economic environment.

The longitudinal survey may be of particular use in nursing research as certain phenomena from these professions lend themselves to being studied over a long period of time. Parahoo (1997) used the example of people coming to terms with the loss of a spouse and the different phases that they may go through. It is obvious that in this case the collection of data on one isolated occasion would not be as beneficial as the collection of data at regular intervals over several years.

A cohort study is a form of longitudinal survey that uses a specific group of respondents for the entire study. Cohort studies chart the development of these groups from a particular time point either prospectively or retrospectively. Such studies are concerned with life histories of sections of populations. They provide information on developmental changes across stages of life in any domain including employment, education, housing, family and health.

Cohort studies have been used to study nurses. The most notable of these studies is the American Nurses Cohort Study. (*www.channing.harvard.edu/nhs/index. html*). The original Nurses Cohort Study was established by Dr Frank Speizer and was funded by the National Institute of Health. The primary idea behind the survey was to investigate the potential long-term consequences of oral contraceptives, diet and lifestyle risk factors. Over 170,000 nurses completed baseline questionnaires for this study. Questionnaires are administered to the cohort every four years.

Box 17.2   British Household Panel Survey.

The British Household Panel Survey began in 1991 and has followed the same group of respondents over the last 24 years. The main aim of the survey is to gain insight into social and economic change at the individual and household level. The survey is a resource for a wide range of social science disciplines and supports interdisciplinary research in many subject areas. It is a household-based study interviewing every adult member of a sampled household. It contains representation from different social groups such as the elderly. The original panel consisted of 5500 households from 250 areas of Great Britain. This equated to 10 300 individuals. In 1999, 1500 households were added from Scotland and 1500 households were added from Wales. In 2000 a further sample of 2000 households were added from Northern Ireland.

(www.statistics.gov.uk/STATBASE/Source.asp?vlnk=1308)

One of the main problems of longitudinal and cohort studies is that the respondents may drop out of the study. This is termed 'mortality' or 'attrition' (Parahoo 1997). It can affect the success of a cohort study. Researchers can also move on to other roles or jobs and it is not uncommon to find that a succession of researchers have worked on the survey over the years.

Another difficulty with longitudinal studies is the effect of the research on the attitudes and behaviours of the respondents. By their very nature longitudinal studies could serve to raise the awareness of the respondents and introduce bias. Time and cost are other inevitable considerations with longitudinal studies. In addition, it may be difficult to ensure continuity among respondents. In some cohort studies, the researchers send Christmas cards and birthday cards to respondents to encourage continued participation.

Sources of data in survey research

Most people will have encountered a survey at some stage either as a respondent to a postal survey or being approached by a market researcher in a supermarket or on the telephone. Organisations carry out surveys for a wide variety of reasons and results are used for different purposes; they include from changing policy to making decisions on a marketing strategy. Social researchers regard surveys as a valuable source of data about respondents' attitudes, beliefs, experience and behaviour.

Questionnaires and interviews

Chapters 22 and 24 describe the main data collection tools for surveys in more depth. Here we will discuss the relative merits of questionnaires and interviews for purposes of a brief comparison of the two methods. There is no universal agreement among researchers about what should be called a questionnaire. It can mean a document containing a list of questions for respondents to complete on their own (the self-completion questionnaire) or it can mean a set of questions that a researcher reads out to a respondent. For the purposes of this chapter, a questionnaire will be considered to be a list of questions contained in a document that respondents complete themselves.

Questionnaires are usually distributed by post although they can be distributed by hand, for example, to patients or visitors in a hospital. More recently, researchers have been distributing questionnaires by e-mail using a distribution list or by simply asking respondents to complete an online questionnaire (Morris *et al.* 2004).

Generally, questionnaires follow a standardised format in which questions are pre-coded to provide a list of responses for selection by the respondent (tick-box questions). However, open-ended questions can be included with space to allow the respondent to provide a written answer. Questions should be easily comprehensible, as the respondent will not be able to seek clarification. For this reason, a questionnaire is often 'piloted' with a small subsection of the target population to ascertain if it is understandable, valid and acceptable. This may result in changes being made to question content or the length of the questionnaire. For a fuller discussion of questionnaires, turn to Chapter 24.

Face-to-face interviews use a list of questions sometimes called an interview guide. This guide may contain either open or closed questions or a combination of both. There is an important distinction between an interview schedule and an interview guide. An interview schedule uses a set of questions in a predetermined order that is adhered to during the interview. An interview guide is a list of areas to be covered, leaving the exact wording and order of the questions to be determined by the interviewer.

As the name implies, structured interviews tend to use an interview schedule with very explicit questions and leave no room for veering off the topic. Semi-structured interviews use the interview guides referred to above and there is room for exploration and for altering the questions based on a respondent's circumstances of replies. In contrast, unstructured interviews are totally open and the researcher has freedom to explore a range of issues around a general subject area. The internet also facilitates opportunities to conduct electronic interactive interviews via e-mail or through the use of chat rooms. However, although electronic technologies are convenient and low cost for the researcher, they are still novel and raise many ethical questions.

Within face-to-face interviews, researchers may record responses by pen or directly onto a laptop computer. This approach is generally reserved for structured interviews that include many closed questions. For interviews using more open-ended questions, the interview is usually audiorecorded. This recording would subsequently be transcribed as an interview transcript. Generally data from questionnaires are analysed using computerised database and statistical analysis software such as the Statistical Package for the Social Sciences (SPSS). Chapter 22 provides a more detailed consideration of interviewing.

Self-completion questionnaires and face-to-face interviews are long established methods of data collection and each have their own strengths and weaknesses (Box 17.3).

Box 17.3 Face-to-face interviews versus self-completion questionnaires.

Face-to-face interviews	Self-completion questionnaires
Costly due to time-intensive nature	Less costly – slower data collection method
Longer and more complex questions are possible	Limited in length and complexity
High response rates	Often associated with poor response rates
Can adapt to include visual materials – e.g. show cards	Excludes the less literate and those who may have a disability e.g. dyslexia, blind
Provides additional opportunities to clarify questions and responses	No opportunity to explain complex instructions, to answer questions or to probe for more detail on open-ended questions
Interviewee is not anonymous	Respondent cannot be connected to their response. As a result, more honest responses may be provided
Can be subject to bias – acquiescence and social desirability bias if not carefully recruited	Respondents have more time to weigh the issues carefully before responding – less prone to acquiescence
Enables interviewer to ensure data is being collected from the correct sample	Researcher cannot ensure the target person completes the questionnaire. For example, a questionnaire aimed at exploring the views of a patient may be completed by a carer

Interview schedules are also used for interviews carried out over the telephone. Telephone surveys have similar benefits to face-to-face interviews, but also facilitate reaching a much wider population at less cost. Telephone surveys are less popular with social researchers than they are with market and commercial researchers. While they may be less expensive to undertake than face-to-face interviews, telephone surveys do not take cognisance of non-verbal cues and surroundings and certain groups may have to be excluded from the survey because they do not have a telephone. The issue of the growing ownership of mobile phones is also creating problems for researchers. Nicolaas (2004) has identified sampling problems in relation to mobile phone users who tend not to be listed in phone directories. Furthermore, mobile phone numbers cannot be linked to a geographical area and they tend to belong to one individual rather than a household.

Secondary data sources

Gilbert (1993) asserted that it is 'a truism of social research that almost all data are seriously underanalysed' (Gilbert 1993:256). This may be one of the reasons that analysis of secondary data sources is continuing to grow in popularity with social researchers. Secondary analysis of data sources implies that the data are being subjected to further analysis than that for which it was originally collected. There are many sources of data that can be used for secondary analysis. Examples include patient or public records such as medical records, audit data, attendance records, nationally available statistics stored in data banks, government data, academic data and research data collected for other purposes. Hospitals retain patient medical records, attendance records, complaints records and other statistical data on both patients and staff.

Census data is also available for secondary analysis. The National Statistics Office is responsible for UK census data. It can provide access to the UK data bank and this can provide large amounts of data on many and varied topics across a lengthy period of time. In the UK, the National Data Archive is located at the University of Essex. It holds mainly UK data but has reciprocal arrangements with other countries for access to their national data. However, the secondary analysis of some of these data may raise ethical questions and may be difficult to access. After all, respondents provide the data for a specific purpose and to use it for another purpose without their consent is potentially problematic.

Observation

Moser and Kalton (1971:245) described observation as 'the classic method of scientific enquiry'. Nonetheless, social researchers use observation relatively infrequently. One type of observation employed in survey research is non-participant observation. Chapter 25 deals in detail with this and other ways of using observation for research purposes.

In terms of practicality and validity, direct observation can have a number of advantages to using a questionnaire or an interview schedule. For example, studies of children may have to rely on observational techniques, as children may not be able to verbalise or write down the answer. Responses provided within questionnaires or interviews may also be inaccurate whereas observation will provide a true picture of the situation. For instance, interview data on how nurses practise may differ from data collected through observing them working.

Observation also has limitations. Non-participant observation does not allow the researcher to explore peoples' attitudes or perceptions. It is also difficult to ensure representativeness using observational techniques. Furthermore, there are obvious ethical issues relating to seeing unsafe practices while being a non-participant observer.

Epidemiology

Epidemiology is the study of how often diseases occur in different groups of people, why they occur (Coggon *et al.* 1997), and the risk factors for these diseases (Bowling 1997). Historically, the impact of epidemiology on the health of the nation has been far-reaching (Whitehead 2000). There has been a long-standing tradition of epidemiology within health care. This is due to the fact that epidemiological research is used to plan and evaluate strategies to prevent illness and as a guide to the management of patients who have already developed a disease (Coggon *et al.* 1997). Epidemiology is concerned with observing, measuring and analysing health-related occurrences in human populations (Trichopoulos 1996). As nursing roles become more involved in preventative care and public health, epidemiology will become increasingly appropriate as a research method. There are five main types of epidemiological surveys.

Descriptive study

Descriptive epidemiology describes the health status of a population or characteristics of a number of patients and attempts to find correlations among such characteristics as diet, air quality and occupation. Box 17.4 gives an example of such a study. As alluded to earlier, descriptive studies may be considered weak because they make no attempt to link cause and effect and therefore no causal association can be determined.

Box 17.4   Descriptive epidemiological survey.

Morize V, Nguyen DT, Lorente C, Desfosses G (1999) Descriptive epidemiological survey on a given day in all palliative care patients hospitalised in a French university hospital. *Palliative Medicine* 13: 105–117

This descriptive study was conducted on one given day on all inpatients requiring palliative care in a French university hospital. In each department, a collaborative team made up of physicians and nurses identified and described the clinical signs, the treatment protocols, the social and family characteristics and the outcome for each patient using a standardised questionnaire. Study subjects were inpatients in the hospital and presented advanced or terminal-stage life-threatening conditions. Two hundred and forty five patients were included in the study. Overall, 66% of subjects suffered from physical discomfort and 80% suffered psychologically. Patients still received specific treatment for their condition in 45% of cases. Social problems were identified principally in medium or long-term care inpatients who made up 36% of the total inpatient population. A request for transfer to another care structure had been completed for 24% of patients. Assistance from the Palliative Care Unit's support team had been requested in 25% of cases, mainly to provide psychological support for the patient and the health care providers. These results have led to reconsideration of the general organisation of palliative care in the health care system.

Cross-sectional studies

A cross-sectional study measures the prevalence of health outcomes or determinants of health, or both, in a population at a point in time or over a short period (Coggon *et al.* 1997). For example, such designs have been used to explore insulin resistance and depression (Timonen *et al.* 2005). However, associations must be interpreted with caution as bias may arise because of selection into or out of the study population.

Case-controlled studies

A case-controlled study is a retrospective comparison of exposures of persons with disease (cases) with those of persons without the disease (controls). In case-controlled studies, such individuals are selected with and without the particular disease and asked about past exposure. Exposure rates within the two groups are compared. Case-controlled studies offer several advantages in that they are quick and relatively inexpensive to conduct and are suitable for studying multiple exposures and rare diseases. However, case-controlled studies present possible biases such as recall bias and interviewer bias.

Box 17.5   Epidemiological cohort study.

Hu BF, Stampfer M, Manson J, Rimm E, Colditz G, Rosner B, Speizer F, Hennekens C, Willett W (1998) Frequent nut consumption and risk of coronary heart disease in women: prospective cohort study. *British Medical Journal* 317: 1341–1345

This study examined the relationship between nut consumption and risk of coronary heart disease in a cohort of women from the Nurses' Health Study, established in 1976, which includes detailed information on the medical history and lifestyle of 121 700 registered female nurses aged between 30 and 55 years. Every two years the participants receive a follow up questionnaire so that information on potential risk factors for diseases can be updated, and newly diagnosed diseases such as coronary heart disease can be identified. This prospective cohort study involved 86 016 participants between 34 and 59 years of age without previously diagnosed coronary heart disease, stroke, or cancer at baseline in 1980. It was found that the frequent nut consumption was associated with a reduced risk of both fatal coronary heart disease and non-fatal myocardial infarction. These data, and those from other epidemiological and clinical studies, support a role for nuts in reducing the risk of coronary heart disease.

Cohort studies

A cohort study is a study in which a healthy group of people are followed over time to measure their exposure to certain conditions or receive a particular treatment and are compared with another group who are not affected by the condition under investigation. As with general cohort studies they are expensive, time-consuming and logistically difficult; however, the design is less subject to bias because it measures exposure before researchers learn the health outcome. Box 17.5 provides an example of a cohort study among nurses.

Conclusion

This chapter has set the survey in its historical context and outlined the main types of surveys used within nursing research. The sources of data have been discussed and the pros and cons of self-completion questionnaires, face-to-face interviews and telephone interviews considered. Other methods used within survey research have also been explored, including secondary data analysis and observations. Epidemiological research and its applicability to nursing research was also outlined. Due to the fact that nursing's body of knowledge continues to be in the early stage of development there is every indication that survey research will continue to be popular for some time to come.

References

Booth C (ed) (1889–1902) *Labour and Life of the People of London*, 17 volumes. London, Macmillan

Bowley AL, Burnett-Hurst AR (1915) *Livelihood and poverty: a study in the economic conditions of working-class households in Northampton, Warrington, Stanley and Reading*. London, Bell

Bowling A (1997) *Research Methods in Health: investigating health and health services*. Buckingham, Open University Press

Coggon D, Rose G, Barker DJP (1997) *Epidemiology for the Uninitiated*, 4th edition. London, BMJ Publishing

Dublin R (1978) *Theory Building*. New York, The Free Press

Fitch MI, Gray RE, Franssen E (2001) Perspectives on living with ovarian cancer: older women's views. *Oncology Nursing Forum* 28:9 1433–1442

Gilbert N (1993) *Researching Social Life*. London, Sage

Hu BF, Stampfer M, Manson J, Rimm E, Colditz G, Rosner B, Speizer F, Hennekens C, Willett W (1998) Frequent nut consumption and risk of coronary heart disease in women: prospective cohort study. *British Medical Journal* 317: 1341–1345

Morris DL, Fenton MV, Mercer ZB (2004) Identification of national trends in nursing education through the use of an online survey. *Nursing Outlook* 52: 248–254

Morize V, Nguyen DT, Lorente C, Desfosses G (1999) Descriptive epidemiological survey on a given day in all palliative care patients hospitalized in a French university hospital. *Palliative Medicine* 13: 105–117

Moser C, Kalton G (1971) *Survey methods in social investigation*. London, Heinemann

Nicolaas G (2004) *Sampling Issues for Telephone Surveys in Scotland*. Survey Methods Unit, National Centre for Social Research. *www.bioss.ac.uk/rss/gerry_nicolaas.ppt*.

Parahoo AK (1997) *Nursing Research: principles, process and issues.* London, Macmillan

Roethlisberger EJ, Dickson WJ (1939) *Management and the Worker.* Cambridge, Harvard University Press

Rossi P, Wright J, Anderson A (1983) *Handbook of Survey Research.* New York, Academic Press

Sim J, Wright C (2000) *Research in Health Care: concepts, designs and methods.* Cheltenham, Stanley Thornes

Timonen M, Laakso M, Jokelainen J, Rajala U, Meyer-Rochow BV, Keinänen-Kiukaanniemi S (2005) Insulin resistance and depression: cross-sectional study. *British Medical Journal* 330: 17–18

Trichopoulos D (1996) The future of epidemiology. *British Medical Journal* 313: 436–437

Walczak JR, McGuire DB, Haisfield ME, Beezley A (1994) A survey of research-related activities and perceived barriers to research utilization among professional oncology nurses. *Oncology Nursing Forum* 21: 710–715

Weisberg H, Krosnick J, Bowen B (1996) *An Introduction to Survey Research, Polling and Data Analysis,* 3rd edition. Thousand Oaks, Sage

Whitehead D (2000) Is there a place for epidemiology in nursing? *Nursing Standard* 14: (42) 35–38

Further reading

Alreck PL, Settle RB (1995). *The Survey Research Handbook: guidelines and strategies for conducting a survey.* 2nd edition. New York, McGraw-Hill

Benevelo L (1980) *The History of the City.* Cambridge, MIT Press

Chang CL, Donaghy M, Poulter, N (1999) Migraine and stroke in young women: case-control study. *British Medical Journal* 318: 13–18

Dupont WD, Plummer ED Jr (1996) Understanding the relationship between relative and absolute risk. *Cancer* 77: 2193–2199

French S, Peterson CB, Story M, Anderson N, Mussell MP, Mitchell JE (1998) Agreement between survey and interview measures of weight control practices in adolescents. *International Journal of Eating Disorders* 23: 45–56

Jinks MA, Lawson V, Daniela R (2003) A survey of the health needs of hospital staff: implications for health care managers. *Journal of Nursing Management* 11: 343–350

Kiecolt KJ, Nathan LE (1985) *Secondary Analysis of Survey Data.* Thousand Oaks, Sage

Salant P, Dillman DA (1994) *How to Conduct Your Own Survey.* New York, John Wiley & Sons

Levine S, Lilienfield AM (1987) *Epidemiology and Health Policy.* London, Tavistock

Mulhall A (1996) *Epidemiology, Nursing and Healthcare: a new perspective.* Houndsmill, Palgrave Macmillan

Websites

dmsweb.badm.sc.edu/grover/survey/MIS-SUVY.html – a tutorial on survey research from constructs to theory *www.amstat.org/sections/srms/brochures/survwhat.html* – American Statistical Association Series: What is a Survey?

www.worldvaluessurvey.org/ – comprehensive measurement of all major areas of human concern including religion, politics, economic and social life

18 Action Research

Julienne Meyer

Key points

- Action research is a research approach that involves interpreting and explaining social situations while implementing a change intervention.
- Action researchers adopt a participatory approach, involving participants in both the change and the research process.
- There are three broad types of action research; *technical-scientific and positivist action research, mutual-collaborative and interpretivist action research*, and *critical and emancipatory action research*.
- Both qualitative and quantitative methods of data collection may be employed during the three phases of action research: exploration, intervention and evaluation.
- Action researchers act as agents of change and need skills not only in research, but also in change management.
- Although sometimes criticised as unscientific, action research has a real world focus and directly seeks to improve practice.

Principles of action research

Much research is disseminated through the publication of research reports, theses and articles, which ultimately may (or may not) influence practitioners to improve the way they work. Action research is different, as it is centrally concerned with the lessons learnt from practice development. It thus focuses on the 'D' end of 'Research & Development'. Given that in applied disciplines, the purpose of research is to understand and improve practice, it is surprising that more funding is not allocated for this type of research.

Action research is an approach to research, rather than a specific method of data collection. The approach involves doing research *with* and *for* people (users and providers of service), in the context of its application, rather than undertaking research *on* them. The action researcher is seen as a facilitator and evaluator of change, whether the focus is on their own practice or the practice of others. Typically in health and social care settings, action researchers begin by exploring and reflecting on patient and/or client experience and, through a process of feeding back findings to providers of services (formal and informal), go on to identify gaps in care that those engaged in the research would like to improve. Through an ongoing process of consultation and negotiation that gives democratic voice to all participants about the best way forward, the action researcher then works to support and systematically monitor the process and outcomes of change. An eclectic approach to data collection is taken, using whatever methods best address the problem being researched, although often action research is written up in its rich contextual detail as a case study.

From case studies of action research, two types of knowledge can be generated – theoretical and practical. In contrast to other forms of research, the action researcher cannot predetermine the nature of the study, as it is dependent on the views and wishes of those with whom they are collaborating. Action researchers thus have to work in a flexible and responsive way to deal with issues as they naturally occur in practice. In so doing, they have to rely as much on their inter-personal skills as their research skills. This requires special thought to be given to how those involved in the research can be protected from harm. Gaining formal ethical approval for the study is not enough. It is important to agree a code of ethical practice at the start of the study that allows participants control over what change happens, how it is researched and how the findings are shared with others.

Action research thus blurs the boundaries between education, practice and research. If nothing else is gained as a result of the research, at least participants in the study should learn and develop from the process of being actively involved with it. As a nurse, I am particularly attracted to the underlying principles of action research namely, its participatory character, its democratic impulse, and its simultaneous contribution to social science (knowledge) and social change (prac-tice) (Carr & Kemmis, 1986). Too much research is built around the researcher as expert with a 'hit and run' approach to data collection, at least this approach aims to give something back (social change), at the same time as contributing to social knowledge.

Common models of working with action research in nursing

Action research is not easily defined, as there are many different models of action research, largely influenced by the level of focus (own practice, collective practice of others, wider political events), degree of participation, and vision of knowledge (Whitelaw *et al.* 2003). Waterman *et al.* (2001) suggest that existing definitions of action research within the literature tend to focus on the description of its charac-teristics. However, following extensive investigation and reflection on the litera-ture, they came up with the following definition:

'Action research is a period of inquiry, which describes, interprets and explains social situations while executing a change intervention aimed at improvement and involvement. It is problem-focused, context-specific and future-oriented. Action research is a group activity with an explicit value basis and is founded on a partner-ship between action researchers and participants, all of whom are involved in the change process. The participatory process is educative and empowering, involving a dynamic approach in which problem identification, planning, action and evaluation are interlinked. Knowledge may be advanced through reflection and research, and qualitative and quantitative research methods may be employed to collect data. Different types of knowledge may be produced by action research, including practical and propositional. Theory may be generated and refined, and its general application explored through cycles of the action research process.' (Waterman *et al.* 2001:11)

Although wordy, this definition deliberately does not specify a particular underlying philosophical perspective in order that it may encompass the variety of approaches in health care action research and not limit its potential. But what are these different types of action research? Whitelaw *et al.* (2003) highlight three broad types of action research in the literature:

- technical-scientific and positivist
- mutual-collaborative and interpretivist
- critical and emancipatory

Technical-scientific and positivist action research

In the technical-scientific model the action researcher sees themselves as expert and primarily draws on traditional scientific methods to investigate a problem in practice. The main aim of the research is to 'test' the effectiveness of a particular type of intervention. While participants in the study may provide 'on the ground' feedback, they are not seen as being sufficiently expert to get involved in the process of research. This model is often associated with management consultancy and is used a lot by health service managers. The tendency for a top-down approach endangers ownership of both the problem and solution, by staff. However, nurses have also utilised this type of action research (Box 18.1).

Mutual-collaborative and interpretivist action research

This model is most often used by nurses (Box. 18.2) and is more firmly based on the underlying principles of action research identified above. It involves the bringing together of policy makers, researchers, service users and health care providers (practitioners and their managers) to identify potential problems, try out solutions and monitor the process and outcomes of change. It relies on open channels of communication and there being a consensus among participants as to what is needed for change, a willingness to make change happen and joint engagement in the process of research. It is sometimes criticised for being too idealistic and in danger of being too dependent on the presence of the action researcher. Change can be short lived, when those who brokered or supported the change leave.

Personally, I feel this misunderstands the learning that can be gained from attempts to change practice. The success of action research does not depend on

Box 18.1   Example of technical-scientific and positivist action research.

McKenna HP, Parahoo KA, Boore JP (1995) The evaluation of a nursing model for long-stay psychiatric patient care Part 1: literature review and methodology. *International Journal of Nursing Studies* 32: 79–94

McKenna HP, Parahoo KA, Boore JP (1995) The evaluation of a nursing model for long-stay psychiatric patient care Part 2: presentation and discussion of findings. *International Journal of Nursing Studies* 32: 95–113

In this study, a modified action research approach was used to implement a selected nursing model on a long-stay psychiatric ward in Northern Ireland. Within a broader quasi-experimental design, specific quality of care indicators were appraised before and after the implementation of the model. These dependent variables were also monitored on a control ward and data were collected on both wards at one pre-test and two post-test points. Planned change theory was used as a guiding framework for the implementation of the model. Researchers acted as consultants for the participants (ward managers). Results demonstrated that on the experimental ward there were statistically significant improvements in audits of quality of care, patients' and staff's perception of ward atmosphere, patient satisfaction, staff's views about nursing models, and patient dependency levels. However, there were no significant changes noted in nurse satisfaction levels, nor nurses' perception of patients' behaviour.

Box 18.2   Example of mutual-collaborative and interpretivist action research.

Meyer J, Johnson B, Bryar R, Procter S (2003) Practitioner research: exploring issues in relation to research-capacity building. *NT Research* 8: 407–417

This three-year collaborative initiative between City University, Central and East London Education Consortium (CELEC – funding body) and seven NHS trusts (four acute, two primary care and one mental health) involved the development and evaluation of seven lead R&D Nurses in Care for Older People (LN) appointed to assist trusts take forward the National Service Framework for Older People (Department of Health 2001). The LNs used action research to work collaboratively with their trusts (service users, providers and managers) to explore ways of improving evidence-based nursing care for older people. The researchers' role at the university was to help the postholders to identify what support and development they needed in their change agent and research roles and to provide evaluative data for the funder. Findings provide concrete evidence of positive change over time in each of the action research sites. Perceived benefits were highlighted, together with a number of lessons learnt from the process. Overall the project was seen as an effective way to commission nurse education.

whether the intended goals are achieved or the change sustained. Intended goals are often linked to policy initiatives and much can be learned from trying to put policy into practice. Further, it is unrealistic to assume that change will be sustained in ever-changing health care contexts. It can take a long time for new ideas to become embedded in practice.

Critical and emancipatory action research

Research is sometimes naïvely seen as apolitical. The very choices we make about what research approach to take and what data collection methods to use are culturally bound and influenced by those in power (funding bodies and academic élites). This action research model is explicit in its political and critical expression and, as such, not always favoured by funding bodies. It challenges the forces that profit from maintaining particular viewpoints; and values notions of participation, empowerment and emancipation (Box 18.3). The Royal College of Nursing Institute Practice Development Unit advocates the use of critical and emancipatory approaches to changing practice, identifying seven important emancipatory processes (Box 18.4). They also stress the importance of facilitation, clinical supervision and action learning, critical companionship, transformational leadership processes, creative arts and using and developing evidence.

Much of the language used to describe practice development is borrowed from the action research literature and it is sometimes difficult to set it apart. For me, the fundamental difference between practice development and action research lies in the extent to which the process and outcomes of change are systematically and rigorously monitored and in relation to whether the findings are published within

---

Box 18.3   Example of critical and emancipatory action research.

McCormack B, Illman A, Culling J, Ryan A, O'Neill S (2002) 'Removing the chaos from the Narrative': preparing clinical leaders for practice development. *Educational Action Research* 10: 335–351

This study involved ward leaders working with a facilitator over a six-month period, to develop knowledge, skills and experience in leading practice developments. A variety of integrated developmental and data collection techniques were used, including reflection on practice, observation of practice, discussions with practitioners, 360-degree feedback and the use of a variety of creative arts. The project focused on self-awareness, the identification of problems in practice, and the introduction of a way of learning that was active and participatory. However, this project was only successful in engaging four ward leaders and, without the commitment of whole ward teams, transformation of practice was not possible. The authors suggest that raising consciousness alone is not enough to sustain change.

Box 18.4   Royal College of Nursing's seven emancipatory processes for practice development.

- using self-reflection and fostering reflection in others
- development of critical intent of individuals and groups
- developing moral intent
- working with values, beliefs and assumptions
- focusing on the impact of the context on practice
- seeing the possibilities
- fostering widening participation and collaboration by all involved

For further details, and more references: *www.rcn.org.uk/resources/practicedevelopment/about-pd/processes/emancipatory/*

the context of a wider body of knowledge. If systematic rigour is applied and findings are to be shared with an audience outside the study's context then this constitutes 'research' and the usual systems of research governance and ethical approval apply. While practice development can involve many of the same processes as action research, it is primarily undertaken for local improvement and, as such, does not need the same formal quality and ethical assurance mechanisms to be applied. However, both practice development and action research require management permission to take place.

The majority of literature on action research advocates critical and emancipatory approaches. However, paradoxically, its exponents have recently been challenged for generally being affirmative and therefore uncritical in their portrayal of action research, thus ignoring the potential of other models to influence practice (Whitelaw *et al.* 2003). Action research is complex and it is not easy to categorise neatly any specific study into a particular type. For me the value of typologies (*see* Hart and Bond 1995 for a most accomplished example) is to explain this complexity, rather than to label.

The role of the researcher in action research

Critics suggest that action research is no different to what goes on in every day practice, for example, practice development, medical audit, clinical governance, and good management. However, as stated before, the essential difference is the focus on systematically evaluating the process and outcomes of change and reflecting on, and disseminating, findings in relation to what is already known about the topic under study. If, as Stringer (1999) suggests, research is

'systematic and rigorous inquiry or investigation that enables people to understand the nature of problematic events or phenomena' (Stringer 1999:5) then the role of the researcher in action research is to make this happen. Modifying ideas from Mills (2003) in relation to teaching, I would argue it involves a process of working with participants to:

- Describe the problem and area of focus.
- Define the factors involved (e.g. community and agencies involved, health care setting within its historical and sociopolitical context, current practice, patient, practitioner and practice outcomes).
- Develop research questions.
- Describe the intervention or innovation to be implemented.
- Develop a timeline for implementation.
- Describe the membership of the action research group.
- Develop a list of resources to implement the plan.
- Describe the data to be collected (qualitative and quantitative).
- Develop a data collection and analysis plan.
- Gain ethical approval and permission to undertake the study.
- Select appropriate tools of inquiry.
- Carry out the plan (implementation, data collection, data analysis).
- Reflect on and report the results (e.g. final report, professional and academic journals, local newsletters).

Not all practitioners have the skills to undertake research and it is important that they seek adequate levels of support. Action research is often undertaken as part of academic study and supervised by colleagues in higher education. Given its emphasis on learning, action research provides an ideal opportunity for the different agencies involved to personally benefit from the process, for example, submitting work in relation to the study to contribute to academic qualifications. However, academic study is not for all and other types of support might be more appropriate. On the market and internet there are a number of toolkits for action research (*see* Hart and Bond (1995) for a good example).

Ethical issues

An important role of the researcher in action research is to ensure the well-being of participants. This is normally assured by going through a process of formal ethical approval. However, the non-predictive nature of action research means that it is additionally important to mutually agree an ethical code of practice, at the start of the study. Winter and Munn-Giddings (2001) highlight a number of ethical issues and principles of procedure. First they emphasise the importance of maintaining a professional relationship, guided by a duty of care and respect for the individual regardless of gender, age, ethnicity, etc., along with a respect for cultural diversity and individual dignity, as well as protection from harm. This last principle is part of any social researcher's role, in addition to the need for informed consent and honesty. However, Winter and Munn-Giddings (2001) suggest that there are other principles of procedure that should be followed in action research (*see* Box. 18.5).

Box 18.5 Ensuring ethical practice – principles of procedure for action research.

- Make sure discussions are fully documented.
- Establish procedures for taking joint decisions.
- Ensure the work of the project remains 'visible' to all participants
- Check back and get any interpretations authorised before wider circulation.
- Enable participants to amend their contribution before its circulation.
- Ensure progress reports and invite suggestions on future developments.
- Differentiate between what is confidential to participants and intended for wider publication.
- Negotiate acceptable rules of confidentiality.
- Give participants the right to withdraw material containing any reference that may identify them.
- Negotiate in advance how disagreements will be resolved.
- Ensure participants seek the group's permission to use material for academic study.
- Draw up clear statement of principles of procedure, early in the work.

Adapted from Winter R, Munn-Giddings C (2001) *A Handbook for Action Research in Health and Social Care*. London, Routledge pp220–224

Having an ethical code of practice does not negate the additional need for research governance and formal ethical approval for action research. However, these quality processes are made all the more complex by the action researcher not being able to say in advance what the research will do. Action research proposals need to be written in collaboration with participants, often as co-applicants, with an inbuilt degree of flexibility. The action researcher should indicate the likely course of the study, specify the need for flexibility and enter into open and ongoing dialogue with funders and ethical committees to seek approval for emergent changes in design.

Methods of data collection

While action research is often written up as a case study and tends to draw on qualitative methods (Meyer 2000), an eclectic approach to data collection is taken. Usually data collection focuses on three stages of the inquiry (exploration, intervention and evaluation) and, where possible, involves participants, as co-researchers, in the design and execution of the study.

Exploration phase

In the exploratory phase of the study, action researchers gather data to explore the nature of the problem and focus of the study. Data are typically generated through questionnaires, interviews and focus groups in order to seek participant opinion as to what needs to change. If the action researcher is an outsider, this phase often includes some participant observation, in order that the researcher can familiarise themselves with the context and establish good working relationships with participants. It helps if the action researcher has some familiarity with the setting, as the clinical credibility of the action researcher can aid entry into the field. Through a process of feeding back findings to participants, the focus of the study (action) is negotiated. The end of the exploration phase usually involves gathering data in relation to the focus of the study in order to establish a baseline from which to measure change over time. Typically this involves data being generated from audits of practice.

Intervention phase

During this phase, a number of action research cycles usually emerge, as spirals of activity. Each action research cycle comprises a period of planning, acting, observing, reflecting and re-planning. Action research should offer the capacity to deal with a number of problems at the same time and often spirals of activity lead to other spin-off spirals of further work. It would be wrong to give the impression of order and linearity, although action research is often written up in this way so as not to confuse the reader! During this period of intense activity, it is important to monitor the process of change and reflect on learning being gained.

Data are thus usually generated through participant observation methods, reflective journals, diaries, fieldnotes and narratives of practice. Throughout the intervention phase, interim findings are fed back to participants to guide their action. Meanwhile, the action researcher should keep self-reflective fieldnotes throughout the study in order to acknowledge their own subjectivity and demonstrate freedom from bias. It is important that they not only represent the views of all participants, including their own, but that they are also clear about whose voice they are representing and when.

Evaluation phase

There is no neat end to an action research project, as often participants wish to continue with the change processes. However, action researchers need to withdraw from the field to analyse and reflect on what has been learnt, in the context of the wider body of knowledge. Before leaving the field, they typically repeat baseline measures to see if change has occurred over time and invite participants to reflect on what has been achieved (or not) and their explanations for this. In the evaluation phase, it is possible to analyse existing documents and protocols to enhance findings and further set the study in context. Most importantly, all findings should be shared with participants to allow them to comment critically on whether they feel their views have been represented adequately and for them to check that they are happy for the material to be shared with a wider audience.

In the Central and East London Education Consortium (CELEC) Action Research Project (Box 18.2) a variety of data collection methods were used to evaluate the process and outcomes of change. The exploration phase involved establishing a baseline from which to measure change over time in each of the seven Trusts. This was done using the audit instruments Monitor 2000, a tool to measure quality of nursing care (Fearon & Goldstone 1995); and SQUIS, a tool to measure quality of social interaction between nursing staff and patients (Dean *et al.* 1993). Stakeholders (lead R&D nurses, Trust and university staff and representatives of the funder) were also interviewed to explore potential areas in need of development and to determine how to take the project forward. During the intervention phase, a large volume of documentary evidence was collected, including minutes of meetings and internal reports (e.g. annual reports) and, with their agreement, data were also gathered about the issues and concerns that the lead R&D nurses presented in monthly action learning sets.

At the end of each year, the lead R&D nurses were invited to design their own evaluation of the project and to report findings in whatever way they chose. In addition, the project co-ordinator and each of the seven lead R&D nurses kept reflective fieldnotes to capture achievements and lessons learnt. Finally, in the evaluation phase, the baseline measures (Monitor and SQUIS) were repeated and stakeholders re-interviewed to ascertain their views on what had been achieved, problems they had encountered and what had been learnt from the experience. Using these data collection methods, it was possible to demonstrate: concrete evidence of improvement over time (improved scores in Monitor and SQUIS); draw attention to other tangible outcomes (e.g. additional funding awarded to extend the way of working into the independent care home sector); describe perceived benefits (e.g. seen as effective way of commissioning nurse education); and describe the lessons learnt (e.g. support needs for change agents). For further details of the project see Meyer *et al.* (2004).

Assessing quality

What makes action research data trustworthy? Waterman *et al.* (2001) provide key guidance for assessing action research proposals and projects. These criteria were later modified by Greenhalgh *et al.* (2004), but others would question the value of even having such standards or criteria (Lyotard 1979). Bradbury and Reason (2002) engage in this debate and conclude with the need to consider five overlapping issues of quality:

- Was the action research group set up for maximal involvement?
- Was the action research useful?

- Did the action research study acknowledge different ways of viewing the world?
    - ensure conceptual-theoretical integrity?
    - embrace ways of knowing beyond the intellect?
    - intentionally choose appropriate research methods?
- Was the action research perceived to be worthwhile?
- Did the action research lead to significant change in understanding or practice?

Bradbury and Reason (2002) suggest that while these issues deserve our attention, they should only be seen as checkpoints to engage in further dialogue about our work. They recognise that different people will wish to place different emphasis on each issue and, rather than aiming to judge action research as being 'good' or 'bad', these five issues of quality should be used to assess whether action researchers have been explicit about their work.

In addition to addressing trustworthiness of data, it is also important to consider their transferability. Action research is often written up as a case study. As such, the findings are reported in their rich contextual detail in order that the reader can judge the relevance to their own practice situation. Sharp (1998) suggests that case studies also lend themselves well to theoretical generalisation, but acknowledges this is not always attempted. This opens up debates about whether there is any general learning to be gained from specific cases. Bassey (1999) advocates that case study researchers should have more confidence in making fuzzy generalisations about their work. By clearly stating from single cases what researchers consider to be 'possible', 'likely', or 'unlikely' in similar contexts, they protect themselves from the charge of being engaged in trivial pursuit. Meyer *et al.* (2000), drawing on findings that compared a single case of action research with those generated by a systematic review of action research, caution against ignoring the findings from the single case. They argue that the findings from a single case of action research more closely reflect reality and are potentially more valid and meaningful to others. These issues relating to case study research are examined in more detail in Chapter 20.

Research as an agent of change

It could be argued that the ultimate aim of all research is to improve practice. However, most research relies on practitioners to implement findings. Slowly the limitations to this segregated approach of research and development are being recognised. A recent report, describing a systematic review of the literature on the spread and sustainability of innovations in health service delivery and organisation (Greenhalgh *et al.* 2004) recommended 'participatory action research' along with 'realistic evaluation' as the way forward. They saw these approaches as being based on a 'whole-systems' approach, in as much as they are:

- theory-driven
- process rather than 'package-oriented'
- participatory
- collaborative and co-ordinated
- addressed using common definitions, measures and tools
- multidisciplinary and multimethod
- meticulously detailed
- ecological (relational to people and context)

Whole-systems approaches to change management are now favoured, as they recognise the complexity and inevitability of change.

Clearly in action research, research is being used as an agent of change. This implies that the action researcher not only needs research skills, but also an understanding of change and skills in change management. The literature about change management is large and not easy to access. Sometimes change is deliberate, a product of conscious reasoning and actions. This type of change is called 'planned change'. In contrast, change sometimes unfolds in an apparently spontaneous and unplanned way. This type of change is known as 'emergent change'.

According to Isles and Sutherland (2001) change can be emergent in two ways: first, managers can make decisions based on unspoken, and sometimes unconscious, assumptions about the organisation, its environment and the future; and second, external factors (such as the economy, competitors' behaviour, and political climate) or internal features (such as the relative power of different interest groups, distribution of knowledge, and uncertainty) can influence the change in directions outside the control of managers. This highlights the need to identify, explore and if necessary challenge the assumptions that underlie decisions. Further, it is important to understand that organisational change is a process that can be facilitated. Isles and Sutherland (2001) conclude that it is vital to recognise that organisation-level change is not fixed or linear in nature but contains an important emergent element. Gibbons *et al.* (1994) suggest that there is a need to break away from linear thinking to more flexible and creative systems that allow true expertise to flourish. As can be seen from what has already been written above, action researchers take account of these issues in both the design and execution of their studies. Indeed, it has been argued that nurses are leading these developments in the field of health services research (Meyer 1997).

Advantages and disadvantages of action research

Waterman *et al.* (2001) identify eight categories of pivotal factors that can be used to demonstrate the strengths and limitations of action research:

- participation
- key persons

- action researcher-participant relationship
- real-world focus
- resources
- research methods
- project process and management
- knowledge

They argue that for each of these factors, there are opposing aspects that help to provide possible avenues for reconceptualising understanding of the process of action research in health care and that offer ideas for its further development. For me, these issues can be summarised into a number of advantages and disadvantages, which are summarised in Box 18.6.

Box 18.6   Advantages and disadvantages of action research.

Advantages	Disadvantages
In situations where:	
• no evidence exists to support or refute current practice	• not viewed as science
• poor knowledge, skills and attitudes to carry out evidence-based practice	• findings not generalisable
• gaps have been identified in service provision	• vulnerability of participants
• services are underused or deemed inappropriate	• depends on collaboration
• new roles are being developed and implemented	• difficult to achieve and sustain change
• work across traditional conflicting boundaries	• feedback can be threatening
	• change hard to measure
	• poor development of theory

Conclusion

This chapter has explored the nature of action research and demonstrated its value at the 'D' end of the 'Research and Development' spectrum. It has identified common models of working with action research in nursing and suggests caution in adopting any one particular model. It has reflected on the role of the action researcher in action research, highlighting the need for a mutually agreed ethical code of practice. In addition it has described the methods of data collection in relation to three phases of action research (exploration, intervention and evaluation) and given some consideration to the idea of research being an agent of change. Finally, consideration has been given to the advantages and disadvantages of action research. In conclusion, it would appear that action research has much to offer health services research, and it is suggested that nurses are leading the way.

References

Bassey M (1999) *Case Study Research in Educational Settings*. Buckingham, Open University Press

Bradbury H, Reason P (2002) Conclusion: broadening the bandwidth of validity: issues and choice-points for improving the quality of action research. In Reason P, Bradbury H (eds) *Handbook of Action Research: participatory inquiry and practice*. London, Sage pp447–455

Carr W, Kemmis S (1986) *Becoming Critical: education, knowledge and action research*. London, Falmer

Dean R, Proudfoot R, Lindesay J (1993) The quality of interaction schedule (QUIS): development, reliability and use in the evaluation of two domus units. *International Journal of Geriatric Psychiatry* 8: 819–826

Department of Health (2001) *The National Service Framework for Older People*. London, Department of Health

Fearon MM, Goldstone LA (1995) Monitor 2000. *An audit of the quality of nursing care for medical and surgical wards*. Newcastle upon Tyne, Unique Business Services Ltd

Gibbons M, Limoges C, Nowotny H, Schwartzman S, Scott P, Trow M (1994) *The New Production of Knowledge: the dynamics of science and research in contemporary societies*. London, Sage

Greenhalgh T, Robert G, Bate P, Kyriakidou O, Macfarlane F, Peacock R (2004) *How to Spread Good Ideas: a systematic review of the literature on diffusion, dissemination and sustainability of innovations in health service delivery and organization*. Report for the National Co-ordinating Centre for NHS Service Delivery and Organisation R & D (NCCSDO). London, London School of Hygiene and Tropical Medicine

Hart E, Bond M (1995) *Action Research for Health and Social Care: a guide to practice*. Buckingham, Open University Press

Isles V, Sutherland K (2001) *Managing Change in the NHS. Organisational Change: a review for health care managers, professionals and researchers*. Report for the National Co-ordinating Centre for NHS Service Delivery and Organisation R & D (NCCSDO). London, London School of Hygiene and Tropical Medicine

Lyotard JF (1979) *The Postmodern Condition: a report on knowledge*. (trans. Bennington G, Massimi B). Manchester, Manchester University Press

McCormack B, Illman A, Culling J, Ryan A, O'Neill S (2002) Removing the chaos from the narrative: preparing clinical leaders for practice development. *Educational Action Research* 10: 335–351

McKenna HP, Parahoo KA, Boore, JP (1995) The evaluation of a nursing model for long-stay psychiatric patient care Part 1: literature review and methodology. *International Journal of Nursing Studies* 32: 79–94

McKenna HP, Parahoo KA, Boore, JP (1995) The evaluation of a nursing model for long-stay psychiatric patient care Part 2: presentation and discussion of findings. *International Journal of Nursing Studies* 32: 95–113

Meyer J (1997) Action research in health-care practice: nature, present concerns and future possibilities. *NT Research* 2: 175–184

Meyer J (2000) Using qualitative methods in health related action research. *British Medical Journal* 320: 178–181

Meyer J, Johnson B, Bryar R (2004) CELEC Action Research Project: care for older people. Unpublished report, London, City University

Meyer J, Johnson B, Bryar R, Procter S (2003) Practitioner research: exploring issues in relation to research-capacity building. *NT Research* 8: 407–417

Meyer J, Spilsbury K, Prieto J (2000) Comparison of findings from a single case in relation to those from a systematic review of action research. *Nurse Researcher* 7:2 37–53

Mills GE (2003) *Action research: a guide for the teacher researcher*. Upper Saddle River, Merrill/Prentice Hall

Sharp K (1998) The case for case studies in nursing research: the problem of generalisation. *Journal of Advanced Nursing* 27: 785–789

Stringer E (1999) *Action Research*, 2nd edition, London, Sage

Waterman H, Tillen D, Dickson R, de Koning K (2001) Action research: a systematic review and guidance for assessment. *Health Technology Assessment Monograph* 5: 23. London, Department of Health

Whitelaw S, Beattie A, Balogh R, Watson J (2003) *A Review of the Nature of Action Research*. Welsh Assembly Government, Sustainable Health Action Research Programme

Winter R, Munn-Giddings C (2001) *A Handbook for Action Research in Health and Social Care*. London, Routledge

Further reading

Reason P, Bradbury H (2002) *Handbook of Action Research: participative inquiry in practice*. London, Sage

Susman GI, Evered RD (1978) An assessment of the scientific merits of action research. *Administrative Science Quarterly* 582–603 (Dec 23).

Websites

www.did.stu.mmu.ac.uk/carn/ – Collaborative Action Research Network, based at Manchester Metropolitan University, provides a network of action researchers linked to the international journal Educational Action Research

www.uea.ac.uk/care/ – Centre for Applied Research in Education (CARE), a UK action research site at the University of East Anglia offering resources and links to other websites

www.bath.ac.uk/carpp/ – Centre for Action Research in Professional Practice (CARP)

www.parnet.org/ – Participative Action Research Network (PARnet), an action research site in North America offering valuable resources and links to other sites

www.scu.edu.au/schools/gcm/ar/arr/links.html – action research resources at Southern Cross University, Australia provides a list of sites offering links and resources to action research, and related topics

19 Evaluation Research

Colin Robson

Key points

- Evaluation is an inescapable feature of modern life in general, and nursing in particular.
- Evaluation research is different from other forms of research in terms of purpose rather than the methods used.
- There is a range of models of evaluation research available, and selection of the model, and type of data collection, are largely dependent on the type of question to which answers are sought.
- Evaluations that combine different models and/or methods are to be preferred.
- The objective in all evaluations should be to improve the service or practice evaluated.

What is evaluation?

An evaluation seeks to assess the worth or value of something. Newspapers, magazines, television and other media are awash with evaluations of cars, household goods, restaurants, films, theatre productions, concerts, investments and sports performances, to name but a few. Those working in hospitals and other health-related settings and services are not immune to evaluation pressures, as many nurses are only too aware. Such pressures are part of a drive to make both public and private services accountable, to seek reassurance that the resources devoted are achieving the results hoped for, and that there is value for money.

On balance, I regard this as a good thing. Resources are not limitless, and we need to make the best use of them. There is considerable satisfaction in finding out that you are providing a valued and effective service. And – if things are not working well – to know this; and to have suggestions about how improvements might be made. However, evaluations are not necessarily benign. They may be carried out for questionable motives; to give spurious authenticity to a decision made to close a service or to cut costs. They can be carried out incompetently or insensitively. They can engender a climate of fear and suspicion, even in situations where the evaluation is being carried out in good faith.

Why evaluation research?

This is where evaluation research comes in. Evaluation research is a type of research. It is distinguishable from other types or forms of research because of its purpose, which, as indicated above, is to assess the worth or value of whatever is evaluated. In nursing, and other health-related areas this is typically a service, programme, innovation, or intervention, but it can be any aspect of what nurses and other health professionals get involved in. Bringing it under the umbrella of research provides certain safeguards. As discussed in Chapter 1, for a study to qualify as research, not only are certain competencies in the researcher called for, but there is also a commitment to the study being carried out in accordance with stringent ethical guidelines (*see* Chapter 3).

The position taken here is that, while evaluation research has a distinctive purpose, it is not restricted in any way as to the type or style of research that can be used. Evaluation research can use an experimental design and can rely on methods producing quantitative data. But it can 'in appropriate circumstances' be purely qualitative; indeed any of the approaches in Section 3 of this text; and by no means excluding action research or case study.

How do you decide which is appropriate? The choice is largely determined, as in other forms of research, by the questions to which you are seeking answers. The rest of this chapter is mainly concerned with introducing a range of possible approaches. To make a start let us consider the type of evaluation that seems to spring to many people's mind when first asked to evaluate.

The satisfaction questionnaire

In its simplest form this tries to find out what people who have been involved with a service, or whatever, thought about it. It is typically a short self-completion questionnaire concentrating on areas such as usefulness and relevance, mainly consisting of questions with a fixed set of possible answers, and one or two open questions where the response is up to them. As with all methods of collecting data this can be done well or poorly. Careful attention needs to be given to the wording of questions as discussed in Chapter 24. It is crucially important that a high response rate is achieved as, logically, you do not know what non-respondents would have said. When questionnaires are completed in your presence, you should be able to set up the situation so that non-response is rare. However, with postal questionnaires this can be a real problem, calling for sustained efforts to achieve acceptable response rates.

This type of simple evaluation has its value, and continues to be both used and published. Recent examples include Carnwell and Baker (2003) who used a postal questionnaire to women with breast cancer who had experienced specialist nursing services in North Wales; Espeland and Indrehus (2003) who used standardised

questionnaires to assess students' satisfaction with nursing education in Norway;
Gambles *et al.* (2004) who used a simple semi-structured questionnaire to elicit the
views of patients receiving palliative care about a course of reflexology sessions;
and Rollison and Carlsson (2002) who evaluated next-of-kin's experiences of the
'advanced home care' provided during the palliative care and death of a family
member. Somewhat more complex designs can be used, as in Allinson (2004) who
incorporated a control group (Box 19.1)

Box 19.1   Example of an evaluation of satisfaction.

Allinson V (2004) Breast cancer: evaluation of a nurse-led family history clinic. *Journal of Clinical Nursing* 13: 765–766

A study based on a convenience sample of 46 women who were to attend the clinic within a three-month period. A two-part questionnaire was used. The first part, given to the patients before their consultation, asked about the service they had received in the symptomatic clinic the previous year. It was anticipated that this might cause problems with recall; therefore, a control group of 15 women who had yet to be allocated to the nurse-led clinic was also recruited. This group saw the doctor alone and completed the first part of the questionnaire the same day. The second part of the questionnaire was given after the consultation with the nurse. The response rate was very high (44 out of 46; and all 15 in the control) 'as women were asked to complete the questionnaires before leaving the department'. Very similar responses were received from the two groups on the first part, suggesting that the time delay was not affecting responses. Very high satisfaction rates for the nurse-led clinics were obtained and key elements (particularly discussion of family history) isolated. It was acknowledged that 'positive skew is a recognised flaw in patient satisfaction surveys' and possibly that 'patients may have been unwilling to complain about this new service thinking it might be withdrawn'.

Evaluation of satisfaction with services need not be confined to questionnaires,
nor to the views of one group. Turner *et al.* (2004) used semi-structured interviews
in evaluating a pilot client attachment scheme in mental health nursing education
and included students', supervisors' and clients' perceptions of the scheme.
Satisfaction studies are not necessarily small-scale either. For example, Jönsson
and Petersson (2003) in a large-scale, interview-based study evaluated and compared the process of planning and preparing reorganisation at two Swedish hospitals, and evaluated the new organisation in one of the hospitals where it had
been in effect for four years. Their main focus was on the satisfaction of different
groups including nurses, nurse assistants and physicians, and on whether goals
set by planning teams in areas such as personnel development and quality
improvement in nursing care had been achieved.

Beech and Leather (2003) castigate the use of immediate subjective responses
to satisfaction questions, which they refer to as 'happy sheets'. In evaluating a
management of aggression course unit for student nurses they, among other

things, use aggression scenarios, which are presented to students who have to identify risk factors within the scenario. Their demonstration of increases in factors identified, from before, to during, to after the course, provides one route to assessing more objectively the effects of the course on those involved.

It will, I hope, be clear from these examples that evaluations can focus on a variety of things in addition to, or instead of, the satisfaction of those involved. The following section discusses some possible foci.

Models of evaluation

Evaluations can focus on many different things, and answer many different questions, including:

- Finding out if needs are being met – answering questions such as: 'Are clients' needs being met?' or 'Are we reaching the target group?'
- Assessing the outcomes – 'Is the service effective?' 'What happens to clients using the service?'
- How the service is operating – 'What is actually happening?' 'Is it operating as planned?'
- Assessing efficiency – 'How do costs compare with benefits?' 'How does its efficiency compare with possible alternatives?'

Note that, for 'service' read 'procedure', or 'programme', or 'intervention', or 'innovation', depending on the situation.

The different approaches are sometimes referred to as *'models of evaluation'*.

Needs-based evaluation

When the focus is on client needs, it is necessary to establish what these needs are. While the needs that many nursing services seek to meet may appear self-evident to those providing the service, a strong principle behind this approach is that, because it is the client or recipient of the service who has the needs, they should have a strong voice in saying what they are. For example, Chiu *et al.* (2004) sought to establish the needs of family members who had a relative admitted to an intensive care unit (ICU) of a Hong Kong regional hospital, through the use of a version of the Critical Care Family Needs Inventory (Lee *et al.* 2000). The evaluation produced evidence that sessions based on the assessed needs did in fact meet these needs. Note that this study was also outcomes-based (*see* below). A quasi-experimental design showed that an experimental group who had the needs-based programme when compared with a control group who followed had a standard introduction to the ICU environment, had reduced anxiety and an increase in satisfaction of family needs.

A needs assessment can provide the means of finding out needs. It is not an evaluation of an existing service, but a way of determining in advance what type of service would be found valuable. Carrying out an initial needs assessment before developing the service helps to tailor the service to these needs. It makes it less likely that resources are wasted on a service, and also provides a useful agenda to focus an evaluation when the service is up and running. Houston and Cowley (2002) show a way of using needs assessment in the context of health visiting to provide a means of empowering clients. Simons and Petch (2002) describe an example where the needs of patients discharged from psychiatric units in Scotland are assessed, together with the associated needs of community staff providing their community care.

Outcome-based evaluation

This is a traditional form of evaluation, which many, including administrators and service-providers, assume (mistakenly) to be the only valid approach. Undoubtedly, assessing the outcomes of a service, intervention or whatever, is often the main priority. However, outcomes can mean many things. If the service has specified goals or objectives then an obvious outcome is to assess whether they have been achieved. A serious shortcoming of this tight objectives-linked approach is that services and interventions involving people are notorious for having unintended and unanticipated consequences (either in addition to, or instead of, the planned ones). Hence there is advantage in spreading the net wide when considering the possible outcomes of involvement with a service.

The simple satisfaction questionnaire is one form of outcome evaluation. As discussed above, it has serious limitations. However, if the patients find something an unsatisfactory experience, this outcome is likely to have an adverse effect on other aspects.

Weze *et al.* (2004) carried out an outcome evaluation of 'gentle touch' in clients with cancer at a centre for complementary care in the north west of England. Their outcome measures included pre- to post-treatment changes in physical and psychological functioning. While statistically significant improvements were seen on several self-report indices, the design (single group pre-post) is inadequate as an evaluation of the effectiveness of the intervention (*see*, for example, the discussion in Robson 2002:137). This is acknowledged by the authors, who advocate subsequent more rigorous evaluation using a randomised controlled design. Armstrong and Edwards (2004) provide an example of such a study (Box 19.2).

The randomised controlled trial is considered in some influential quarters as the 'gold standard' for evaluation (and other) research, but it is not without its critics (*see* the discussion in Robson 2002:116–23). Lindsay (2004) analyses 47 published randomised controlled trials in the field of nursing research that were published in 2000 or 2001. He identifies bias and unreliability in all of the studies suggesting that inadequate study design is widespread in such trials of nursing interventions.

> **Box 19.2** Evaluation example using a randomised controlled trial.
>
> Armstrong K, Edwards, H (2004) The effectiveness of a pram-walking exercise programme in reducing depressive symptomatology for postnatal women. *International Journal of Nursing Practice* 10: 177–194.
>
> A 12-week randomised trial was set up investigating the effects of an exercise intervention group (a pram-walking programme for mothers and their babies) compared to a non-structured social support group (similar to a playgroup). Comparison between measures of physical fitness and responses to structured questionnaires pre- and post-intervention showed that the primary objectives were achieved. Mothers following the exercise programme showed reduced depressive symptoms and improved fitness as compared to the social support group. Assessment of social support levels showed no changes in either group. A direct association between improvement in fitness and reduction in depression in the pram-walking group is claimed. They also suggest that other factors in combination with improvements in fitness influenced improvements in depression levels.

Process evaluation

This style of evaluation seeks to find out how the programme or service works in practice. What is the experience of those involved? What actually happens on the hospital ward or wherever? Outcome evaluation is typically (though not necessarily) based on methods of data collection that yield quantitative data. Process evaluations typically rely on methods such as observation and interviews, where the data are commonly qualitative. If it has been planned that the service should be delivered in a particular way, one concern for a process evaluation is for possible discrepancies between the planned and the actual.

Wynaden *et al.* (2003) carried out a study evaluating staff perception of a three-month clinical trial of an emergency health triage and consultancy service. This was based on interviews of 11 night duty emergency department staff (both nurses and doctors). It was characterised methodologically as a descriptive, qualitative, exploratory study. High standards of qualitative data analysis were observed in coding, finding categories, clustering, etc., independent checking of transcripts, and establishment of audit trails. The major themes that emerged from the analysis are discussed and there is strong confirmation that the trial demonstrated that this was a highly successful way of working.

When the net is cast wider to include the views of several different groups (or 'stakeholders'), this is sometimes referred to as a 'pluralistic evaluation' (Hall 2004). Duxbury (2002) provides an example (Box 19.3).

Box 19.3   Example of a pluralistic evaluation.

Duxbury J (2002) An evaluation of staff and patient views of and strategies employed to manage inpatient aggression and violence on one mental health unit: a pluralistic design. *Journal of Psychiatric and Mental Health Nursing* 9: 325–337

The views of 80 patients, 72 nurses and 10 medical staff, on three acute mental health wards, were explored. Data were gathered using an incident form, a questionnaire and interviews. The main finding was of a clear distinction between the way staff and patients view both the problem and the response. Patients' views presented staff approaches as 'controlling' with the belief that environmental and poor communication factors underpin aggressive behaviour. Staff, however, attributed aggressive behaviour to internal patient and external factors. A substantial majority of the incidents reported involved verbal aggression as opposed to violent behaviour. Despite this, almost half the responses incorporated medication, restraint or seclusion. Patients viewed such traditional methods as part of the problem. Models were developed to explain the complex nature of patient aggression from different perspectives. Resulting from this, proposals were made for approaches to deal with the problem that are more meaningful and subsequently effective.

Cost-benefit valuation

Assessment of the costs expended in running a service in relation to the benefits accruing is of obvious interest and importance. In cost-benefit analysis the costs measured in monetary terms (pounds, euros, dollars or whatever) are compared with the benefits, also in monetary terms. This is not an easy task in practice, as difficult decisions have to be made, both about what to include, and how to reach the monetary values. Yates (1997) considers problems with the common assumption that outpatient care is far less expensive than inpatient care. For example, the fact that families who play a part in that care will typically have reduced opportunities for employment, in addition to restrictions on their private and social life, could reasonably be entered into the 'costs' side of the equation. In general, however, the relative costing of two or more services or variants of services, is somewhat more straightforward and conclusions about the 'best buy' easier to make. Robson (2000, appendix B) provides an introduction to carrying out these analyses.

Jester and Hicks (2003a; b) use cost effectiveness analysis to compare 'Hospital at Home' and inpatient interventions. The first paper showed hospital at home to be significantly more effective in terms of patient satisfaction and reduced joint stiffness, and at least as effective as inpatient care on a range of other indicators. The second paper is essentially a worked example of how a variety of approaches, including cost-benefit and cost effectiveness analyses, can be used. It is practical and lucid, and is strongly recommended to nurses and others interested in carrying out these types of analyses. Figure 19.1 presents a useful framework, which could be readily adapted to other nursing interventions.

Formative and summative evaluations

A formative evaluation seeks to promote the development of the service or intervention evaluated. A summative evaluation seeks to describe what effect a service or intervention has had on those involved. Outcome evaluations are sometimes characterised as summative, and process evaluations as formative. However the distinction is not clear-cut.

A process evaluation provides information about one aspect of the effects that the intervention is having; i.e. it is in that sense summative. The outcomes of a service or intervention can have a formative influence. Positive outcomes can lead to its continuation and possible extension. Equivocal ones may hasten closure.

A common aphorism is that 'the purpose of evaluation is to improve rather than prove'. Indeed, it could be argued that all evaluations should have a concern for the improvement of whatever is being evaluated. Outcome evaluations are deficient in this respect. Whatever the outcomes, they give little or no direct guidance about what could or should be changed to lead to improvement. Put in other terms, few evaluations (and, in particular outcome evaluations) ask, or seek answers to, the 'why' question. Why does the service or intervention have the effects that it does?

An approach called 'realistic evaluation' (Pawson & Tilley 1997) follows this route. They argue in favour of adopting a realist philosophy, where the task is to identify the mechanisms operating in a situation that led to the observed effects. Building on the finding that most social interventions produce weak overall group effects they set the task as 'finding what works, for whom, in what situations'. Their highly polemical text, which includes a swingeing critique of the utility of randomised control group methodology in evaluation research, has been influential. McEvoy and Richards (2003) make a strong case for a particular form of realism, known as critical realism, providing a basis for a way forward for evaluation research in nursing. They stress the importance for nursing interventions being properly understood if they are to be used effectively in the context of clinical practice. To date, however, there is a dearth of evaluations following this approach in the nursing context.

Quantitative or qualitative?

The examples discussed above incorporate both quantitative and qualitative data collection methods. It is worth reiterating the point made previously, that the choice of quantitative or qualitative methods should be largely dependent on the questions to which you seek answers when doing evaluation research. Pragmatically, it is the case that some audiences find numbers and statistical analysis persuasive.

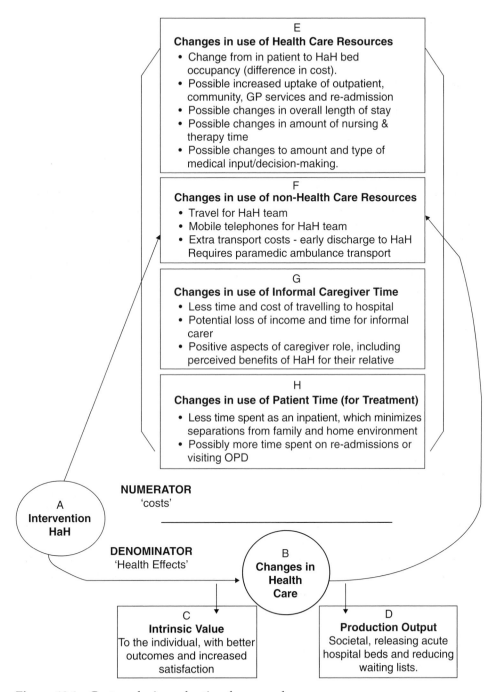

Figure 19.1 Cost-analysis evaluation framework.
Reproduced by permission of Blackwell Publishing from Jester R, Hicks C (2003) Using cost-effectivness analysis to compare Hospital at Home and in-patient interventions. Part 2. *Journal of Clinical Nursing* 12: 20–27
©Blackwell Publishing Ltd, 2003

These audiences, including many administrators and managers, typically call for outcome evaluations, which almost inevitably incorporate the collection of quantitative data. Conversely, some audiences, including practitioners and client groups often more readily empathise with vivid accounts and other forms of qualitative data analysis.

This does not have to be an either/or decision. There can be advantage in asking a range of evaluation questions and using a corresponding range of both quantitative and qualitative data collection methods. Such designs are sometimes referred to as mixed method. The benefits of such an approach are illustrated in a study by Morgan and Stewart (2002). They describe how the use of quantitative (quasi-experimental) and qualitative (grounded theory) methods in an evaluation of new dementia special care units led to a better understanding of how the nursing home environment affects residents with dementia. This study also emphasises the valuable point that evaluation research cannot be perfectly preplanned. It is a process that involves ongoing decisions and management of unexpected events. They describe the sequence of key methodological decisions made during the planning, implementation, and integration phases of the study, conducted over a 21-month period.

The political nature of evaluation

Evaluations inevitably impinge in various ways on those involved. They can affect people's lives, primarily through the ways in which the findings and recommendations are acted upon. But the mere fact that an evaluation is taking place increases the sensitivity of all involved. As a researcher you can try to make it clear that it is the service, innovation or whatever, which is the focus of the evaluation. Staff will still suspect it is their performance that is being assessed.

In other words, evaluations always take place in a political context. The various interest groups, including politicians, administrators, medical staff, nurses, patients, etc. are likely to be influenced or affected by policy decisions arising from the research. Each of these groups may seek to influence the evaluation to best serve their interests.

This poses problems for an evaluator. Are you the 'hired hand' in the pay of those in powerful positions? Or representing the interests of the relatively powerless? The former is ethically dubious, particularly if the choice of evaluation questions is limited to those that the sponsor is comfortable with. The latter is advocated by some and, in seeking to redress inequalities, has its attractions. However, an evaluation which has a concern for all stakeholders, as well as being ethically sound, is likely to be most useful and most likely to be used.

Evaluation research and evidence-based practice

Evaluation research and evidence-based practice (as discussed in Chapter 31) have similar concerns. They are both in the business of assessing value, and both fall within an accountability, value-for-money agenda. As currently conceived evaluation research would seem to have the wider remit; anything and everything is grist to the evaluation mill, whereas evidence-based practice is self-evidently restricted to practice.

Early evaluation research was firmly within the experimental, comparison groups, paradigm. Later developments have a much more broad church view, which this chapter has sought to reflect. To a relative outsider, evidence-based practice shows signs of moving on a similar journey. A quantitative and statistical view where the best, to some the only, evidence comes from randomised controlled trials, appears to be now under question, with wider views of what is meant by 'evidence'.

Conclusion

A central aim of this chapter is to make it clear that evaluation research can come in many forms and styles. It can vary from the one-off small-scale study by someone evaluating a situation or practice with which they are directly involved, to the multi-site extended evaluation of national initiatives by a large research team. Newell (2003) in an editorial for the journal *Clinical Effectiveness in Nursing* sought to encourage the incorporation of evaluations routinely into nursing practice developments, pointing out that in the *Making a Difference* programme (Department of Health 1999), which proposes new nursing, midwifery, and health visiting roles and activities in the UK NHS, an evaluation element is conspicuous by its absence.

Finally, do remember that evaluation research is inevitably political (in that it is likely to affect the interests of one or more groups) and partly because of this is always sensitive. Make sure that you have given serious attention to the ethical issues involved.

References

Allinson V (2004) Breast cancer: evaluation of a nurse-led family history clinic. *Journal of Clinical Nursing* 13: 765–766

Armstrong K, Edwards H (2004) The effectiveness of a pram-walking exercise programme in reducing depressive symptomatology for postnatal women. *International Journal of Nursing Practice* 10: 177–194

Beech B, Leather P (2003) Evaluating a management of aggression unit for student nurses. *Journal of Advanced Nursing* 44: 603–612

Carnwell R, Baker SA (2003) A patient-focused evaluation of breast care nursing specialist services in North Wales. *Clinical Effectiveness in Nursing* 7: 18–29

Chiu YL, Chien WT, Lam LW (2004) Effectiveness of a needs-based education programme for families with a critically ill relative in an intensive care unit. *Journal of Clinical Nursing* 13: 655–656

Department of Health (1999) *Making a Difference: strengthening the nursing, midwifery and health visiting contribution to health and health care.* London, Department of Health

Duxbury J (2002) An evaluation of staff and patient views of and strategies employed to manage inpatient aggression and violence on one mental health unit: a pluralistic design. *Journal of Psychiatric and Mental Health Nursing* 9: 325–337

Espeland V, Indrehus O (2003) Evaluation of students' satisfaction with nursing education in Norway. *Journal of Advanced Nursing* 42: 226–236

Gambles M, Crooke M, Wilkinson S (2004) Evaluation of a hospital based reflexology service: a qualitative audit of patient perceptions. *European Journal of Oncology Nursing* 6: 37–44

Hall JE (2004) Pluralistic evaluation: a situational approach to service evaluation. *Journal of Nursing Management* 12: 22–27

Houston AM, Cowley S (2002) An empowerment approach to needs assessment in health visiting practice. *Journal of Clinical Nursing* 11: 640–650

Jester R, Hicks C (2003a) Using cost-effectiveness analysis to compare Hospital at Home and in-patient interventions, Part 1. *Journal of Clinical Nursing* 12: 13–19

Jester R, Hicks C (2003b) Using cost-effectiveness analysis to compare Hospital at Home and in-patient interventions, Part 2. *Journal of Clinical Nursing* 12: 20–27

Jönsson AC, Petersson H (2003) Participation of professional categories when reorganizing two hospitals – a comparative study and an evaluation. *Journal of Nursing Management* 11: 234–241

Lee IYM, Chien WT, Mackenzie AE (2000) Needs of families with a relative in a critical care unit in Hong Kong. *Journal of Clinical Nursing* 9: 46–54

Lindsay B (2004) Randomized controlled trials of socially complex nursing interventions: creating bias and unreliability? *Journal of Advanced Nursing* 45: 84–94

McEvoy P, Richards D (2003) Critical realism: a way forward for evaluation research in nursing? *Journal of Advanced Nursing* 43: 411–420

Morgan DG, Stewart NJ (2002) Theory building through mixed-method evaluation of a dementia special care unit. *Research in Nursing and Health* 25: 479–488

Newell R (2003). Evaluating and disseminating practice development. *Clinical Effectiveness in Nursing* 7: 1–2

Pawson R, Tilley N (1997) *Realistic Evaluation.* London, Sage

Robson C (2000) *Small-Scale Evaluation: principles and practice.* London, Sage

Robson C (2002) *Real World Research: a resource for social scientists and practitioner-researchers,* 2nd edition. Oxford, Blackwell

Rollison B, Carlsson M (2002) Evaluation of advanced home care (AHC). The next-of-kin's experiences. *European Journal of Oncology Nursing* 6: 100–106

Simons L, Petch A (2002) Needs assessment and discharge: a Scottish perspective. *Journal of Psychiatric and Mental Health Nursing* 9: 435–445

Turner L, Callaghan P, Eales S, Park A (2004). Evaluating the introduction of a pilot client attachment scheme in mental health nursing education. *Journal of Psychiatric and Mental Health Nursing* 11: 414–421

Weze C, Leathard HL, Grange J, Tiplady P, Stevens G (2004) Evaluation of healing by gentle touch in 35 clients with cancer. *European Journal of Oncology Nursing* 8: 40–49

Wynaden D, Chapman R, McGowan S, McDonough S, Finn M, Hood S (2003) Emergency department mental health triage consultancy service: a qualitative evaluation. *Accident and Emergency Nursing* 11: 158–165

Yates BT (1997) Formative evaluation of costs, cost-effectiveness, and cost-benefit: toward cost-procedure-process-outcome analysis. In Bickman L, Rog DJ (eds) *Handbook of Applied Social Research Methods*. Thousand Oaks, Sage pp285–314

Further reading

Chen HT (2004) *Practical Program Evaluation: accessing and improving planning, implementation and effectiveness*. Thousand Oaks, Sage

Hall I, Hall D (2004) *Evaluation and Social Research: introducing small-scale practice*. Basingstoke, Palgrave Macmillan

Robson C (2000) *Small-Scale Evaluation: principles and practice*. London, Sage

Websites

http://nmap.ac.uk/ – Nursing, Midwifery and Allied Professions (NMAP) site, a major UK gateway to internet research in nursing, midwifery, and allied health areas. Search on 'evaluation research' for a wide range of useful links to relevant sites. They include full evaluation reports not available as journal articles, all of which have been quality-assessed

www.york.ac.uk/inst/crd/ – Centre for Reviews and Dissemination includes databases on NHS Economic Evaluations (NHSEED), and of abstracts of reviews of effects (DARE)

gsociology.icaap.org/methods/ – free resources for anyone carrying out evaluation research (particularly those without easy access to academic libraries). The focus is on 'how-to-do' evaluation research, and the methods used, covering, for example, surveys, focus groups, sampling and interviews. Most of these links are to resources that can be read over the web.

www.policy-evaluation.org/ – site devoted to evaluation with extensive links to resource guides and databases. There are also links to mailing lists including EVALTALK (a general and lively discussion group on issues involved with doing evaluation research) and GOVTEVAL (which focuses on public sector evaluations). It can be fascinating to 'lurk' on these lists (i.e. to join but not make contributions yourself), and members are typically very helpful to new evaluators with queries

www.jameslindlibrary.org/ – for a broader, historical, perspective on evaluation research, I recommend marking the 250th anniversary of James Lind's evaluation of different treatments for scurvy, which details the evolution of tests of treatment effects, ranging from an Old Testament (Daniel, chapter 1:16) description of a controlled test of diets, through an 11th century Chinese evaluation of the effects of ginseng, to the present day

20 Case Study Research

Charlotte Clarke and Jan Reed

Key points

- Case study research explores a phenomenon in its context and assumes that this context is of significance to the phenomenon.
- It is a flexible and holistic approach to research design in which data collection is shaped by the boundaries of the case being studied.
- A critical step is to define the case, making sure that it illustrates the issue under investigation.
- Insider knowledge of the context, or at least the ability to access it, is important in shaping the sampling and data collection methods.
- The ability to transfer knowledge beyond the case is important in developing high-quality case study research.

Introduction

For many practitioners the idea of case study methodology strikes several chords. As practitioners have become more aware of the importance of taking a holistic and individualised approach to care, a research method that is in tune with these ideas seems a natural fit. Case study methodology has a connection with the ways in which nurses and other health care practitioners think about practice, in terms of 'cases' or individual service users. This connection between research and practice is perhaps most clearly demonstrated by the use of the 'case study' in health care practice. The medical profession, for example, have a long tradition of using 'cases' as a method of exploring practice, from the case conference where people gather to assess and plan care, to the case study publication in professional journals, where an example of a patient's history and treatment is presented.

As such, case study research offers a valuable means of exploring a phenomenon in its context and assumes that the context is of significance to understanding the phenomenon. Phenomena may be conceptual (such as vulnerability), or people, or organisational depending on the focus of the research being undertaken. This emphasis on knowing the phenomenon in its context and as it occurs in practice characterises case study research and even those forms of case study that are single-case clinical trials (e.g. testing within a single individual whether a new medication improves their health) assume the need to understand the impact of the context on the establishment, processes and outcomes of the phenomenon.

Using case studies in research, then, has a resonance with professional practice. It offers the opportunity of learning in a way that pays attention to and respects the individuality and unique nature of service users and services. In addition it is a way of exploring the dimensions of each case in a holistic way, where key factors or variables can be investigated as their relevance becomes evident in each case, rather than to a preset research design.

This flexibility and individuality, however, leads to the main difficulties of case study research. First, there is the problem of relevance to other cases, sometimes expressed in other traditions as 'generalisability'. In other words there is a question about how the phenomena observed in one case can have any relevance to other cases – after all, if it has no relevance then the effort to learn has very little benefit for wider practice. The second difficulty is one of structure and design, that is if case studies are too flexible and data can be collected in an *ad hoc* way as and when it looks interesting or becomes available, then there is a danger of the original questions being lost in a sea of data, producing findings which do not go very far in addressing the issues which gave rise to the study.

Both of these points have been raised in the literature discussing case study research (*see* for example, Corcoran *et al.* 2004; Meyer 2003; Yin 1994). Writers have either dismissed case studies as a useful approach because of perceived methodological limitations, or argued that its potential has not been realised because researchers have had only a superficial understanding of the methodology, seeing it simply as a convenient label to describe their small-scale studies. Writers have exhorted case study researchers to pay more attention to the theoretical and methodological aspects of case studies in order to move beyond these limitations. As Corcoran *et al.* (2004) have argued:

> 'case study research . . . falls short of its promise due to a lack of theorising about the research methodology or an understanding about the methodology' (Corcoran *et al.* (2004:7)

It is useful to outline some of the measures that allow case study research to confidently challenge these criticisms and ensure high-quality research. In principle, the measures are no different from those needed of high-quality research of any design, namely that the researcher should:

- Have an effective conceptualisation of the issue under study and the research questions. For case study research this means knowing how to define 'the case', something that is somewhat harder to achieve than may at first appear.
- Have a good understanding of the research philosophy that is being used. This will ensure that data is collected that 'fits' together, it all contributes to addressing the question and helps to avoid the risk of collecting whatever data is to hand (the magpie effect).
- Think through carefully what is being learnt from the case study and how this can contribute to learning that is beyond the specific case. For example, case study methods may be best at answering questions about processes, and the

notion of a population from which a sample is drawn may be very different to that of other research approaches.

It is important to emphasise that case study research is complex and tackles real-life issues in their full glory in practice! The scale and scope of case studies is very variable and they can be very substantial multi-site studies. It is certainly not a way of adding gloss to a poor quality and poorly developed research design, whether small or large-scale. This chapter includes illustrations from several studies that we have been involved with which use case study approaches, either as part of a larger study or as the primary research design.

Definitions of case study methodology

One of the most commonly quoted definitions of case study methodology is that by Yin (1994) who described the case study as an approach to empirical enquiry that:

'investigates a contemporary phenomenon within its real-life context, when the boundaries between phenomenon and context are not clearly evident' (Yin 1994: 13).

There are, of course, other definitions, but this one is used frequently, perhaps because it comes from one of the key writers on case studies, whose book, first published in 1984, has become an important resource for researchers. It also points to some of the features of a research question that would make case study methodology appropriate. First there is the emphasis on the contemporary nature of the phenomenon, second there is the importance placed on its 'real-life' nature, and finally, and most importantly, there is the idea that a division between setting and phenomenon is difficult to draw: the phenomenon is intimately connected to the context, and to research one without the other would be to produce only a partial account of what is happening.

Case study research, then, is about treating the phenomenon being researched as a distinct entity or case, and exploring it in the context in which it occurs. This, however, does not explain what a case is, or how this can be demarcated, so further clarification is needed. This is quite a difficult move to make, paradoxically, because the links between phenomena and context that are so integral to the justification of using a case study approach make it difficult to put boundaries around a case for the purposes of definition.

One way to approach this is to eschew an overall definition of a case which could be applied across studies, and to see this definitional process as one which each researcher needs to engage with: in other words that the definition of a case needs to be thought through carefully in the light of the research goals of the study. For example, if the goal is to understand the experiences of an individual service user, then the case can be defined around that service user, their experiences and thoughts. If the study is about how an organisation responds to change, then the case can be defined as an organisation. This is not to say that the case needs to be defined as an inviolable unit that cannot be thought of in different ways: there may be a utility in breaking down a case into subunits for the purpose of data collection and analysis. A case study of a family, for example, may be broken down at some point into parents and children as sub-units, depending on the questions being asked. Matching the boundaries of the case study to the research questions being asked enables the data collection and analysis to be focused and relevant. Defining the case, then, can be seen as a process not reliant on textbook terminology but on the specific aims and focus of the research.

Defining the case depends much on the 'pre-understanding' of the researcher (Gummesson 1998). Meyer (2003) has described this pre-understanding as potentially arising from:

> 'general knowledge such as theories, models and concepts or from specific knowledge of institutional conditions and social patterns' (Meyer 2003:331)

Researchers come to projects from a range of different experiences and debates about the researched topic. Building on 'pre-understanding' leads to the definition of the case and its boundaries, the processes of data collection, and the process of data analysis. As Gummesson (1998) has argued, the challenge for researchers is not to split their pre-understanding from their research, but to be:

> 'able to balance on a razor's edge using their pre-understanding without being its slave' (Gummesson 1998:58)

Pre-understandings lead to research aims and questions, which then lead to specific definitions of what a case is for a particular study.

Nurses and other health care practitioners have a particular advantage in pre-understanding the issues and contexts they seek to research as they possess considerable 'insider' knowledge from their practice experiences (Reed et al. 1996). The challenge lies in using this insider knowledge effectively to shape research questions and design.

Much like grounded theory, case study approaches to research may integrate sampling with data collection and with data analysis, each informing the other. For example, the analysis of one piece of data may suggest that the study could be informed by data collected from a different part of an organisation. This allows for structured and defensible flexibility in the research and maximises the ability of the study to respond to the theoretical sensitivity of the researcher.

Research questions

A fundamental part of carrying out a case study is to identify the research questions. This is pertinent, of course, in any study, but because of the individual nature of the case study, the research questions and the ways of answering them are correspondingly individual, and need careful thinking through: methodology cannot be simply 'off the peg' i.e. standardised and pre-determined. Bergen and While (2000) describe how case study method has derived from a wide variety of disciplines, each with their own methodological orientation (e.g. pure science through to sociology) and implications for the research questions asked. Case study methodology can be either quantitative or qualitative, that is the research questions can be about exploring the case, either in words or numbers. In addition case studies may have goals or questions that are about describing phenomena or making links (often causal between aspects of phenomena). These different aims give rise to questions as follows:

> How does this family deal with and manage the implications of this family member's health problem?

> How are services for people with this health problem organised?

> How do staff manage appointments in this clinic?

> Has the re-organisation of the system for making appointments reduced non-contact time for the staff?

These questions are a mix of the descriptive, 'what is happening here?', and the inferential, 'how are these things linked here?' They will vary according to the research aims and how it is hoped they will inform and contribute to debates about practice, policy or theory. There should be a logical flow from the research question to the selection of the case and the process of data collection and analysis.

Selection of cases

Discussions of sampling in case study methodology are somewhat different from those of other research approaches. They go back to the pre-understanding of the researcher and what they want to do with their research, and are therefore about how a case can be defined, its constituents, and its boundaries. Some approaches, for example, Soft Systems Methodology (SSM) (Checkland & Scholes 1999) can work well with case study methodology, because they have a theoretical framework that is specific about the dimensions of the phenomena being studied. Soft Systems Methodology focuses on the communication patterns within and between organisations, and provides a framework for identifying what the constituents of a system might be. It is based on the idea that the way to understand organisational activity is to think of it as being part of a communication system, and that exploration should focus on the way that communication happens across the system. Soft Systems Methodology has an inherent set of research goals, and a way of defining a case as the system of communications between and within organisations. Starting off with one point in the system, the boundaries of the case can be mapped out by asking who communicates with whom at this point. The identification of the sample is shaped by the theory underpinning the study. An example of Soft Systems Methodology in a case study design is given in Box 20.1.

Box 20.1   Using soft systems methodology in practice development research.

Clarke CL,Wilcockson J (2001) Professional and organisational learning: analysing the relationship with the development of practice. *Journal of Advanced Nursing* 34: 264–272

Clarke CL, Wilcockson J (2002) Seeing need and developing care: exploring knowledge for and from practice. *International Journal of Nursing Studies* 39: 397–406

The study aimed to understand how developments in practice spread and were sustained within an organisation. Three case study sites were identified as NHS organisations with a good level of practice development. Approximately 15 people in each organisation were interviewed about the ways in which they develop practice and why. The Soft Systems Methodology guided questions about the social and political aspects of practice development as well as organisational structures and allowed theory to be developed and explored with the participants.

Where a theoretical framework is not so clear, however, researchers need to think through their definition of the phenomena under study very carefully in order to map out its dimensions. It may be necessary for some preliminary work to be done to make sure that the cases chosen will help to answer the research questions. This issue arose in a study being undertaken by the authors at the time of writing that was examining specialist services for older people. It began with a national survey to identify the scope and range of specialist services, and then explored the processes of development in more detail, focusing on the development of specialist nursing roles. The sampling matrix shown in Table 20.1 was circulated to the research steering group so that the variables identified by the project team could be ranked by steering group members in order of importance to the project aims (the final ranking is given in the right-hand column).

The ranking of the variables was based on the research objectives and was translated into a sampling matrix (Reed *et al.* 1996). Matrix sampling is a process where the key variables of interest in a study are laid out in a matrix form. Possible cases for inclusion in a study are entered into the matrix, so that the characteristics are set out in a way that makes selection processes visible to researchers and readers. This allowed the team to match up case study sites with the research priorities and ensure that there was a range of cases that would explore key issues and reflect the range of models of specialist services that had been developed.

A further concern is whether a sample should be homogenous or heterogeneous, in other words whether the case study should include similar or dissimilar phenomena. Again this is a product of the study aims: it may be that a case study will seek out a range of phenomena in order to broaden the understanding of

Table 20.1 Sampling criteria for case study sites for specialist services and older people survey.

Sampling criteria	Rank
Roles of specialised staff (i.e. whether they are used as advisors to other staff, or have a direct role in care provision),	1
How does the service utilise user opinion/feedback/advocacy groups (e.g. in-service development or service audit).	2
Integration and partnership of trust activity across the whole system of service provision (i.e. whether the role is restricted to the trust or has the potential to impact on other agencies)	3
How the client group has been demarcated (i.e. whether older people are explicitly identified as a group, or whether this is subsumed under other headings, such as medical speciality or type of provision)	4
How the service/post has been developed	5
How does the service offer services for older people of diverse ethnic backgrounds/or cater for older people of all ethnic backgrounds?	6
Which National Service Framework-Older Person themes and/or standards does this service contribute to?	7

difference, or it may be that a study would select similar examples in order to increase the amount of data available over a narrower range.

This discussion of sampling echoes the earlier discussions about the definitions of a case. Case study approaches can involve 'sub-units' where a case may have different components, so a case study of an organisation may involve a number of different departments or partners or clients, which may be chosen because of their similarities or differences. Moving up a level of unit of analysis, the sampling strategy for the study as a whole may involve multiple case study sites, which might, as with case sub-units, be selected in order to provide contrasting examples or similar ones.

The context dependency of case study research leads to the need for local knowledge to ensure that sampling reflects this context. As a result sampling in case study research for researchers who are unfamiliar with the area can be particularly complex. One approach that we have developed and used in a number of studies takes a multistage approach to sampling. For example, Box 20.2 illustrates the sampling flow from issue to unit of data collection within a case. Boxes 20.3 and 20.4 describe studies that illustrate this process in practice.

Research design

The idea of flexible sampling is linked to the idea of a flexible research design. The design, for example, can have a built in facility for inductive sampling (where subsequent samples are based on previous analysis of data and intended to allow deeper analysis of the phenomenon), as an initial case study leads to a need to

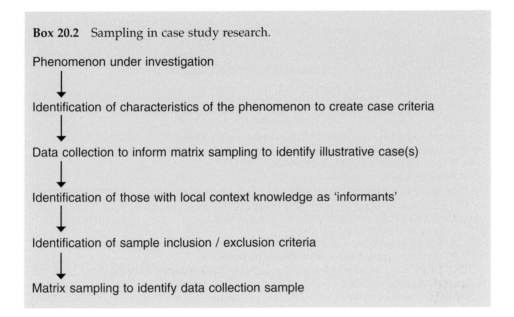

Box 20.2   Sampling in case study research.

Phenomenon under investigation

Identification of characteristics of the phenomenon to create case criteria

Data collection to inform matrix sampling to identify illustrative case(s)

Identification of those with local context knowledge as 'informants'

Identification of sample inclusion / exclusion criteria

Matrix sampling to identify data collection sample

explore the research question with further cases chosen for their utility in exploring key issues. Alternatively, the design can be planned from the outset. Yin (1994) has talked about multiple case studies, where parallel investigations can be carried out, again, either to explore differences or similarities as indicated in the research question.

There are, though, challenges to achieving consistency across multiple case study sites. Box 20.5 describes a study into Help the Aged voluntary sector schemes that tackled some of these problems. Appreciative inquiry gave the research a coherence, which could have been missing given the diversity of the schemes and the differences in background and experience of the researchers. Appreciative inquiry is an approach to organisational evaluation and learning which begins by identifying and examining examples of successful working, and further explores ways of building on these (Reed *et al.* 2002). This allowed the analysis to identify the unique developments in the study sites, and the lessons to be learned across sites.

Data analysis

This chapter began by pointing out the criticism levied at case studies regarding the failure of the methodology to reach its potential because of the lack of rigour in analysis. As case studies are so embedded in particular contexts, it is tempting

Box 20.3 Case study sampling in a leadership course evaluation.

Clarke C, Reynolds J, McClelland S, Reed J (2004a) *Evaluation of the NHS Leading Modernisation Programme*. Final Report. Northumbria University, Newcastle

In an evaluation of a leadership course for modernisation leads in Strategic Health Authorities (SHAs) that was commissioned by the NHS Modernisation Agency:

- The phenomenon was defined as the processes of modernisation activity in SHAs.
- The case criteria (identified after various forms of data collection and analysis) were:
    - gender of SHA modernisation lead
    - geographical location
    - doctoral level registration status of SHA modernisation lead as part of the leadership course
    - whether posts had been held outside the NHS
    - level of academic qualification
    - pre-course profile of individual in relation to leadership and modernisation activity
    - general management and/or clinical background
- Five SHAs were selected as case study sites following matrix mapping of all 28 SHAs against the case criteria.
- The informants were identified as the SHA modernisation leads who were participants in the leadership course.
- The sample criteria within each SHA sought to identify a sample of stratified maximum variation, which is designed to maximise the generation of information rather than seeking generalisation.
- Using the sampling criteria the informants each identified 24 people in their SHA (e.g. 'people who have most influenced the way that I modernise', 'people who I think have implemented modernisation activities across boundaries and/or agencies') and mapped them on a further sampling matrix against various criteria (e.g. 'this person has been particularly involved with leadership/care delivery systems/improvement science', 'this person is employed by NHS/other organisation'). From this pool of nominated people, the research team selected 15 for interview in each site, ensuring diversity and breadth in the sample.

to produce an analysis with only local relevance. There is a huge difference between simply saying 'this is what happened in this case' and extending this to discuss the relevance of this case to broader issues.

There are three approaches that can be taken to consider the way in which case study research can contribute to broader issues. First, this needs to be built into the research questions and study design from the outset. Appropriate modelling and theorising of the phenomenon from its conception will ensure that the study is set up to produce data amenable to analysis that can make a wider contribution. For example, the project described in Box 20.3 was commissioned as an evaluation of a leadership course, but was also designed to contribute to a knowledge base about the processes of practice and service development. As much was learned

Box 20.4 Case study sampling in dementia care research.

Clarke CL (1999) Family caregiving for people with dementia: some implications for policy and professional practice. *Journal of Advanced Nursing* 29: 712–720

In this case study, the issue concerned the experiences of someone with dementia and so the case was that of an individual who had dementia and their family and non-family carers. Each of the nine cases was identified through services to which they were known and these people with dementia in turn nominated a family member and identified non-family carers who could be approached for interview. In this way, each case involved data collection with the person with dementia, one family member and up to three non-family carers.

Clarke C, Luce A, Gibb C, Williams L, Keady J, Cook A, Wilkinson H (2004b) Contemporary risk management in dementia: An organisational survey of practices and inclusion of people with dementia. *Signpost* 9: 1 27–31

In a study exploring how people with dementia construct and manage risk the 56 people with dementia (who were interviewed twice over two months) each nominated a family member and a non-family carer for interview. In this way many case studies were created and this high number of cases to explore the issue under investigation poses particular challenges at the point of analysis.

about the ways in which people and services modernise as was learned about the leadership course. To achieve this, the research team needed to possess or know how to access local on-the-ground knowledge to ensure context sensitivity. They also had to be sufficiently aware of the contemporary knowledge base and philosophical options to allow theoretical sensitivity to inform the project development.

Second, having collected the data there is a need to analyse it in two ways. Initially, the internal patterns in the data must be carefully teased out and confirmed, whether through qualitative or quantitative data analysis methods. This is the level of analysis that is most often described and concerns getting to grips with the detail of the data itself and organising it in a way that allows those patterns to be described. In the second way, which may be concurrent with the first or most often will follow it, the results of the data analysis need to be analysed in relation to the external knowledge base generated by other research and the practice and policy environment. This can be best described as external patterning. In this way, the contribution of the internal data analysis can be explored in relation to the external knowledge environment and the study's contribution to that knowledge base carefully articulated.

Third, there needs to be careful consideration of the transferability of the results of the study from one context to another. This has some similarities to the process of generalising from a sample to a wider population in that the researcher needs

Box 20.5   Using appreciative inquiry to guide data collection.

Reed J, Jones A, Irvine J (2005) Appreciating impact: evaluating small voluntary organisations in the United Kingdom. *Voluntas: International Journal of Voluntary and Non-profit Organisations* 16: 123–141

This study was commissioned by Help the Aged to explore the achievements of local voluntary sector schemes. The 10 schemes selected by Help the Aged for the evaluation were each very different, in systems, goals and structures. In addition, the data were collected by a team of researchers with various backgrounds, experiences and skills. A case study approach was used to capture the unique characteristics of the schemes, but the same methodological model, appreciative inquiry, was used to ensure that the data collected were consistent, to allow the synthesis of findings across cases (Quinn Patton 2003).

Each scheme was visited by a designated researcher from the team when appreciative inquiry interviews (with users, volunteers, staff and stakeholders) were carried out, and the background information was collected about the schemes. Participants were invited to share their experiences and describe what they valued about those experiences. They were asked to give an example from their experience of when the scheme worked really well for them. Then the 'miracle question' was posed: 'Suppose one night a miracle occurred and everything is in place to make this scheme better – what would the miracle be?' The next stage – 'dialoguing what should be' – focused on ideas and actions to achieve the vision identified during stage two. The interviewees were asked about the steps or recommendations that would help the scheme to develop in the way they had envisioned.

This framework was used for all of the interviews. For the individual interviews, the researcher led the participants through the stages. For large groups, where the participants were willing and able to interview each other, they worked in pairs. The researcher facilitated the group session by introducing each stage of the process, allowing time for discussion to take place. Where the participants were not willing or able to divide into pairs, the researcher facilitated a group discussion using the appreciative inquiry framework. Written notes were made during the interviews by the researcher, and by the interviewees where they were able to do this. Particular attention was given to the recording of apposite statements and quotes. This captured the key issues and experiences of the participants as they moved through the appreciative inquiry process.

to know what characteristics of the sample need to be present in the wider population to legitimately claim that the results can be generalised from one to the other. In case study research there needs to be an examination of the factors that reside in the context, and which can be found in other contexts, in order that claims of transferability may be made with some credibility. The classic example is a case study of some innovative development that is perceived to have happened 'only because Mary is here' and that if others had a Mary then they would achieve the same development. It is important to move beyond the 'Mary factor' and analyse just what it is about the way in which Mary works and has been able to work within the organisation that has allowed an innovation to occur. In this way, having examined and analysed data within its context, there is a step required of

de-contextualising the issue, transferring it to another context and re-contextualis-
ing it there. In other words, the analysis of context needs to identify the critical
aspects of context that would allow something to be used elsewhere so long as
certain critical aspects of context were (or were not) present.

One important consideration in the analysis of data in multiple case study
research is the extent to which data are analysed within or across cases. It may be
that the cases have been purposefully selected to reflect different dimensions of
the phenomenon. In this situation, analysis across case is necessary to ensure that
all dimensions are taken into account in developing the findings from the data.
Cross-case analysis can be used to emphasise commonality or difference between
cases. Within case analysis, where each case is taken in turn and analysed as an
interdependent set of data, this will maximise identification of the context dependent aspects of the phenomenon. For example, Stake (1995) refers to seeking to
refine an understanding of an issue by searching for patterns across a number of
cases. For most studies, some analysis at both 'within' and 'across case' level is
appropriate. In the study of care management conducted by Bergen and While
(2000), Yin's (1994) ideas of designating a unit smaller than the case for the purposes of analysis was adopted: the case was care management and the unit of
analysis was individual community nurse's practice.

Data analysis in case study research requires attention to the analytical demands
of the very wide range of data sources that may be involved. Yin (1994) refers to
documentation, archival records, direct observation, participant observation,
interviews and physical artefacts as of equal relevance to case study research.
Many of these, such as documentary analysis, are a way of using pre-existing
materials as data sources (Reed 1992). While such data has the advantage of being
relatively 'untouched' by the research process, as it was written for other reasons,
it has been produced for particular audiences, and these need to be borne in mind
when analysing these data.

Presentation and reporting

The presentation and reporting of any research study requires consideration of
the audience. In case study research this is coloured in particular by issues such
as maintaining confidentiality and the plurality of audiences. As case study
research is context-dependent, it is necessary to describe organisations and people
in considerable detail and even if anonymity of names is maintained this level of
context description may make it quite easy for people and places to be identified.
This should be acknowledged with participants at the start of the research and it
may be necessary for some forms of reporting to obscure the association between
place/person and reported detail. This may be most easily achieved through
cross-case reporting which does not seek to portray each case individually. On the
other hand, people and organisations can become very involved in case study
research and naturally wish to see their role profiled appropriately. They may also

wish to learn what they can from the work and in this instance they may find it most helpful to receive the research presented in a way that is very explicit about each case. For example, in the Help the Aged study described earlier, brief reports were written for each case study site that were in addition to the overall (and more public) report of the research in which only the cross-case analysis was presented.

In addition, reporting to people and organisations in a way that is accessible for their practice needs to be complemented by making the findings of the research accessible to the wider academic and practice communities through publication and presentations. To achieve this effectively will require the work to have relevance beyond the local case study sites, as described above. There also needs to be a level of theoretical analysis in presenting and disseminating the work so it can be transferred to other settings and that has the catalytic ability to make people think about their current knowledge and practice.

Conclusion

In conclusion, case study research is unique in the emphases it places on the importance of the context and the impact of the context on the phenomenon under investigation. The design, sampling and data collection methods reflect this emphasis on context dependency. There is however, a need to analyse the data and articulate the findings in a way that is both respectful of this context and that allows the research to be transferred to other environments. It is a form of research that is attractive to researchers and practitioners alike and that draws on the knowledge base of both.

References

Bergen A, While A (2000) A case for case study studies: exploring the use of case study design in community nursing research. *Journal of Advanced Nursing* 31: 926–934

Checkland P, Scholes J (1999) *Soft Systems Methodology in Action*. Chichester, Wiley

Clarke CL (1999) Family caregiving for people with dementia: some implications for policy and professional practice. *Journal of Advanced Nursing* 29: 712–720

Clarke CL, Wilcockson J (2001) Professional and organisational learning: analysing the relationship with the development of practice. *Journal of Advanced Nursing* 34: 264–272

Clarke CL, Wilcockson J (2002) Seeing need and developing care: exploring knowledge for and from practice. *International Journal of Nursing Studies* 39: 397–406

Clarke CL, Reynolds J, McClelland S, Reed J (2004a) *Evaluation of the NHS Leading Modernisation Programme, Final Report*. Newcastle upon Tyne, Northumbria University

Clarke C, Luce A, Gibb C, Williams L, Keady J, Cook A, Wilkinson H (2004b) Contemporary risk management in dementia: An organisational survey of practices and inclusion of people with dementia. *Signpost* 9:1 27–31

Corcoran PB, Walker KE, Wals AEJ (2004) Case-studies, make-your-case studies, and case stories: a critique of case-study methodology in sustainability in higher education. *Environmental Education Research* 10:1 7–21

Gummesson E (1988) *Qualitative Methods in Management Research*. Lund, Norway, Studentlitteratur, Chartwell-Bratt

Meyer CB (2003) A case in case study methodology. *Field Methods* 13: 329–352

Quinn Patton M (2003) Inquiry into appreciative evaluation. *New Directions for Evaluation* 100:4 85–89

Reed J (1992) Secondary data in nursing research. *Journal of Advanced Nursing* 7: 877–883

Reed J, Procter S, Murray S (1996) A sampling strategy for qualitative research. *Nurse Researcher* 3:4 52–68

Reed J, Pearson P, Douglas B, Swinburne S, Wilding H (2002) Going home from hospital: – an appreciative inquiry study. *Health and Social Care and the Community* 10: 36–45

Reed J, Jones A, Irvine J (2005) Appreciating impact: evaluating small voluntary organisations in the United Kingdom. *Voluntas: International Journal of Voluntary and Non-profit Organisations* 16: 123–141

Stake RE (1995) *The Art of Case Study Research*. Thousand Oaks, Sage

Yin RK (1994) *Case Study Research: design and methods*, 2nd edition. Thousand Oaks, Sage

21 Systematic Reviews and Secondary Research

Catherine Beverley, Mary Edmunds-Otter and Andrew Booth

Key points

- Secondary research, in particular systematic reviews, contributes to evidence-based practice by using explicit methods to identify, select, critically appraise and summarise large quantities of information to aid the decision-making process.
- The three main types of secondary research are systematic reviews, practice guidelines and economic evaluations.
- Regardless of the type of secondary research, several discrete, but interconnected, stages are followed: writing a research protocol, systematically searching the literature, selecting relevant studies, assessing the quality of the literature, extracting key information from the selected studies, summarising, interpreting and presenting the findings, and writing up the research in a structured manner.

Introduction

This chapter builds upon Chapters 7 and 8 to provide a practical introduction to conducting secondary research (i.e. reanalysing existing research), with specific reference to systematic reviews. Readers are advised to refer to these two earlier chapters regarding the skills required to access and appraise research literature. A worked example relating to antibiotics and antiseptics for venous leg ulcers (taken from a Cochrane protocol on the Cochrane Library) is used throughout (Box 21.1).

Background to secondary research

The knowledge base for any evidence-based profession is founded on secondary research. By reanalysing previously collected data from original (primary) studies in research syntheses, it is possible to summarise large volumes of information in a succinct manner. This not only increases the precision of the overall result, but also assists in establishing generalisability of findings, and examining conflicting results. It also provides an opportunity to identify gaps in the current knowledge base, and hence suggest future primary research areas.

Box 21.1 A Cochrane protocol for a systematic review.

O'Meara S, Ovington L. (2002) Antibiotics and antiseptics for venous leg ulcers (protocol). *The Cochrane Database of Systematic Reviews* 2002, Issue 2. Chichester, John Wiley

Background: Chronic venous leg ulceration is a recurring condition affecting 0.1% of the general population at any point in time. A range of interventions may be considered for the treatment of patients with chronic venous leg ulcers, including compression bandaging, various types of dressings and topical applications, debriding agents, vasoactive drugs, fibrinolytic therapy and physical therapies.

Objectives: To determine the effectiveness of topical and systemic antibiotics and antiseptics for the healing of venous ulcers.

Criteria for considering studies for this review: Prospective randomised controlled trials (RCTs) or non-randomised clinical controlled trials with a concurrent control group (CCTs) evaluating topical or systematic antibiotics or antiseptics in the treatment of venous ulcers will be included.

Search strategy for identification of studies: RCTs and CCTs will be identified from the Cochrane Wounds Group Specialist Trials Register.

Methods of the review: Titles and abstracts of studies identified will be assessed in terms of their relevance and design, according to the selection criteria. Details of the studies will be extracted and summarised using a data extraction sheet. A narrative summary of results will be presented.

Systematic reviews

A *'systematic review'* (or *'overview'*) is:

> 'a review of the evidence on a clearly formulated question that uses systematic and explicit methods to identify, select and critically appraise relevant primary research, and to extract and analyse data from the studies that are included in the review' (Khan *et al.* 2001:4)

Whereas 'review' (sometimes referred to as a narrative or traditional review) is a general term used to describe a synthesis of the results and conclusions of two or more publications on a given topic, a systematic review strives to comprehensively identify and synthesise all literature on a given topic. A systematic review, aims to be:

- systematic (e.g. in its identification of literature)
- explicit (e.g. in its statement of objectives, materials and methods)
- reproducible (e.g. in its methodology and conclusions) (Greenhalgh 2000)

The term *'meta-analysis'* is often used interchangeably with 'systematic review'. However, it describes a statistical technique used to combine the results of several studies into a single estimate (Khan *et al.* 2001).

Examples of systematic reviews in nursing include reviews on home care by outreach nursing for chronic obstructive pulmonary disease (Smith *et al.* 2003), specialist nurses in diabetes mellitus (Loveman *et al.* 2004), and nursing record systems (Currell & Urquhart 2003). All these examples can be found on The Cochrane Library (*www.nelh.nhs.uk/cochrane*).

Practice guidelines and economic evaluations

Other examples of secondary research are practice guidelines and economic evaluations. Practice guidelines are:

'directions or principles presenting current or future rules of policy for the health care practitioner to assist him in patient care decisions regarding diagnosis, therapy, or related clinical circumstances . . . The guidelines form a basis for the evaluation of all aspects of health care and delivery' (Clinical Practice Guidelines, National Library of Medicine, MeSH Browser)

Many evidence-based guidelines, such as those produced in the UK by the National Institute for Health and Clinical Excellence (NICE), have implications for nursing. Recent examples at the time of writing included:

- *Antenatal care – routine care for healthy pregnant women*
- *Infection control*
- *Prevention of health care-associated infection in primary and community care*
- *Pressure ulcers – risk assessment and prevention*

These can be accessed on the NICE website (*www.nice.org.uk*).

An *economic evaluation* entails drawing up a balance sheet of the advantages (benefits) and disadvantages (costs) associated with different health care options so that choices can be made (Robinson 1993). Published examples include an economic evaluation of patient education models for diabetes (Loveman *et al.* 2003) and a cost effectiveness analysis of inhaler devices used in the routine management of chronic asthma in older children (Peters *et al.* 2002).

Advantages of secondary research

Well-conducted secondary research studies offer several advantages over single primary research studies (Mulrow 1995; Greenhalgh 2000). For example:

- Large amounts of information can be assimilated quickly and efficiently, thereby assisting in the decision-making process.
- The use of explicit methods helps to limit bias in identifying and excluding studies.

- The results of different studies can be formally compared to establish generalisability of findings and consistency of results.
- Reasons for inconsistency in results across studies can be identified and new hypotheses generated.
- Quantitative techniques, such as meta-analysis, increase the precision of the overall result.
- Conclusions are thus considered to be more reliable and accurate.

Stages in conducting secondary research

For each of the above types of secondary research, the researcher typically follows discrete, but interconnected, stages:

- writing a research protocol, outlining the purpose and methods of the research
- systematically searching the literature
- selecting relevant studies
- assessing the quality of the literature
- extracting key information from the selected studies
- summarising, interpreting and presenting the findings
- writing up the research in a structured manner

This chapter focuses on systematic reviews, the most common of research syntheses, but the described methods apply, to varying degrees, to other types of secondary research.

Writing a systematic review protocol

The first step in undertaking a new systematic review is to establish whether there is sufficient need for a review. This starts with a comprehensive search for existing reviews addressing the same (or similar) research question(s), and critically appraising any potentially relevant reviews. Existing and ongoing systematic reviews can be identified by searching:

- The Cochrane Database of Systematic Reviews (CDSR) (*www.nelh.nhs. uk/cochrane*)
- The Database of Reviews of Effects (DARE) (*www.york.ac.uk/inst/crd/darehp. htm*)
- Major health-related databases, such as MEDLINE, using methodological search filters designed to retrieve systematic reviews. Box 21.2 provides an example of such a filter. Local health care librarians can provide advice and support in identifying and using search filters.

Box 21.2 Methodological search filter designed to retrieve systematic reviews in MEDLINE (Dialog).

The following search filter, originally designed by Ann McKibbon at McMaster University in Canada, can be added to any subject search in MEDLINE (Dialog interface).

1. review-academic.pt.
(pt means publication type)
2. review-tutorial.pt.
3. systematic NEAR review.ti,ab,de.
(NEAR means the two words must be within five words of each other)
(ti,ab,de looks for the words in the title, abstract and MeSH heading (descriptor) field)
4. systematic NEAR overview.ti.ab.de.
5. (metaanaly$ OR meta analy$ OR meta-analy$).ti,ab,de.
($ is the truncation symbol)
6. meta-analysis.pt.
7   1 or 2 or 3 or 4 or 5 or 6

If existing reviews are outdated, or of poor quality, it may become necessary to update them or to conduct a new review from scratch. The key to a successful systematic review lies in the reviewer's ability to be precise and specific when stating the problems to be addressed. A structured approach to framing questions should be used. These components include the populations, interventions (or exposures) and outcomes related to the problem posed in the review, and the designs of studies that are suitable for addressing it (Khan *et al.* 2004). This stage in the systematic review process is perhaps the most difficult, yet most important task to get right. A review protocol is drawn up specifying the plan that the review will subsequently follow. It is a key reference document throughout the review process. Modifications should only be made to the protocol if there is a genuine reason (for example, if an additional outcome measure is identified upon closer examination of the literature).

A review protocol typically includes:

- *Background and rationale to the review.* This includes a justification for the review being undertaken, as well as a preliminary assessment of potentially relevant literature and its size.
- *Review question(s).* The review question(s) should be well focused in terms of the population, intervention and outcome(s).
- *Inclusion criteria.* These should follow on logically from the review question(s), and cover any restrictions regarding study design or publication type, language or year of publication. Any exclusion criteria should be stated explicitly

and reasons for them given. Where feasible, these criteria should be applied to the studies by two independent reviewers.

- *Literature search strategy*. This should outline details of the sources to be searched and a sample search strategy.
- *Quality assessment strategy*. This should provide details of the critical appraisal checklist or scale (preferably validated) used to assess the quality of the included studies.
- *Data extraction strategy*. Where possible, a sample data extraction form (Box 21.5) indicating the information to be collected from each study (e.g. details about the participants, methods, interventions, results, etc.) should be included.
- *Proposed analysis*. This should document the type of data that are likely to be found (e.g. quantitative or qualitative), and the proposed data synthesis and presentation strategy (e.g. meta-analysis).
- *Plans for reporting and dissemination*. This should describe the strategy for reporting and disseminating the findings to relevant audiences.
- *Members of the review team*. Ideally a systematic review should be undertaken by a review 'team', although many smaller reviews are written by lone researchers. Members of a review team should include an information specialist to identify, locate and store relevant references; someone to review the literature; a methodologist (such as a statistician); and content experts, possibly in the form of an advisory group.
- *Project timetable*. Include a draft timetable outlining each stage in the systematic review.
- *Proposed costings*. Even small-scale reviews entail costs (e.g. staff time, obtaining articles, etc.). It is important to be aware of these costs at the outset and, if necessary, apply for additional funding.

Systematically searching the literature

The aim of a systematic literature search is:

'to provide a list as comprehensive as possible of primary studies, both published and unpublished' (Khan *et al.* 2001:21)

Refining the review question

The search starts by refining the review question and translating it into a search strategy that can be used to interrogate electronic bibliographic databases. As well as searching the literature to identify existing systematic reviews, 'scoping' searches will ensure that the final strategy reflects all components of the review question(s). Chapter 7 introduced the PICO (patient-intervention-comparison-outcome) framework, which is a useful tool for focusing research questions. Box 21.3 applies this to the review of antibiotics and antiseptics for venous leg ulcers.

Selecting relevant sources to search for a systematic review

A review team should search a wide variety of sources for published, as well as unpublished, literature including:

- large electronic bibliographic databases, such as Medline, CINAHL, EMBASE and Science Citation Index
- subject-specific electronic bibliographic databases, such as AMED (for allied health literature), PsycINFO (for psychological and psychiatric literature), AgeINFO (for literature relating to older people), etc.
- research and trials registers, such as CENTRAL, Current Controlled Trials, National Research Register, Research Findings Register, Index to Theses and Dissertation Abstracts

Box 21.3   A refined review question: antibiotics and antiseptics for venous leg ulcers.

	Components	Keywords	Synonyms (i.e. alternative search terms)
P	Patient/Problem/ Population	venous leg ulcers	varicose ulcer (MeSH) leg ulcer (MeSH) venous ulcers
I	Intervention	antibiotics	exp antibacterial-agents (MeSH) antibiotics penicillin cephalosporin aminoglycosides gentamicin quinolones ciprofloxacin clindamycin metronidazole trimethoprim
C	Comparison	antiseptics	exp anti-infective agents, local (MeSH) antiseptics disinfectants
O	Outcomes	wound healing	wound healing (MeSH) ulcer healing wound size wound duration

O'Meara S, Ovington L. (2002) Antibiotics and antiseptics for venous leg ulcers (protocol). *The Cochrane Database of Systematic Reviews* 2002, Issue 2. Chichester, John Wiley

- grey literature databases, such as HMIC and SIGLE
- the internet, including generic search engines (e.g. Google) and subject-specific search engines (e.g. OMNI)
- handsearching the table of contents of key journals in the field
- checking the reference lists of selected articles
- contacting experts and organisations in the field
- conducting citation searches on key articles and authors using Science Citation Index and Social Sciences Citation Index

Note: while some database names originated as meaningful acronyms it is common practice to identify and to refer to these resources by their abbreviated forms.

Developing sensitive search strategies

Systematic literature searches use highly sensitive search strategies to ensure that no relevant studies are overlooked. This means that the reviewer will look through a larger set of references (usually hundreds, or even thousands) to minimise the chance of missing relevant items. Using 'specific' search strategies means that the search retrieves fewer, highly relevant references, but the reviewer runs the risk of missing relevant studies. The reviewer, therefore, aims to achieve the right balance between *'sensitivity'* and *'specificity'* when designing search strategies.

The sensitivity of a search strategy can be increased by:

- including more search terms and thesaurus terms (identified from previously retrieved references)
- using truncation (* or $) or wildcards (? or #) in free text searches
- using 'OR' to combine terms within the same concept
- using 'NEAR' to retrieve terms within the same sentence
- utilising a combination of free text and thesaurus search terms
- 'exploding' thesaurus search terms
- selecting 'all subheadings' for thesaurus search terms
- searching only on the 'population' and 'intervention', i.e. not introducing 'outcomes' or 'comparisons' into the strategy
- not applying date, language, or study design limits to the search strategy
- using 'sensitive' methodological search filters (*see* below)

Methodological search filters

Methodological search filters are strategies that are added to the subject search and are designed to retrieve different types of evidence from the search. Filters have been developed for the major types of question (i.e. therapy, prognosis, diagnosis and aetiology). Sample filters can be found within the 'Searching' section of *Netting the Evidence* (*http://www.shef.ac.uk/scharr/ir/netting*).

Addressing publication bias

Publication bias means that studies with significant results are more likely to be published (Khan *et al.* 2004). Debate centres on whether systematic reviews should identify and include non-English language or unpublished research (Egger *et al.* 2003; Easterbrook *et al.* 1991). For example, McAuley *et al.* (2000) have shown that if unpublished studies are not included in meta-analyses the effectiveness of an intervention may be overestimated. However, even the most comprehensive literature search cannot eliminate the possibility of publication bias. For example, most studies are published years after the research was conducted; other studies are never published; there is a tendency towards 'selective reporting', i.e. where only studies which show statistically significant results are published; and multiple publication of the same results from a single study in several different journals is common. Techniques to address 'publication bias' are given under 'Summarising, interpreting and presenting the findings' below.

Managing large sets of references

It is essential to use a reference management system to manage the large numbers of references. Chapter 7 introduced electronic reference management software packages such as Reference Manager, EndNote and Procite. These packages allow the reviewer to:

- store and maintain references (journals, books, reports, websites, theses, etc.)
- import references directly from major electronic bibliographic databases, such as MEDLINE
- keep track of references ordered from libraries
- assign keywords to references (e.g. the keyword 'RCT' can be applied to all references retrieved from a clinical trials search)
- retrieve sets of references by author, publication year, title, keywords, etc.
- insert personal notes and comments relating to individual references
- automatically create reference lists in the reviewer's preferred journal style
- insert references directly into word-processed research reports

Documenting a systematic literature search

The review team should keep an accurate record of the search strategy used. This helps to avoid duplicated effort and provides a basis for updating the review in the future. Information to be recorded includes the date of the search, the sources searched, the search terms used and the number of references retrieved.

Selecting relevant studies

When selecting studies for inclusion the aim is to identify those articles that address the question(s) being posed. It is important to screen all the references retrieved and obtain the full text of studies that potentially meet the inclusion criteria. These criteria should stem directly from the review question(s) and relate to the core components of the question, i.e. participants, interventions, outcomes and study design. Box 21.4 lists the criteria for considering studies for inclusion in the antibiotics and antiseptics for venous leg ulcers example.

Criteria should be set in advance and piloted to check that they can be applied consistently. Final decisions about inclusion and exclusion are made after reading the full text of articles. Reasons for exclusion are recorded. Errors of judgement in study selection can be reduced by using two independent reviewers. However, this is not always feasible and it is often acceptable to assess a sample of studies independently.

Assessing the quality of the literature

Study quality refers to the degree to which a study takes steps to minimise bias and error in its design, conduct and analysis (Khan *et al.* 2004). Once studies of a minimum acceptable quality (based on the study design) have been selected, an in-depth critical appraisal is required. It is important to determine whether there is a quality (or study design) threshold that defines the weakest acceptable study to be included. For example, many Cochrane reviews only include RCTs.

Detailed quality assessment of studies within a systematic review (Khan *et al.* 2004) aims to:

- simply describe the quality of studies included in the review
- explore whether different effects in different studies can be explained by variations in their quality
- help decide whether to pool the effects observed in included studies
- aid in determining the strength of inferences from the data
- recommend how future studies should be conducted

When conducting a systematic review, it is essential to identify suitable checklists for each study design that will meet the inclusion criteria. If a checklist does not exist, then using existing tools that reflect generic issues relating to validity, reliability and applicability is preferable to developing an unvalidated checklist.

Extracting key information from the selected studies

Data extraction involves identifying and recording important items (such as details of the author, the setting, the participants, the interventions, the outcomes, and the main results) from each study. Data extraction forms are used to facilitate this; these should be piloted so as to reduce errors and minimise bias. For example, the

Box 21.4 Criteria for considering studies for review: Antibiotics and antiseptics for venous leg ulcers.

O'Meara S, Ovington L. (2002) Antibiotics and antiseptics for venous leg ulcers (protocol). *The Cochrane Database of Systematic Reviews* 2002, Issue 2. Chichester, John Wiley

Types of participants
Trials recruiting patients described in the primary studies as having venous leg ulcers will be included. Trials recruiting participants with different types of wounds (e.g. arterial ulcers, ulcers due to mixed arterial/venous disease, and diabetic foot ulcers) will be included only if the results for patients with uncomplicated venous disease are presented separately.

Types of intervention
The primary intervention will be topical or systemic antibiotics or antiseptics prescribed for venous leg ulceration. Systemic preparations can be given orally or intravenously and may be administered singly or in combination. Control regimens can include placebo, an alternative antibiotic or antiseptic, any other therapy, or no treatment.

Types of outcome measures
Primary outcomes
Trials reporting any of the following outcomes at any endpoint will be included:

- time to complete ulcer healing
- proportion of ulcers completely healing during trial period
- objective measurements of change in ulcer size

Secondary outcomes
Where reported, the following outcomes will also be recorded:

- changes in signs and/or symptoms of clinical infection
- changes in bacterial flora
- development of bacterial resistance
- ulcer recurrence rates
- adverse effects of treatment
- patient satisfaction
- quality of life
- costs

Studies will only be eligible for inclusion if they report the primary outcome since those reporting secondary outcomes only are likely to introduce reporting bias.

Types of studies
Prospective randomised controlled trials (RCTs) or non-randomised clinical controlled trials with a concurrent control group (CCT) evaluating topical or systemic antibiotics or antiseptics in the treatment of venous ulcers will be included.

data extraction form must accommodate different study designs and ensure that the researcher consistently collects the same type of data from each study. Sample data extraction forms are provided in the CRD Centre for Reviews and Dissemination (CRD) Report Number 4 (Khan *et al.* 2001) *(www.york.ac.uk/inst/crd/ pdf/crd4_app3.pdf)*. Box 21.5 documents the proposed data extraction strategy for the antibiotics and antiseptics for venous leg ulcers example.

Summarising, interpreting and presenting the findings

Having extracted all relevant data, this information must then be synthesised. In many cases this entails providing a descriptive summary *('narrative commentary')*, possibly supported by a tabular presentation *('summary tables')*. Where possible, quantitative data are combined in a 'meta-analysis' to quantify the benefits (or harms) of an intervention. Before undertaking such an analysis it is important to

Box 21.5 Data extraction strategy: Antibiotics and antiseptics for venous leg ulcers.

O'Meara S, Ovington L. (2002) Antibiotics and antiseptics for venous leg ulcers (protocol). *The Cochrane Database of Systematic Reviews* 2002, Issue 2. Chichester, John Wiley

Details of the studies will be extracted and summarised using a data extraction sheet. If data are missing from reports, then attempts will be made to contact the authors to obtain missing information. Studies that have been published in duplicate will be included only once, ensuring that all relevant data from all publications are included. Data extraction will be undertaken by one reviewer and checked for accuracy by a second reviewer.
  Types of data extracted will include:

- study details (i.e. study authors, year of publication, country where study performed)
- methods (i.e study design (e.g. RCT), method of randomisation or allocation, unit of randomisation/allocation, overall sample size and methods used to estimate statistical power, statistical methods used for data analysis)
- participants (i.e. setting of treatment, participant selection criteria)
- interventions (i.e. duration of treatment, specific antibiotics and antiseptics used) per study group
- outcomes measured (including methods used for identifying micro-organisms)
- baseline characteristics of participants per treatment group (e.g. gender, age, ethnicity, wound size, wound duration, prevalence of co-morbidities, etc.)
- results (i.e. numbers per study group, results per group for each outcome, withdrawals (per group) – numbers and reasons)

establish whether it is appropriate to do so. For example, there is no point pooling the results if:

- Only one study has estimated the effect of an intervention.
- There are significant differences in the participants, interventions, and/or setting that could substantially affect the outcomes *(clinical heterogeneity)*.
- There is excessive variation in the results of the studies *(statistical heterogeneity)*.
- The outcome(s) have been measured in different ways in each study.
- The studies do not contain the required information.

In simple terms, a meta-analysis involves taking individual results for the same outcome from several studies and calculating a 'single summary statistic' (sometimes referred to as an *effect measure*). Standard effect measures include 'odds ratio', 'relative risk', 'risk difference', 'number needed to treat', 'standardised mean difference' and 'weighted mean difference'. The *relative risk* (RR) is the most widely used measure. It represents the proportion of participants who are observed to have the risk of an event in the intervention group as a ratio to the proportion of participants with the same risk in the control group. An RR of one indicates no difference between the comparison groups (Khan *et al.* 2001).

Where studies examine 'similar' groups, effect sizes across studies should be compared and an overall effect calculated by taking a weighted average of the individual study effects. However, not all readers will feel comfortable in interpreting the statistical measures involved. The results of a meta-analysis can be presented graphically as a *Forest plot*, sometimes referred to as a 'blobbogram' or 'odds ratio diagram'. This represents the individual study results within the review together with the combined meta-analysis result. An example is provided in Figure 21.1.

The vertical line represents the line of no effect, i.e. where the group receiving the intervention are no better or worse off than the control group or, in other words, where the odds ratio (OR) is equal to 1. The small 'blobs' represent the results of individual trials. The area of each 'blob' represents the weight given to each study in the meta-analysis. Larger, higher-quality studies receive more weight than smaller, lower-quality ones. The larger diamond-shaped 'blob' next to the 'Total' row represents the overall meta-analysis result when all the studies are pooled together. The horizontal lines associated with each 'blob' represent the confidence interval (in this case, 95%) for each result.

The confidence interval tells us how much uncertainty is associated with each result. Narrow confidence intervals indicate that the same result is likely to occur were we to repeat the study many times. Wider confidence intervals mean that different results would be more likely to occur. In the above example comparing respiratory outreach nurses with a control the overall pooled result indicated by the diamond lies to the left of the line of no effect. This indicates less of the outcome (mortality) in the treatment (respiratory outreach nurse) group. However, the horizontal points of the diamond, indicating the confidence interval when all

Review: Home care by outreach nursing for chronic obstructive pulmonary disease
Comparison: 01 Respiratory outreach nurse vs control
Outcome: 05 Mortality

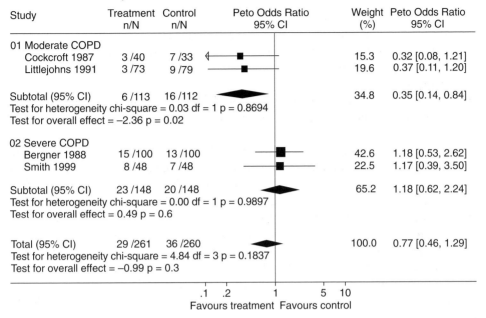

Study	Treatment n/N	Control n/N	Peto Odds Ratio 95% CI	Weight (%)	Peto Odds Ratio 95% CI
01 Moderate COPD					
Cockcroft 1987	3 /40	7 /33		15.3	0.32 [0.08, 1.21]
Littlejohns 1991	3 /73	9 /79		19.6	0.37 [0.11, 1.20]
Subtotal (95% CI)	6 /113	16 /112		34.8	0.35 [0.14, 0.84]
Test for heterogeneity chi-square = 0.03 df = 1 p = 0.8694					
Test for overall effect = −2.36 p = 0.02					
02 Severe COPD					
Bergner 1988	15 /100	13 /100		42.6	1.18 [0.53, 2.62]
Smith 1999	8 /48	7 /48		22.5	1.17 [0.39, 3.50]
Subtotal (95% CI)	23 /148	20 /148		65.2	1.18 [0.62, 2.24]
Test for heterogeneity chi-square = 0.00 df = 1 p = 0.9897					
Test for overall effect = 0.49 p = 0.6					
Total (95% CI)	29 /261	36 /260		100.0	0.77 [0.46, 1.29]
Test for heterogeneity chi-square = 4.84 df = 3 p = 0.1837					
Test for overall effect = −0.99 p = 0.3					

.1   .2   1   5   10
Favours treatment Favours control

Figure 21.1   An example of a Forest plot.
From Smith B, Appleton S, Adams R, Southcott A, Ruffin R (2001) Home care by out-reach nursing for chronic obstructive pulmonary disease. *The Cochrane Database of Systematic Reviews*, Issue 3
© Copyright Cochrane Library, reproduced with permission

the studies are pooled together, cross the line of no effect, which means that the result is not significant. Closer examination of the plot and the text of the review reveals that, because the authors have pooled studies including people with both moderate and severe chronic obstructive pulmonary disease, the overall effect 'mixes up' people most likely to benefit from the treatment with those who are less likely to benefit.

A meta-analysis is a complex mathematical calculation often requiring input from a statistician. Fortunately several software packages, such as Review Manager (*www.cc-ims.net/RevMan*) are available to facilitate this process.

Even rigorously conducted systematic reviews cannot eliminate the risk of *publication and related biases*. Therefore a formal assessment of such risks should be incorporated into the review. Statistical and modelling techniques, such as *funnel plots*, exist to assist in highlighting these biases. These plot individual effects from studies against some measure of study information (e.g. study size). If the resulting inverted funnel is asymmetrical this may indicate the presence of bias, although this could also be due to chance.

Writing up the review

A succinct report of the review allows readers to judge its validity and the implications of its findings (Khan *et al.* 2001). All Cochrane reviews are reported in a consistent manner that includes a structured abstract, background, objectives, criteria for considering studies, search strategy, methods of the review, description of studies, methodological quality, results, summary of analyses, discussion, reviewers' conclusions (including implications for practice and research) and references. A similar structure should be adopted when writing up any systematic review. The QUOROM (**QU**ality **O**f **R**eporting **O**f **M**eta-analyses) sets a standard for the quality of reporting of systematic reviews of RCTs (Moher *et al.* 1999).

Systematic reviews of qualitative research

Recent years have seen the rapid evolution of techniques for identifying and synthesising qualitative research although there is little consensus as to which methods should be used for searching, appraising and synthesising good quality studies (Booth 2001). Part of this complexity stems from the diversity of qualitative research. Some argue that a particular method of appraisal or analysis may privilege specific types of qualitative research. Evans and Pearson (2001) provide a good overview of the main issues for qualitative systematic reviews for nurses. They characterise these under six stages of the review process:

- defining the focus
- locating studies
- selecting studies for inclusion in review
- critical appraisal
- data extraction
- data synthesis

The stages of the systematic review process are thus common to both quantitative and qualitative research. It is at the point of data extraction and synthesis that the paths most clearly diverge.

Approaches to syntheses of qualitative research tend to divide into those that regard reviews of qualitative research as broadly equivalent to those for quantitative research and those that state that secondary qualitative research is, in fact, conceptually aligned to primary qualitative research. The former assumes that comprehensive searches of the qualitative literature are required to eliminate possible sources of bias while the latter aims for a sampling strategy that arrives at theoretical saturation. Both approaches work from the premise that systematic reviews of qualitative research should be systematic, explicit and reproducible but other concepts, strongly associated with quantitative systematic reviews, such as the requirement to be 'comprehensive' mark the battle lines.

The increasing interest in systematic reviews of qualitative research stems from a broadening of review questions beyond effectiveness to examine such issues as patient views, compliance and acceptability of health care (Khan *et al.* 2001). By conducting a thematic analysis the reviewer identifies key themes from individual studies and then seeks to establish whether any themes map or 'translate' from one study to another. This process requires that the reviewer follows published methods for appraising qualitative research studies.

Early attempts at systematic review of qualitative research have been limited by trying to impose a rigid template from quantitative reviews that has been adjusted slightly to accommodate qualitative research. More recently has come recognition that methods from qualitative research can not only inform the conduct of qualitative reviews but can also benefit systematic reviews in general. For example the iterative approaches typically used to develop and refine interpretation of qualitative data can be used to challenge the prescriptively sequential model of reviews perpetuated by the quantitative model. Similarly, approaches to handling potential investigator bias, reduced to a token declaration of interest statement in quantitative reviews, can be enhanced through reference to the key qualitative research concept of reflexivity.

Examples of syntheses of qualitative research include a review of the experiences of those with diabetes (Box 21.6) (Thorne & Paterson 1998) and an examination of compliance with medication to construct a model of barriers and enablers (Britten *et al.* 2002). It should be recognised that there is a fundamental difference between quantitative and qualitative systematic reviews as the former aim to be aggregative (in bringing the evidence together in an additive way) while the latter aim to be interpretative (in broadening our understanding of a specific phenomenon) (Noblit & Hare, 1988).

Conclusion

Secondary research, in the form of systematic reviews, practice guidelines and economic evaluations, provide the opportunity to generate a synthesis of research evidence to inform practice. Explicit methods are used to identify, select, critically appraise and summarise large quantities of information. Irrespective of the type of secondary research, several discrete, but interconnected, stages are followed.

These include:

- writing a research protocol
- systematically searching the literature
- selecting relevant studies
- assessing the quality of the literature
- extracting key information from the selected studies
- summarising, interpreting and presenting the findings
- writing up the research in a structured manner.

Box 21.6 A qualitative systematic review of published experiences of diabetes.

Paterson BL, Thorne S, Dewis M (1998) Adapting to and managing diabetes. *Image: Journal of Nursing Scholarship* 30: 57–62

Question: What is the 'lived experience' of people who have diabetes mellitus?

Data sources: Six databases (Sociofile, PsycLit, Dissertation Abstracts, CINAHL, Medline, and Allied Health) were searched for dissertations, theses, articles, and book chapters together with refereed journals and books (1980–July 1996).

Study selection: Included studies were qualitative interpretive research reports of first-hand experience of living with diabetes.

Data analysis: Meta-ethnographic synthesis was used and individual studies were reviewed by multiple researchers.

Main results: 38 studies were identified employing a variety of qualitative methods. Participants were mainly white women with insulin-dependent diabetes mellitus. The prevailing metaphor was the concept of *balance*. Learning to balance involves making the decision to assume control and then actually assuming control. Assuming control involves *knowing one's body*, *learning how to manage diabetes*, and *fostering supportive, collaborative relationships* with others.

Conclusion: Patients with diabetes mellitus focus on learning to *balance* management of their disease with the desire for a normal life by deciding to assume control and then following through.

References

Booth A (2001) *Cochrane or cock-eyed? How should we conduct systematic reviews of qualitative research?* Presented at the Qualitative Evidence-based Practice Conference, Taking a Critical Stance. Coventry University, May 14–16 2001 *www.leeds.ac.uk/educol/documents/00001724.htm*

Britten N, Campbell R, Pope C, Donovan JL, Morgan M, Pill R. (2002) Synthesis of qualitative research: a worked example using meta-ethnography. *Journal of Health Services Research and Policy* 7: 209–215

Currell R, Urquhart C (2003) Nursing record systems: effects on nursing practice and health care outcomes (protocol for a Cochrane Review). *The Cochrane Database of Systematic Reviews* Issue 3. Chichester, John Wiley

Easterbrook PJ, Berlin JA, Goplan R, Matthews DR (1991) Publication bias in clinical trials. *The Lancet* 337: 867–872

Egger M, Juni P, Bartlett C, Holenstein F, Sterne J (2003) How important are comprehensive literature searches and the assessment of trial quality in systematic reviews? Empirical study. *Health Technology Assessment* 7: 1 *www.ncchta.org/execsumm/summ701.htm*

Evans D, Pearson A (2001) Systematic reviews of qualitative research. *Clinical Effectiveness for Nursing* 5: 111–119

Greenhalgh, T (2000) *How to Read a Paper: the basics of evidence based practice*, 2nd edition. London, BMJ Publishing

Khan KS, Kuna R, Kleijnen J, Antes G (2004) *Systematic Reviews to Support Evidence-Based Medicine*. London, Royal Society of Medicine

Khan KS, ter Riet G, Glanville J, Sowden AJ, Kleijnen J (eds) (2001) *Undertaking Systematic Reviews of Research on Effectiveness. CRD's guidance for carrying out or commissioning reviews*, 2nd edition. CRD Report No. 4. University of York, NHS Centre for Reviews and Dissemination

Loveman E, Cave C, Green C, Royle P, Dunn N, Waugh N (2003) The clinical and cost-effectiveness of patient education models for diabetes: a systematic review and economic evaluation. *Health Technology Assessment* 7:22

Loveman E, Royle P, Waugh N (2004). Specialist nurses in diabetes mellitus (protocol for a Cochrane Review). *The Cochrane Database of Systematic Reviews*, Issue 3. Chichester, John Wiley

McAuley A, Pharm B, Tugwell P, Moher D (2000) Does the inclusion of grey literature influence estimates of intervention effectiveness reported in meta-analyses? *The Lancet* 356: 1228–1231

Moher D, Cook DJ, Eastwood S, Olkin I, Rennie D, Stroup DF (1999) Improving the quality of reports of meta-analyses of randomised controlled trials: the QUOROM statement (Quality of Reporting of Meta-analyses). *The Lancet* 354: 1896–1900

Mulrow C (1995) Rationale for systematic reviews. In Chalmers I, Altman DG (eds) *Systematic Reviews*. London, BMJ Publishing

National Library of Medicine, Medical Subject headings (MeSH) from PubMed, MeSH browser. *www.ncbi.nlm.nih.gov/entrez/query.fcgi?db=mesh*

Noblit GW, Hare RD (1988) *Meta-Ethnography: synthesizing qualitative studies*. Paper series on qualitative research methods, Volume 11. Newbury Park, Sage

O'Meara S, Ovington L (2002) Antibiotics and antiseptics for venous leg ulcers (protocol for a Cochrane Review). *The Cochrane Database of Systematic Reviews* Issue 2. Chichester, John Wiley

Paterson BL, Thorne S, Dewis M (1998) Adapting to and managing diabetes. *Image: The Journal of Nursing Scholarship* 30: 57–62

Peters J, Stevenson M, Beverley C, Lim JNW, Smith S (2002) The clinical effectiveness and cost-effectiveness of inhaler devices used in the routine management of chronic asthma in older children: a systematic review and economic evaluation. *Health Technology Assessment* 6:5

Robinson R (1993) Economic evaluation and health care: What does it mean? *British Medical Journal* 307: 670–673

Smith B, Appleton S, Adams R, Southcott A, Ruffin R (2003). Home care by outreach nursing for chronic obstructive pulmonary disease (protocol for a Cochrane Review). *The Cochrane Database of Systematic Reviews Issue 3*. Chichester, John Wiley

Thorne S, Paterson B (1998) Shifting images of chronic illness. *Image: The Journal of Nursing Scholarship* 30: 173–178

Further reading

Bero LA, Grilli R, Grimshaw JM, Harvey E, Oxman AD, Thompson MA (1998) Closing the gap between research and practice: an overview of systematic reviews of interventions to promote the implementation of research findings. The Cochrane Effective Practice and Organization of Care Review Group. *British Medical Journal* 317: 465–468

Chalmers I, Altman DG (eds) (1995) *Systematic Reviews*. London, BMJ Publishing

Egger M, Davey-Smith G, Altman DG (eds) (2001) *Systematic Reviews in Health Care. meta-analysis in context.* London, BMJ Publishing *www.systematicreviews.com*

Glaziou P, Irwig L, Bain C, Colditz G (2001) *Systematic Reviews in Health Care: a practical guide*. Cambridge, Cambridge University Press

Mulrow CD, Cook D (eds) (1998) *Systematic Reviews: synthesis of best evidence for health care decisions*. Philadelphia, PA, American College of Physicians

Torgerson C (2003) *Systematic Reviews*. London, Continuum International Publishing Group

Websites

www.campbellcollaboration.org – Campbell Collaboration

www.cochrane.org – Cochrane Collaboration

www.nelh.nhs.uk/cochrane – Cochrane Library

www.shef.ac.uk/scharr/ir/netting /– Netting the Evidence, links to methodological search filters, critical appraisal checklists, etc.

www.york.ac.uk/inst/crd/report4.htm – NHS CRD Report No. 4, Undertaking Systematic Reviews of Research on Effectiveness

Section 4
Collecting Data

This section contains five practical chapters dealing with the common methods used in nursing research to collect data. A generic approach has been maintained, with several of the methods, such as interviewing and observation, being used in both qualitative and quantitative research.

Chapter 22 begins by tackling interviews, a versatile data collection method widely used in nursing research. This is followed by Chapter 23 describing focus groups, increasingly popular as an adjunct to individual interviews or as a tool in themselves. Both these chapters deal with the purposes to which the methods are best suited, the essential preparation for, and conduct of, the interview or focus group, and practical and ethical issues raised.

Chapter 24 then deals with questionnaires, perhaps the most widely used method of data collection in health care research. The art and science of questionnaire design and administration is not as simple as it first seems, however, and this chapter will help the reader to avoid some common pitfalls.

Observation, structured or unstructured, participant or not, is a powerful tool for data collection that is used less often than it might be, perhaps because of the demands made upon the researcher. Observation, as used in quantitative and qualitative research, is very different, and Chapter 25 discusses each approach carefully. Ethical issues raised are considered, as are the problems of ensuring validity, reliability and trustworthiness of the data.

Lastly Chapter 26 deals with physiological measurement as a research tool. Many nurses have traditionally been employed to collect data for clinical trials, and such researchers will find this chapter valuable for its attention to the detail of reliable and valid measurement. The chapter will also be of value for any nurse researcher who wishes to include physiological and clinical measures in her research, and those using scales for such phenomena as pain, quality of life and physical dependency.

22 Interviewing

Angela Tod

Key points

- Interviews can be used to collect qualitative and quantitative data, and can vary in their degree of structure. The degree of structure is dictated by the research design and purpose.
- Key skills in conducting rigorous interviews include developing a well-designed data collection tool, selecting a suitable environment, establishing rapport, and balancing the direction and flexibility of questioning.
- Interviews can generate rich data reflecting the perspective of participants. Interviews can be of particular value when the research focus is a sensitive area.
- Interviews are labour intensive, expensive and can introduce bias.
- Interviews provide a unique opportunity to gain insight into a range of subjects and experiences related to nursing and health services.

Introduction

This chapter considers some of the key issues confronting the researcher in conducting a research interview. Brief attention is paid to the purpose and nature of the research interview. This is followed by an overview of different types of interview and some of the advantages and disadvantages of the different forms. The main issues to reflect on when undertaking research interviews are reviewed, followed by an outline of some factors relating to validity, reliability and ethics.

The purpose of the research interview

Conducting a research interview is one of the most exciting and fascinating methods of data collection in nursing and health care research. This may explain why it is one of the most commonly used data collection methods. Interviews are used in both qualitative and quantitative research as the primary data collection method or as a supplementary method in mixed method studies.

Reasons for undertaking interviews

The purpose of undertaking a research interview varies widely. The research aim will dictate the exact nature and form of the interview in terms of structure, direction and depth. Generally the more that is known about a topic beforehand, the more structured and less in-depth the exploration.

A structured interview approximates to a standardised interviewer-administered questionnaire. Structured interviews normally generate quantitative data. Some include limited open questions and have some capacity to produce qualitative data. Structured interviews would be used for a survey in order to measure variables in a specific population. The inclusion of open questions facilitates the collection of data to illuminate survey responses.

The majority of interview-based studies in nursing are qualitative in nature and so adopt a less structured, more 'in-depth' approach. Such methods are recommended when the research purpose is to:

- explore a phenomenon about which little is known
- understand context
- generate a hypothesis or theory to explain social processes and relationship
- verify the results from other forms of data collection, for example, observation
- illuminate responses from a questionnaire survey
- conduct initial exploration to generate items for questionnaires

Interviews, therefore, have the capacity to describe, explain and explore issues from the perspective of participants.

Boxes 22.1, 22.2, and 22.3 illustrate different uses of the research interview. Kamphuis *et al.* (2004) (Box 22.1) use semi-structured interviews to explore the experience of patients living with an implantable cardioverter defibrillator (ICD). This study demonstrates how interviews can generate qualitative data to inform caregivers of the physical and psychosocial implications of having an ICD.

Tod *et al.* (2003) (Box 22.2) used interviews in the qualitative component of a multimethod interventional study exploring the use of the internet in a ward environment. It demonstrates how interview data can explain responses to an intervention in an experimental study.

Laws (2004) (Box 22.3) uses structured interviews to collect quantitative data from doctors and nurses on obesity management.

The difference between a clinical and research interview

Nurses are trained to use interviews to obtain information from patients in clinical settings. While this clinical experience may be a good preparation, the research context and purpose is different and requires different skills. In research interviews the data collection requirement is broad as it is necessary to understand meanings regarding the area of study from the participants' viewpoint.

Box 22.1   Using interviews as a single method of data collection in a qualitative study.

Kamphuis HCM, Verhoeven NWJM, de Leeuw R, Derksen R, Hauer RNW, Winnubst JAM (2004) ICD: a qualitative study of patient experience the first year after implantation. *Journal of Clinical Nursing* 13: 1008–1016

In this study 21 patients with an implantable cardioverter defibrillator (ICD) were interviewed one, six and 12 months post discharge. The aim was to explore patients' experience of life with an ICD. The semi-structured interviews were conducted and audiotaped. The tapes were transcribed and analysed using content analysis. The study revealed the nature of situations caused by the ICD and patients' physical and psychosocial experiences of them. These include physical and cognitive deterioration and confrontation with mortality.

The authors report that the methods provided a rigorous and insightful means of exploring an area about which little is known. It allowed experiences to be categorised and better understood by caregivers. It provided a platform for experiences to be studied further in both quantitative and qualitative research.

Box 22.2   A study using interviews in a multimethod study.

Tod AM, Harrison J, Morris Docker S, Black R, Wolstenholme D (2003) Access to the internet in the clinical area: expectations and experiences of nurses working in an acute care setting. *British Journal of Nursing* 12: 425–434

This multimethod 'before-and-after' study aimed to evaluate the impact of open, ward-based access to the internet on the clinical practice of nurses and allied health professionals. Three methods of data collection were employed, each for different reasons. A questionnaire survey captured participants' attitudes to the internet, barriers and facilitators to access and use, views of its use and training needs. Continuous monitoring data of participants' use of the intervention was collected. This indicated the nature of actual use over the study period.

The semi-structured qualitative interviews of 16 participants were conducted prior to and after the intervention. The interviews were audiotaped, transcribed and analysed to generate themes related to expectations and experiences of the internet at work.

The study illustrates how interviews can be used to illuminate questionnaire responses and results from monitoring data.

In the clinical context, data collection is focused on identifying a problem, fitting it into a predetermined category e.g. diagnosis, and deciding a management or intervention strategy (Britten 1995). This means the clinical situation lends itself to being more controlled by the clinician. In addition a nurse would freely respond to patients' questions related to the clinical situation. In a research interview, this is not appropriate. To respond to questions may deviate away from the interview focus and may bias responses by changing the participant' knowledge base. Judgements made by researchers therefore differ from those of the nurse.

Box 22.3   A study using interviews to collect data in a quantitative study.

Laws R (2004) Current approaches to obesity management in UK primary care: the Counterweight Programme. *Journal of Human Nutrition and Dietetics* 17: 183–190

This study aimed to examine obesity management in 40 primary care practices in the UK. 141 general practitioners and 66 practice nurses were interviewed using a structured approach. A researcher-administered questionnaire was used to establish which of five obesity management approaches participants used. The approaches were based on time spent with patients and the nature of advice given. Referral practice and attitudes to obesity management were also recorded. Reported practice in the interviews was compared to recorded practice in the clinical notes.

The approach revealed that obesity was under-reported and under-recognised in primary care. However, it demonstrated the challenge of collecting data from busy clinical staff as one third of the participants did not complete the questionnaire/interview.

Types of interview

Structure

Robson (2002) states that the most common distinction made between different types of interview is the degree of structure and standardisation. A continuum exists from completely structured to unstructured interviews (Figure 22.1). In general, the less structured an interview the more in-depth and flexible the ques-

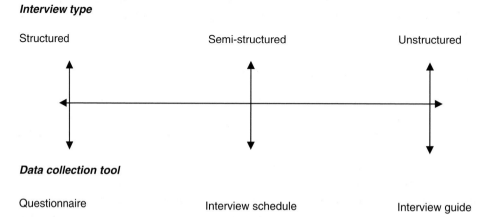

Interview type

Structured   Semi-structured   Unstructured

Data collection tool

Questionnaire   Interview schedule   Interview guide

Figure 22.1   The continuum of interview structure and data collection tool required.

tioning. An unstructured interview is likely to be led more by the informant agenda rather than the interviewer. It will generate qualitative data.

In structured interviews the balance of control lies with the interviewer. Such an approach would be adopted for survey purposes. Structured interviews are also used if it is not possible for the participant to self-administer a questionnaire, for example, if the participant does not have the ability or concentration to read.

In many qualitative studies semi-structured and unstructured interviews are used. Semi-structured interviews will have predetermined topics and open-ended questions laid down in an interview schedule. They retain the flexibility necessary to follow issues raised by participants that had not been anticipated. Control and direction of interviews of this nature still lies with the researcher but there will be capacity to be responsive to the interviewee's agenda and views. Semi-structured interviews are widely used in qualitative studies adopting a number of methodological approaches in nursing research.

Unstructured interviews are the most in-depth and least directive. The aim here is often to explore in great detail a general area of interest or a phenomenon. A few themes may guide the interview, but it will be led by the participant's perspective and viewpoint. Interviews of this nature are very informal and can appear more like a conversation than an interview. The interview guide will comprise a list of topics rather than predefined questions. This approach is more commonly adopted in qualitative research methodologies where little previous knowledge exists regarding the area of study.

The degree of structure employed in an interview will depend on the purpose of the study and the depth of inquiry required. It will also vary according to the resources available. With structured interviews, questioning techniques are standardised to ensure the reliability of the data. Unstructured interviews can be labour-intensive and expensive. Their informal and unguided structure means they can take a long time to conduct and also to transcribe and analyse. As is always the case with research, it is important to choose the right tool for the job and to make sure the approach adopted is achievable within the time and cost restraints of a study.

Face-to-face versus telephone interviews

The vast majority of individual interviews are conducted face-to-face. The researcher is able to probe and investigate hidden and suppressed views and experiences. The ability to observe body language and have eye contact helps to interpret what is being said. It also helps to interpret emotion, distress, anxiety and silence, and to respond accordingly. For example, if a respondent displays emotion it may provide an appropriate opportunity to collect data on a sensitive and upsetting experience of great value to the study. On the other hand, it may be appropriate to appraise the situation with regard to stopping the interview. Making this judgement is difficult if the interview is not face-to-face.

Telephone interviews are increasingly being used to conduct structured and semi-structured interviews. In some circumstances it may be a cheaper, more convenient mode of inquiry. Telephone interviews are limited in their ability to detect detailed information, misinformation and the emotional implications and subtext relating to the interview topic. However, there are situations where telephone interviews have clear advantages, particularly for structured interviews. Midanik and Greenfield (2003) compared the use of telephone and in-person interviews to collect data for a national survey on alcohol use. They found no differences in the number and quality of responses and so advocate the use of telephone interviews for national surveys. Telephone interviews are cheaper, requiring less travel and the equipment needed is minimal (a simple connecting cable between the phone and tape recorder).

In a qualitative research project, Garbett and McCormack (2001) were able to capture the views of 26 nurses working in different roles and settings across the UK by using telephone interviews. To undertake face-to-face interviews would have been expensive and required long distances to travel. Using the telephone also helped to ensure participants were not under any pressure to participate as they found it easier to refuse.

Telephone interviews can offer a more sensitive and less threatening approach when the nature of the research topic may create a risk of participants thinking they would be judged. It also provides a more convenient option if people are busy and have conflicting commitments.

One-off or longitudinal interviews

Numerous studies use interviews as a one-off strategy of data collection where interviews are collected at one point in time. Longitudinal or sequential interviews include the ability to collect data at different time points, for example, during the course of a patient's illness. This captures the evolving experience of the participant and tracks changes and gaps, for example in expectations and experiences or in health status.

Sequential interviews can generate richer data. Field and Morse (1985) claim that it is often impossible to collect good quality data at the first interview. The increased trust that develops over time between researcher and interviewee will also facilitate more in-depth and better quality data.

Undertaking an interview

On the surface an interview may appear to be a process of asking a few questions. In reality conducting a sound and rigorous interview can be a testing and complex enterprise (Robson 2002). The researcher has a responsibility to master certain techniques in order to produce results that are meaningful, useful and ensure that the interviewees' generous contribution is not in vain.

Developing the data collection tool

A structured interview will require a questionnaire. An unstructured interview will have maximum flexibility and often requires a guide comprising only a few core items. With a semi-structured interview a suitable schedule is essential to achieving the right balance of direction and flexibility. This means the central research question will be addressed as well as allowing new and interesting responses to be explored further. A number of factors should be considered in constructing an interview schedule. How important these are may depend upon the purpose of the study (i.e. to generate quantitative or qualitative data) and the nature of the questioning (i.e. level of structure and sensitivity of the subject).

First, it is necessary to be clear about the types of questions to be asked. Six main types of questions have been identified; behaviour or experience, opinion or belief, feeling, knowledge, sensory experience and background information such as demographics (Britten 1995; Patton, 1987). Some are easier to ask about and answer than others. Questions related to behaviour and knowledge may elicit short and specific responses. In comparison, questions about beliefs and feelings are more challenging, complex and potentially sensitive. They may need to be approached gradually and only after non-threatening questions have been asked.

Box 22.4 Sequence of questions in an interview.

Interview sequence	Type of questions
Introduction	• Introduce the study. • Explain the purpose of the interview. • Check the participant understands the purpose and nature of the study. • Obtain or verify consent. • Promote a relaxed atmosphere by making conversation.
Warm-up	• Ask neutral, unthreatening questions. • Ask for factual background information e.g. age, children, job. • Seek clarification or expansion if necessary.
Main interview questions	• Ask questions relating to the main research aim. • Ensure sequence follows some logic and sense. • Start with broad questions followed by more focused ones. • Leave the most sensitive and difficult questions until last. • Use prompts and probes to generate deeper and richer data.
Wind down	• Round off with a few simple questions, especially if the interview has been tense, emotional or sensitive. • Let the interviewee know the interview is winding up, for example say 'to finish with . . .' • Ask if there is anything else they would like to add.
Close of interview	• Check again there is nothing else they want to add. • Check people know and remember what will happen to the data • Thank the participant.

Compiled with reference to Robson (2002); Legard et al. (2003)

It is common for the sequence of the schedule to be divided into sections, for example, introduction, 'warm up' or opening questions, the main interview questions, 'wind down' questions and closing the interview (Box 22.4).

Inappropriate timing of questions can sabotage the interview. If rapport and trust have been established it is possible to ask questions of an extremely sensitive nature. It is necessary continually to judge the appropriateness of an interview question in terms of the timing and how it will be interpreted and received by the interviewee.

Prompts can be built into the interview. These are particularly important in semi-structured interview schedules. Prompts have been described as questions that derive from the researcher (Robson 2002). They are intended to test an *a priori* assumption of the researcher or facilitate the interviewee to reflect on or expand upon a certain theme issue (Legard *et al.* 2003). They can also be used if participants lose their thread as a way of encouraging them to re-engage with the interview.

Tod *et al.* (2001) used a semi-structured interview schedule to explore patients' experience of angina symptoms in order to identify barriers and facilitators in symptom reporting. Box 22.5 provides examples of broad questions used to start the interview followed by more focused questions with predetermined prompts.

Box 22.5   Example of questions used in a semi-structured interview.

Type of question	When/why asked	Example
Broad question	Asked at the beginning of the interview to gain an overview of the patient's experience, develop rapport and influence subsequent questioning	Can you tell me something about your general health?
Focused question	Asked afterwards to elicit information about diagnosis of angina and any other chronic condition	Do you have any longstanding illness or disability?
Structured questionnaire	Administered as a way of verifying the patient has angina	Administer the *Rose Angina Questionnaire* (Rose *et al.* 1977). This is a short questionnaire eliciting information on the patient's chest pain and is an objective measure of angina symptoms.
Prompt	If not mentioned investigate further whether they have angina	Has your doctor told you what is wrong with you, i.e. what causes the chest pain?

The results of this study are found in Tod et al. (2001)

Conducting the interview

Selecting a suitable environment

Maintaining a suitable interview environment will often require a trade-off between accessibility, comfort and level of distraction. If a venue is considered inappropriate or inaccessible people will be reluctant to take part. Common choices are the interviewee's home or workplace. A more neutral location may be required if people are likely to be distracted by or protective of their personal and professional setting.

The comfort of the environment is essential if interviewees are to feel relaxed, at ease and able to concentrate. On occasions, however, it may be necessary to sacrifice some comfort in order to involve participants from certain groups, for example interviewing patients on bedrest or nurses on or near their ward.

Choosing an environment with minimum risk of disruption is also a concern. There are certain things that a researcher can do to facilitate this, such as turning off telephones and other equipment, or putting up a 'do not disturb' sign.

All best laid plans go astray and sometimes the unexpected occurs, for example a participant having unexpected childcare commitments resulting in a child present at the interview. The researcher then needs to make a judgement about whether to proceed with the interview with the knowledge that the quality may be affected, or whether to cancel the interview and risk offending the participant.

Establishing rapport

A successful interview will be reliant upon developing a sense of trust and rapport. The attitude and demeanour of the interviewer is key and it is essential that they appear genuine and interested in the participant's views. Legard *et al.* (2003) suggest that the researcher displaying confidence, tranquillity and credibility facilitates this. Humour and adaptability are also tools. Being organised, efficient and focused, having a well-planned and paced schedule of questions and being responsive to the mood, body language and priorities of the interviewee all help to develop a good interview relationship. The posture and bearing of the researcher should convey attention and interest.

Questioning technique

Techniques used to facilitate questioning need to maintain a balance between direction and flexibility. Where the balance lies will reflect the research aim, method and level of structure. Techniques include active listening, being clear and unambiguous, not leading respondents towards particular views or beliefs and, again, keeping interested. The tradition is to advise researchers to say as little as possible because of the risk the interviewer may contaminate, influence or confuse the interviewee. Some researchers now argue for more interaction in qualitative interviews on the grounds that it allows the researcher to test out emerging ideas and discussion helps to explore more complex issues (Melia 2000). One approach to being more interactive is what Melia (2000) refers to as 'verbal memo-ing' where the interviewer investigates initial arguments emerging from analysis. Another option that can be used in both qualitative and quantitative research would be to construct vignettes or scenarios from earlier accounts to draw out opinion in subsequent interviews.

The appropriate use of prompts and probes can help achieve the right balance of breadth and depth in the questioning (Legard *et al.* 2003). In structured interviews they may be used to clarify a question if it is misunderstood. In unstructured and semi-structured interviews some questions lead the respondent to broad statements that may set the stage or reveal a range of issues and dimensions. Probes may then be used to uncover layers of meaning. Probing questions have the capacity to amplify, explore, explain or clarify (Legard *et al.* 2003). The astute use of silence to help participants reflect and respond is a valuable interview technique. An interested look, maintaining eye contact, or summarising can all help to prompt a response.

Managing the interview

An interview is a sensitive interaction and needs careful handling. This should start from the outset by considering how the participant perceives the researcher. Difference or similarity in age, ethnicity, gender or social status can all make a difference to how people respond. Demeanour and appearance may vary, therefore, between interviewing a chief executive of a hospital and teenagers. Clarity of introduction both of the researcher and the project itself can also help. This will also minimise any risk of role conflict for a nurse conducting a research interview.

Setting the scene for the respondent is essential. Points to explain include:

- There are no right or wrong answers.
- They have the right to withdraw or stop at any time.
- They can interrupt or ask for explanations whenever they want.
- The interview will be recorded (usually on audiotape) with their permission.

Common pitfalls in conducting interviews

Field and Morse (1985) include the risk of losing the research role and slipping into that of a teacher, preacher or counsellor. This risk is a particular danger in less structured interviews where the discussion is more in-depth. On occasions it is difficult to avoid role conflict, especially for nurses and others with a clinical training. The interviewer must avoid putting his or her own view and perspective forward. This is a particular hazard when the respondent has said something the researcher disagreed with or finds offensive. To explore such views gently will be more productive than challenging them (Legard *et al.* 2003).

Handling a situation that is emotionally charged can be testing if a participant becomes upset, anxious or angry. Sensitive questioning can help, as will communicating empathy and interest with body language and eye contact. However, it is important not to be frightened of such emotional situations. Not only do they often produce the most valuable and insightful data, the participant may find it a positive experience to discuss the issue in this way.

Selecting the most appropriate way of recording an interview is a key factor in its success. The most common form of recording is audiotape, supplemented by fieldnotes. Other media include videorecording, videoconferencing or internet chat rooms. In making a decision it is important to consider how intrusive the technology will appear to the participant, ease of use of the technology, reliability, and ethical aspects regarding confidentiality and privacy. It is always important to check that recording equipment is working well before the interview. Budgeting on the quality of this technology may be a false economy. Following the interview the recording is normally transcribed verbatim ready for analysis.

When taking fieldnotes it is necessary to be aware of how this will be interpreted by the respondent. It is easy to appear as if the researcher is not listening or interested, if they appear more absorbed in scribbling notes than in participating in the interview.

Additional challenges in managing an interview can occur if the researcher and participant do not speak the same language and an interpreter is used. Developing rapport and trust can be more difficult if conducting an interview through a third person. It is therefore necessary to ensure the interpreter is acceptable to the participant and culturally appropriate, in addition to having good language skills. Maintaining accuracy in collecting data is also difficult. The interpreter should be skilled and practised in research interview work and be able to demonstrate accuracy of translation between interviewee and interviewer.

Managing an interview well is a difficult task and needs practice. Piloting is recommended, especially when the researcher is new to the interview process. Piloting allows questions to be tested and refined and practice gained in using recording equipment. A novice interviewer is advised to secure good supervision, not just to support the research design and data analysis, but also to aid reflection of the interview experience. Mistakes are inevitable, but it is always worth reflecting back on these and discussing ways to avoid the same pitfalls in the future.

Advantages and disadvantages of interviews

Interviewing is a flexible and adaptable method of data collection and can be an efficient way of collecting data on a myriad of subjects including participants' views, attitudes, behaviours and experiences. The flexibility of the interview format and structure is one of its greatest advantages. The interview is malleable and can be adapted to fit the needs and purpose of different studies from quantitative surveys to detailed phenomenological explorations of individuals' experiences.

Structured interviews have the capacity to generate a large volume of data from a large sample. They are an excellent means of collecting data that is predominantly quantitative but can incorporate qualitative questioning. It is possible to use structured interviews to test the findings of smaller, in-depth interview studies with a larger population.

Semi- and unstructured interviews have an unrivalled ability to generate data of depth and complexity. The forum of the interview provides the opportunity to explore the intricacy of an issue from the perspective of individual participants.

Interviews may provide the only method of eliciting the views of people who are often 'hard-to-reach' in terms of research and who would be reluctant or unable to participate in research using other methods. There is some indication that, while not intentionally having a direct therapeutic effect, people do find the experience of being interviewed a positive one.

Many of the disadvantages are reflected in the challenges referred to earlier, for example, the risk of introducing bias by inadequate sampling or questioning. Following the advice and techniques above can avoid this. However, one danger to be considered is that the involvement in the interview itself may change the views or perceptions of the participants. The researcher should be continually vigilant of this risk of a 'Hawthorne effect' throughout data collection and analysis.

Finally, interviewing can be expensive in terms of time and funding. Resources may be required to support the researchers or participants' involvement, for example, travel, care of participants' dependants, reimbursement for loss of earnings, refreshments. The costs of reliable technical recording equipment, transcription and the researchers are not insignificant and need to be considered when making the decision to use interviews as a data collection method.

Issues of validity and reliability

The degree of reliability (the accuracy and consistency of the data collection) required from an interview will vary. In a structured interview, high levels of reliability will be sought. Training and a robust schedule will ensure standardised practice between different researchers. With a more in-depth, semi- or unstructured interview reliability is less achievable. Such an interview will be flexible and interactive in order to understand the individual's social construction and representation of the research phenomenon. However, a competent researcher with a consistent approach and well-designed schedule will be able to maximise the rigour of the results (Lincoln and Guba 1985).

The validity of a study considers how 'true' the data are. The challenge is to demonstrate that the findings are an accurate account of the participant's representation of the topic, and not due to bias.

Data collection bias may arise in interviews because of the way the sample has been selected, how the interview is conducted or because of the researchers' influence. In order to protect against these risks it is necessary to monitor and reflect on the following questions:

- Has the sample any inbuilt bias, e.g. are some groups excluded or under-represented?
- Are the questions addressing the participants' concerns, views and experiences?
- Have the interviewees been given the opportunity to adequately present their views?
- Has the researcher led or influenced the participant's responses in any way?

Having clear and well-prepared documentation will help address these questions, for example interview schedules and fieldnotes.

Ethical issues with interviewing

Some of the major ethical issues relating to interview based studies are outlined here.

Consent

Chapter 10 gives details of the procedures that need to be followed to obtain informed consent. Potential interviewees should be approached with sufficient time to reflect on the implications of participation, and not feel pressurised into taking part. A signature is required to indicate informed consent has been given. When this is obtained some time prior to the interview taking place, consent should be verified immediately before the actual interview.

Anonymity and confidentiality

The names and identity of participants should not be revealed as a result of the collection, analysis and reporting of the study, in order to preserve their anonymity and confidentiality. It is important to ensure that first contact with participants about the study is via someone with a legitimate role and right to identify them, for example the consultant or senior nurse involved in patients' care.

There are circumstances when complete anonymity is not possible to guarantee, for example, when reporting the age, gender and medical condition/role would identify a person. In smaller interview-based studies, recruiting from a limited sampling frame this is a real risk. Where this threat occurs it should be pre-empted and included in the informed consent procedure. Sometimes people are prepared to be involved despite the risk of being identified, but they should be given the chance to agree any direct references and quotes from them used in any reports or publications.

In order to protect anonymity, interviewees are sometimes referred to by number or pseudonym. Asking a person to choose their own pseudonym can help them understand the confidentiality implications of participation.

Once an interview tape has been recorded, all identifiable references need to be removed from the tape and transcript. These ought then to be stored in locked, secure storage and in password-protected computers. Tapes are usually destroyed or returned to participants on completion of the study.

Protecting participants' and researchers' rights, and protecting them from harm

Ensuring interviewees' understanding of the study and its requirements is a key concern when protecting them from harm. It is therefore important to make certain people know what subjects will be covered, especially where these are sensitive or distressing in nature. Where necessary, support for the participant may be required and, where available, stated in the information sheet.

When explaining the study, it is important not to raise the expectations of participants regarding its impact on their own care, other people's care or the development of services. People often participate in interviews, where they share their views and experiences, for altruistic reasons. Researchers should endeavour to be realistic in any claims that the study has the capacity to make change.

One major risk in conducting interviews is where a risk to the participant or someone else is revealed. Examples include:

- a patient revealing suicidal thoughts
- a patient or staff member describing an incident of negligence or abuse
- a patient revealing that their medical condition has deteriorated

These challenging dilemmas should be considered on a case-by-case basis. The risk-benefit balance of reporting what the participant has disclosed or remaining silent may vary tremendously. Where possible the risk of this should be pre-empted, a reporting process put in place and made clear in the information sheet. For example, the situation might be discussed with a patient's doctor or nurse.

Finally, researchers have a requirement to protect themselves. If an interview has been particularly emotional, tense or challenging, the availability of experienced, trusted supervision to facilitate reflection is invaluable.

The other main risk for a researcher relates to issues of personal safety. It is standard practice for interviewers to inform an identified person of the time and location of an interview and inform them when it is over and they have left the venue. This is a particular requirement when interviewing in people's own home or unknown environments. A mobile phone and panic alarms are sometimes carried as additional means of communication if the researcher feels exceptionally threatened.

Conclusion

Conducting an interview involves sharing an aspect of someone's life. As such, the decision to employ interviews as a data collection method should not be taken lightly. The practical, procedural, ethical and cost implications all have to be considered. However, if these are addressed, and a researcher has the required expertise and support, conducting an interview can be a vehicle to gaining a unique insight into the area of study and a privilege and pleasure to undertake.

References

Britten N (1995) Qualitative research: qualitative interviews in research. *British Medical Journal* 311: 251–253

Department of Health (2001) *Governance Arrangements for NHS Research Ethics Committees.* London, Department of Health

Field PA, Morse JM (1985) *Nursing research: the application of qualitative approaches.* London, Chapman & Hall

Garbett R, McCormack B (2001) The experience of practice development: an exploratory telephone interview study. *Journal of Clinical Nursing* 10: 94–102

Kamphuis H, Verhoeven N, de Leeuw R, Derksen R, Hauer R, Winnubst J (2004) ICD: a qualitative study of patient experience the first year after implantation. *Journal of Clinical Nursing* 13: 1008–1016

Laws R (2004) Current approaches to obesity management in UK primary care. *Journal of Human Nutrition and Dietetics* 17: 183–190

Legard R, Keegan J, Ward K (2003) In-depth interviews. In Ritchie J, Lewis J (eds) *Qualitative Research Practice.* London, Sage pp138–169

Lincoln YS, Guba E (1985) *Naturalistic Inquiry.* London, Sage

Melia KB (2000) Conducting an interview. *Nurse Researcher* 7: 4 75–89

Midanik LT, Greenfield TK (2003) Telephone versus in-person interviews for alcohol use: results of a 2000 National Alcohol Survey. *Drug and Alcohol Dependence* 72: 209–214

Patton MQ (1987) *How to Use Qualitative Methods in Evaluation.* London, Sage

Robson C (2002) *Real World Research*, 2nd edition. Oxford, Blackwell

Rose GA, McCartney P, Reid DD (1977) Self-administration of a questionnaire on chest pain and intermittent claudication. *British Journal of Preventive and Social Medicine* 31: 42–8

Tod AM (2003) Smoking cessation services in pregnancy: a qualitative study. *British Journal of Community Nursing* 8: 56–64

Tod AM, Harrison J, Morris Docker S, Black R, Wolstenholme D (2003) Access to the internet in the clinical area: expectations and experiences of nurses working in an acute care setting. *British Journal of Nursing* 12: 425–434

Tod AM, Read C, Lacey A, Abbott J (2001) Overcoming barriers to uptake of services for coronary heart disease: a qualitative study. *British Medical Journal* 323: 214–217

Further reading

Graham H (1987) Women's Smoking and Family Health. *Social Science and Medicine* 25: 47–56

Tod AM, Lacey EA (2004) Overweight and obesity: helping patients to take action. *British Journal of Community Nursing* 9: 59–66

23 Using Focus Groups

Claire Goodman and Catherine Evans

Key points

- Focus groups are a useful data collection method when the aim is to clarify, explore or confirm ideas with a range of participants on a predefined set of issues.
- Group interactions are an important feature of focus groups and an integral part of the data collection process.
- It requires considerable preparation and skill to run a successful focus group, ideally one person should act as the moderator of the group while a second researcher acts as observer.
- Analysis of focus group data should ask specific questions about the group process and interaction as well as the content of the discussion.

Purpose of focus groups

A focus group is an in-depth, open-ended group discussion that explores a specific set of issues on a predefined topic. Focus groups are used extensively as a research method in nursing research in two ways:

- To obtain the views and experiences of a selected group on an issue (Goodman *et al.* 2003, Box 23.1; Kevern & Webb 2004, Box 23.2) or
- To use the forum of a group discussion to increase understanding about a given topic (Phillips & Woodward 1999, Box 23.3).

Focus groups seldom aim to produce consensus between participants and are unlikely to be the method of choice if this is the study's aim. The key premise of focus groups is that individuals in groups do not respond to questions in the same way that they do in other settings and it is the group interaction that enables participants to explore and clarify their experience and insights on a specific issue. Participants can share and discuss their knowledge and even revise their original ideas and understanding. This data collection method allows the researcher to expose inconsistency within a group as well as providing examples of conformity and agreement. Focus groups, therefore, have the potential to provide a rich source of data.

Box 23.1   The use of focus groups in the preliminary stages of a study.

Goodman C, Woolley R, Knight D (2003) District nurses' experiences of providing care in residential care home settings. *Journal of Clinical Nursing* 12: 67–76

This study identified that although district nurses spend an increasing amount of time visiting older people in care homes, little is known about their work in these settings or the issues they encounter. Initially, five separate focus groups were held with district nurses and community staff nurses to inform the development of a questionnaire. There were 44 participants in total. To ease participation four of the groups were held either just before or just after a meeting the practitioners were scheduled to attend, so participants could choose to come early or stay later. One group was organised separately. Each group lasted between 40 minutes and an hour, was taped, and had a moderator and an observer.
   The group discussion revealed many shared experiences, but less consensus about what the district nurse role in care homes should be. Although district nurses undertook similar activities they held very different beliefs and rationales for this work. For example, some practitioners offered teaching and support to care home staff as a way of maintaining continuity of care for older people and building relationships with staff, while others represented it as a means of reducing the need to visit so frequently, as care home staff absorbed simple nursing tasks into their work. The authors concluded that staff preoccupations and anxieties about workload demand and boundaries of care appeared to overshadow concerns and awareness of the needs of the older people resident in care homes.

Focus groups were first developed for market research at Columbia University, USA and used to gauge audience responses to propaganda and radio broadcasts during World War II. Twohig and Putnam (2002) in their review of studies that have used focus groups in health care research did not identify any studies cited by MEDLINE before 1985 but noted it has been a widely used method in sociology, education and political science.

Focus groups are not aligned with a particular tradition of qualitative research. It is therefore important that researchers who use this method are sure that it fits with the overall research approach. As the discussion is organised *outside* the everyday experience and there is a preset focus to the interaction there are inevitable tensions in employing focus group methods in studies that have a strong emphasis on naturalistic inquiry and immersion in the participants' lived experience. For example, the researcher would need to justify how the use of focus groups would fit with a study that is based on grounded theory or phenomenology (*see* Chapters 13 and 15 for more detailed consideration of this issue).

There is considerable variation in how focus groups are reported in nursing research literature and little agreement about optimum group size and numbers of groups to include within a study. There is also criticism that focus groups encourage a superficial approach to enquiry and therefore have limited value as a standalone data collection method.

Box 23.2   The use of focus groups to elaborate upon quantitative research findings.

Kevern J, Webb C (2004) Mature women's experiences of pre-registration nurse education. *Journal of Advanced Nursing* 45: 297–306

Government policy in England has targeted the recruitment of mature women into nurse training as a way of addressing the shortage of qualified nurses. This study aimed to follow-up a quantitative study of mature female pre-registration diploma students to gain a deeper understanding of their experiences of higher education and to identify appropriate organisational support systems for them. A purposive sample of mature students (n = 40) were invited by letter to participate in the study. Five focus groups were held involving 32 women. The lead researcher moderated the groups; no observer was present. A list of six agenda items formed the broad framework for the focus groups. The group processes were recorded using audiotape and written notes. From the thematic analysis of the transcripts, the experiences of the mature women nursing students formed three major themes.

'Didn't know what to expect' described the women's uncertainty about entering nurse training.

'Reality shock' encompassed the competing demands of academic study, nursing placements and family commitments.

'Learning the Game' referred to the strategies the women adopted to remain on the course, for example, moderating their academic expectations of themselves.

The authors conclude that ideology and patriarchy restrict women's activities in university. They identified the need to expand the options for women with multiple role demands by providing, for example, more flexible and well-organised student-centred programmes.

Conducting a focus group

It is a misconception to regard focus group interviews as a simple way of gathering data from multiple participants. A focus group requires the researcher to give time to preparation and have skills in facilitating group discussion. It is labour intensive and often involves two researchers, one as moderator of the group discussion and the other as observer. Consideration is given here to sampling strategy and group size, developing a topic guide and how to conduct a focus group, including managing the discussion and recording information.

Sampling strategy and group size

Major challenges to using focus groups include identifying, sampling and recruiting participants, group size and composition, and decisions on how many focus groups should be held.

Box 23.3 The use of focus groups to increase understanding of a given topic.

Phillips K, Woodward V (1998) The decision to resuscitate: older people's views. *Journal of Clinical Nursing* 8: 753–761

This study aimed to explore how older people felt about resuscitation and decisions of Do Not Resuscitate (DNR) for certain patients. The researchers were interested in participants' views on who should be involved in deciding a person's resuscitation status. To obtain a 'healthy' sample of older people, people aged over 50 years attending a local 'drop-in' centre were approached to participate. Participants joined one of two focus groups held in a private room at the centre segmented by age; one group comprising eight people in their 50s and the second comprising nine people in their 70s. A structured topic guide moved from the broad area of 'what does resuscitation mean?' through to specific sensitive questions of 'would you want to be asked whether you wanted to be resuscitated?' A moderator facilitated the group discussion, using audiotape to record group process; no observer was present. Audiotapes were transcribed and subject to thematic content analysis; four principal themes were identified:

- factors in favour of resuscitation
- factors against resuscitation
- when is it appropriate not to resuscitate
- who makes the decision?

Overall, participants agreed that patients and relatives should be involved in DNR decision, but were ambivalent as to whether they would like to be personally involved.

The identification and sampling of members of the target population is guided by the aims, or research questions for the study (*see* Chapter 2). It can be useful to develop a topic-specific sampling strategy to encompass the diversity of people involved in the subject area (Kitzinger & Barbour 1999). For example, Chiu and Knight's (1999) sampling strategy to investigate low uptake of breast and cervical screening by black and minority ethnic women, included women from seven language groups in order to obtain a spread of views and experiences from this varied population.

To gain access to the possible participants from the target population, it is often helpful to approach a stakeholder or group representative. For example, a director of nursing in a health trust is a useful stakeholder to gain access to NHS nurses. Identifying participants from populations not necessarily associated with an organisation, for example, 'healthy' older people, can be assisted by approaching places where they congregate, such as a drop-in centre and advertising the project or recruiting a pre-existing group (Box 23.3).

Non-random sampling techniques such as purposive and convenience sampling (*see* Chapter 12) are normally used because the intention of the focus group is usually to increase understanding of a phenomenon, not provide evidence directly generalisable to a wider population. Moreover, a randomly-selected group may not hold a shared perspective on the research topic, prohibiting meaningful group discussion (Morgan 1997). Purposive sampling is preferable when sampling participants with specific characteristics, experience or knowledge, such as district nurses working within the care home sector (Box 23.1). If the target population is small, difficult to identify or access, convenience sampling can be helpful. When all participants within the target population would be eligible to participate selection can be based upon interest in participating in the study and availability.

Group composition and size are both contentious issues within the focus group literature. Again, decisions are based upon the nature of the enquiry, the study design and the amount of time and funding available. Debates on group composition focus on homogeneity (similar participants) versus heterogeneity (diverse participants) and the use (or not) of pre-existing groups. Homogeneous groups, segmented by, for example, a shared perspective such as age (Box 23.3), language group or professional position (Boxes 23.1 and 23.2) are generally preferable to ensure free discussion and enable cross-group comparisons (Morgan 1997). Differences, however, between participants in a heterogeneous group are often illuminating and the use of pre-existing groups can enable the context to be captured within which ideas are formed and decisions made (Kitzinger 1994). Using pre-existing groups can also be useful in recruiting people unlikely to come forward to participate in a focus group if they feel marginalised by society or are unwilling to participate with people they do not know. However, in groups where participants are very familiar with each other, existing group norms and hierarchies may inhibit the contributions of members (Kitzinger & Barbour 1999).

The size of a focus group varies typically from between five members to no more than 12. The group must be large enough to ensure diversity of perspectives, and be small enough to ensure everybody has a chance to participate. Decisions on group size are informed by:

- the nature of the subject area (the more sensitive the area the smaller the group)
- the level of group structure (the more structure the larger the group)
- the resources available (funding for more than one group, size of room space)
- moderator expertise (less experienced moderator the smaller the group)

Generally, it is advisable to invite more than the required number of group members to counter the inevitable problems of no-shows. Telephoning people who have agreed to participate a few days beforehand can reduce this problem. The focus group needs to be conducted at a convenient time in an accessible venue, and there may be value in interviewing people away from the institution they belong to (Kitzinger & Barbour 1999). In practice, it is often the financial resources and time available for the study that influence venue choices.

Focus groups need more preparation and anticipation than individual interviews. On the day of the focus group the moderator should arrive sufficiently
early to signpost the location; arrange the room and have refreshments for
participants. An ideal room is one that is private, large enough to accommodate
the group, quiet and comfortable. If working with an observer it is important to
talk through the anticipated process and the topic guide, and agree seating
arrangements.

Structuring group discussion and developing a topic guide

The level of group structure depends upon the intention of the focus group. A
structured group using a topic guide is preferable when the research questions
are clear, for example, using focus groups to develop questionnaires for individual
interviews (*see* Box 23.1). A less structured group framed around one or two topic
areas, is useful in exploratory research when little is known about the area of study
(*see* Box 23.2). Both approaches have advantages and disadvantages. The structured approach ensures consistency across groups enabling comparisons to be
made between groups, but a narrow set of questions may limit the discussion and
inhibit contributions on related issues. Less structure often creates a livelier group
discussion. A compromise between the two approaches may also be used (*see* Box
23.3). Morgan (1997) describes this as a 'funnel-based' approach in which:

> 'each group begins with a less structured approach that emphasises free discussion
> and then moves toward a more structured discussion of specific questions' (Morgan
> 1997:41)

The research aims and the literature should inform the development of the topic
guide (McLafferty 2004). The intention of the guide is to create a natural progression through the topic areas and stimulate group discussion without influencing
the responses. A structured guide uses at most five to six questions. A less structured approach is to organise the guide around two or three broad discussion
topics, loosely phrased as questions, like, 'We are interested in . . . ? What can you
tell us about this area? (Morgan 1997). In both instances, the questions are ordered
to move from general to specific and non-sensitive to more sensitive, the aim being
to enable all group members to participate (Kingry *et al.* 1990). The topic area
should be familiar to all, not be intimidating or require personal exposure. More
sensitive or probing questions come nearer the middle of the interview. This provides participants with time to feel safe to speak within the group. Open-ended
questions prefixed by either, *how, what, where* or *why* allow participants freedom
to respond. Too many 'why' questions can be experienced as confrontational and
provoke defensive responses (Nyamathi & Shuler 1990).

Managing the discussion

Sufficient time should be allowed to greet and seat participants. Begin the session
by welcoming participants, introducing yourself and the observer, clarifying the

purpose of the session, and the anticipated finish time. Ensure participants understand how the discussion will be recorded, who has access to these recordings and how confidentiality will be maintained. Ask if participants have any questions about the interview format and agree ground rules. Ground rules are intended to facilitate group discussion, not confine it. The agreed rules should be concise, few in number and displayed for participants (e.g. on flip chart). They may state:

- Issues discussed in the group are confidential to the participants and the researchers.
- Only one person is to speak at a time.

Introductions to the topic should be brief and clear, and instructions kept to a minimum. This helps participants to understand the focus of the session, without directing their thinking, and emphasises that the ownership of the group discussion belongs to both the participants and the moderator. Participant introductions create an opportunity for all to speak and provides identification markers to differentiate participants for the observer and when transcribing the audiotapes. Plan for latecomers and ensure that participants are informed prior to the interview whether or not they will be able to take part if they arrive after the indicated start time.

Moderators should promote debate by asking open questions and probing for more detail on points of interest, reflecting a point made to confirm understanding, and summarising points to check that all areas have been covered, particularly before changing a topic. These techniques reinforce for participants that the points they make are valued, and encourages their participation in the discussion. The discussion should include all areas in the topic guide, particularly if conducting several focus groups. Incomplete data sets restrict comparative analysis between groups and may compromise the aims of the study.

Moderators need to encourage participation by inviting group members to comment on an individual's views especially if someone is dominating the discussion. Avoid expressing personal opinions or correcting participants' knowledge to prevent biasing the discussion towards a particular opinion or position (Gibbs 1997). Correcting or supporting participants' knowledge can be addressed at the end of the interview. For example, Roth et al. (2003) provided a health care worker in HIV at the end of focus group sessions on bilingual health advocacy and antenatal HIV testing to provide further information on HIV.

Group exercises may be used within the session to explore understanding about a particular issue or to indicate preferences. Kitzinger (1994) for example, used cards with statements on them about HIV to explore participants' perceptions of risks. Such exercises encourage participants to focus on each other rather than the moderator.

Timekeeping is essential and shows respect for participants' time. Leave 5–10 minutes to round up the interview. This provides an opportunity for participants to offer further comments and reflect on their experience of participating in the group.

Recording information

Group interactions are the crucial feature of focus groups and mark them as different from individual interviews. Audiotape, videotape and an observer can be used alone, or in combination to record the group interaction. Ideally, transcribed audiotape is preferable, with an observer and/or videotaping. Video tapings can be poor at recording speech and are normally used in combination with an audiotape. An observer is useful for recording, for example, the group's seating arrangement and non-verbal cues of supportive or aggressive behaviour. An observation sheet with headings for particular areas of interest can help to structure the observations.

Audio and video equipment should be reliable and have a high-quality microphone for recording groups, rather than individuals. The quality of the tape recording directly influences the precision of the transcribing and the consequent validity of the transcript analysis. Ensure audiotapes are the correct length for the interview and labelled with an identification number, date and time, to prevent recording over data and as a reference point for transcribing (Bramley 2004).

Analysis

The principles and process of analysis for focus group data are very similar to those applied to qualitative data obtained from individual interviews (see Chapters 22 and 27). When undertaking analysis of a focus group discussion it is important however, to be clear about the purpose of the analysis and whether it is the group discussion as a whole or the range of contributions to that discussion that is of interest. The research question and the rationale for using focus groups guide the analysis, and inform how the data are organised and read.

It is seldom practical to ask focus group participants to check the validity of transcripts or preliminary analysis. It is therefore useful to summarise at the end of the group what the moderator believes to be the main issues to emerge from the discussion for confirmation or clarification by the group. This not only helps understanding but also represents the first stage in analysis where tentative themes can be identified and subsequently tested within the detailed analysis of the group transcripts. At the end of the focus group it is also good practice for the group's moderator to debrief with the observer to record initial impressions of how the group went and to identify issues that may directly affect the analysis. Factors such as dominance of the discussion by particular individuals, impressions of how engaged participants were with the issues raised and whether non-participation in the group indicated disagreement or affirmation with what was being said should be noted. These first impressions are useful as memoranda that can subsequently inform analysis.

In contrast to analysis of individual interviews, an important part of the analytic process is identifying areas of agreement and controversy and how views are modified or reinforced during the group discussion. When coding data it is helpful to think about the data as a group process. It is therefore sensible to organise the data to reflect how the discussion progressed. Most groups will take some time to establish a rapport and there will be some issues and questions that generate more interest and contributions than others. Coding the data into narrative units can be helpful as there will be some major issues identified within the group discussion that either generate the most contributions or the strongest responses. This means that individual responses to a particular issue or question, the asides, challenges and elaborations that occur within the group are coded together and in relation to each other.

Software that supports qualitative analysis is invaluable as it can track individual contributions as well as interactions and responses and allows interrogation of the data in different ways. Furthermore, by tracing the development and sequence of statements of the discussion on an issue it is possible to judge which ideas participants offered as tentative thoughts at the beginning of a focus group became, by the end of the group, established views.

In a review of the use of focus groups as a research method in nursing research, Webb and Kerven (2001) suggest that the approach to analysis of focus group data is often relatively unsophisticated and that the interaction that occurred within groups is rarely reported. They suggest that the analytic procedure should ask specific questions of the group process and interaction to deepen the understanding of the data obtained. In this way the researcher can identify statements that provoked the most emotion, reaction or conflict, how different statements related to each other, if there were discernible alliances that emerged within the group or particular interests that were emphasised over others.

The use of descriptive statistics to summarise the frequency with which issues were raised and the amount of time spent discussing an issue can be helpful, particularly when comparing responses between different focus groups. When marked differences are identified between groups this should prompt another look at what it was about these groups, their membership or setting, that could explain the variation. However, there should be considerable caution in suggesting that a particular subject or issue was more important or significant because it was raised more frequently than something else. Counting statements made on particular topics will generate a list of what participants said, but attributing meaning to this can be problematic unless the analysis also accounts for how people interacted within the group.

Issues of validity and reliability

Validity is the extent to which a procedure actually measures what it proposes to measure. Typically, focus groups have high face validity as a credible method that can directly capture the views of participants in response to the study focus. Threats to face validity are those that threaten the accuracy of the participants' views on the topic areas of interest. These can include research questions that are unsuitable for a focus group because they are concerned with the narrative on individual experience. Idiosyncratic and opportunistic recruitment from the population of interest can make it difficult to interpret findings. A lack of transparency in how the group discussion was organised, the prompts used, the amount of direction given to the group by the moderator and approaches to analysis can also threaten the confidence with which the results from focus group research can be interpreted.

Reliability concerns the degree of consistency in observing the area of interest over time. For focus groups, reliability is most relevant as it relates to the consistency in the data gathered within each respective group. Threats to consistency across groups include the structure and delivery of the topic guide, the impact of moderator bias, differences between the groups' membership, for example regarding gender, the interview environment, and accuracy in transcribing and analysing audiotapes. However, in groups where the emphasis is on discovery, the diversity of the participants may enhance the breadth of understanding.

Advantages of focus groups

Whereas focus groups can appear to be a quick and flexible method of data collection, they are not an inexpensive or time-saving method. Considerable time is required to recruit participants, set up the groups, transcribe and analyse the data generated. There are however, some clear advantages that focus groups methods have over other data collection methods. In the early stages of a study the discussion and data generated by a focus group can identify complex problems and areas that need further exploration and clarification. A group discussion held at the end of the study provides the opportunity for participants to respond to the findings and offer explanations or alternative interpretations. The exploratory and illuminatory function of focus groups can thus extend and challenge how researchers define their research questions and report their findings. Used in conjunction with other methods such as interviews and observation, focus group data can confirm, extend and enrich understanding and provide alternative narratives of events and beliefs.

Focus groups are frequently used when the opinions of lay people are sought. The method does not require participants to be able to read and write, and people can feel safe within a group. If facilitated well participants can express their views in relation to the opinions and experiences of others without feeling pressure to respond all the time. It is participant-driven and enables the language, priorities and attitudes of a group to be expressed. It is one of the few data collection methods that allow people to modify their initial thoughts and ideas as part of the data gathering process. Paradoxically, focus groups can be a good way of researching topics that are taboo or controversial when participants who hold an experience in common can give each other permission to discuss. For example, focus groups may be used to enable people who are HIV-positive to discuss freely their attitudes to sexual health and the issues they encounter as a result of their health status.

The synergy generated from a group discussion often enables participants to consider the topic with more enthusiasm than an individual interview can achieve. However, questions examining feelings or requiring personal reflection may only be suited to a focus group approach when participants have self-selected or they know each other and are comfortable with that level of public self-disclosure such questions require. It is the level of engagement expressed within a group, the range of participation and the ability to develop the discussion around certain issues that are often a good measure of how successful a focus group has been.

Limitations of focus groups

Focus groups can have high credibility and face validity but equally they can be susceptible to researcher manipulation and bias. The limitations of the method are the reliance on the skill of the group moderator, the risk of individual participants dominating discussion and excluding the contributions of others and the possibility that the structure and format of focus groups excludes certain groups from participation.

Focus group facilitation is difficult. The novice researcher should take the opportunity to observe some focus groups before taking on the moderator role, consider training on group dynamics and talk through with an experienced colleague how they will lead the group. The moderator has to maintain a balance between encouraging discussion and participation and being careful not to bias responses by giving preference to speakers whose views are perceived as the most 'interesting'. The moderator also needs the confidence to be able to re-focus the group if participants break into two or three separate discussions at the same time and intervene if the discussion threatens to become destructive or lead to conflict.

Most authors writing on the subject of focus groups raise the spectre of the dominant group member as a major limitation of the method. Participants who are very assertive in their views can discourage participation from those who disagree or who are less certain in their opinions. Where participants have different levels or authority or education this too can affect willingness to participate. Nevertheless, if the focus group is seen as an opportunity to capture how a group expresses their opinions and if certain people can make statements that are unchallenged and allowed to dominate, then the analysis must capture this. Reed and Payton (1997), argue that if one considers focus groups as 'displays of group perspectives' then *how* groups negotiate and develop their views can be as revealing as what is said.

Focus groups can discriminate against an individual's ability to participate. Kitzinger (1994) described including people in a group who had different communication disabilities such as deafness, partial paralysis affecting speech and dementia. They could all converse individually with the researcher, but had diffi-culty communicating with each other precluding meaningful interaction in a group setting. Most focus groups also require people to be able to communicate in the language of the researcher, which may exclude some people from minority ethnic groups who do not share a common language. It is possible to involve translators as an earlier example showed (Roth *et al.* 2003) although this can make the discussion more stilted and mean that the nuances of meaning are harder to identify (Twinn 1998).

The location of focus groups may also affect the ability to participate and exclude some potential participants. For example, where a focus group is held may favour participation by people who have easy access to transport or live close to the proposed venue.

Ethical issues

The particular ethical issues that arise within focus group research are the main-tenance of confidentiality, consent, the management of disclosure and maintaining the respect and feelings of self-worth of each participant. It is important that par-ticipants agree that the discussions held within the group are confidential and not shared outside the group. The moderator needs to ensure that each participant agrees to this, especially in situations where the group know each other.

The discussion format of a focus group can mean that people forget that the reason they are meeting is to participate in a research project. Frequently, discus-sion will prompt disclosures that may not have been made within the context of an interview. Although this can interrupt the flow of the conversation it is the moderator's responsibility to remind group members how the discussion will be used and why.

Consent is more problematic – apart from staying silent it is very difficult for an individual within a group to withdraw their consent to participate. The right to withdraw consent should be discussed prior to the focus group and although silence can be a useful option it may be wrongly interpreted as a form of assent to what others are saying. Researchers should consider offering participants the opportunity to withdraw consent after the group has met if they believe that the discussion did not reflect their views or it was a process they no longer wanted to be associated with. This would mean their contributions could not be reported.

The process of group participation can lead to unanticipated consequences. It can raise consciousness, expose underlying conflicts and falsely create an expecta-tion that something will be done about the issues raised. Owen (2001) has dis-cussed how distinctions between focus groups and therapy groups can become blurred especially if participants share painful personal experiences. She outlines the challenges of facilitating a group where women shared the experience of having lost a child. Ensuring group members felt 'safe' was as important as obtaining the data: she describes taking the decision to sensitively move the discussion on, when participants were becoming distressed.

Although this kind of data is very rich, it is exploitative if people expose their feelings and reveal their needs but there is then no means of offering further support. It is therefore important to have mechanisms in place for individuals to revisit the issues raised and if necessary to discuss them further. As part of this process the moderator also needs to consider their role within the group discussion, ensuring that participants understand it and consider the extent to which they are prepared to disclose their own views.

Finally, the moderator has a responsibility to ensure that participants do not feel devalued by their experience in the group. This can happen when opinions that are expressed are ridiculed or strongly opposed by other group members. In these situations the moderator should reinforce the right of each person to have an opinion and for it to be listened to, even if people are not in agreement. If this is not possible then the moderator should change the focus of the group's discussion or bring it to a close.

Conclusion

This chapter has provided an overview of the purpose and usefulness of focus groups for nursing research. It has emphasised that this method of data collection requires careful preparation and skill in leading and managing group discussion. The method is particularly useful when researchers wish to understand and clarify thinking on a topic from a group perspective. The need to be transparent about the purpose and process of the focus group and sensitive to the particular ethical challenges this method poses has been emphasised throughout. In conclusion, focus groups are a useful and versatile data collection method that can be used within a wide range of study settings and with diverse groups to great effect.

References

Bramley D (2004) Making and managing audio recordings. In Seale C (ed) *Researching Society and Culture*, 2nd edition. London, Sage pp207–223

Chiu L, Knight D (1999) How useful are focus groups for obtaining the views of minority groups? In Barbour RS, Kitzinger J (eds) *Developing Focus Group Research: politics, theory and practice*. London , Sage pp99–112

Gibbs A (1997) *Focus Groups*. Guildford, University of Surrey Social Research Update

Goodman C, Woolley R, Knight D (2003) District nurses' experiences of providing care in residential care home settings. *Journal of Clinical Nursing* 12: 67–76

Kevern J, Webb C (2004) Mature women's experiences of pre-registration nurse education. *Journal of Advanced Nursing* 45: 297–306

Kingry MJ, Tiedje LB, Friedman LL (1990) Focus groups: a research technique for nursing. *Nursing Research* 39: 124–125

Kitzinger J (1994) The methodology of focus groups: the importance of interaction between research participants. *Sociology of Health and Illness* 16: 103–121

Kitzinger J, Barbour RS (1999) Introduction: the challenge and promise of focus groups. In Barbour RS, Kitzinger J (eds) *Developing Focus Group Research: politics, theory and practice.* London , Sage pp1–20

McLafferty I (2004) Focus group interviews as a data collecting strategy. *Journal of Advanced Nursing* 48: 187–194

Morgan DL (1997) *Focus Groups as Qualitative Research,* 2nd edition. London, Sage

Nyamathi, Shuler P (1990) Focus group interview: a research technique for informed nursing practice. *Journal of Advanced Nursing* 15: 1281–1288

Owen S (2001) The practical, methodological and ethical dilemmas of conducting focus groups with vulnerable clients. *Journal of Advanced Nursing* 36: 652–658

Phillips K, Woodward V (1999) The decision to resuscitate: older people's views. *Journal of Clinical Nursing* 8: 753–761

Reed J, Payton V (1997) Focus groups: issues of analysis and interpretation. *Journal of Advanced Nursing* 26: 765–771

Roth C, Ahmed S, Feldman R, Sandall J, Sunderland J (2003) *Bilingual advocacy and HIV testing: an evaluation of service in East London.* London, City University

Twinn S (1998) An analysis of the effectiveness of focus groups as a method of qualitative data collection with Chinese populations in nursing research. *Journal of Advanced Nursing* 28: 654–661

Twohig PL, Putnam W (2002) Group interviews in primary care research: advancing the state of the art of ritualised research. *Family Practice* 19: 278–284

Webb C, Kevern J (2001) Focus groups as a research method: a critique of some aspects of their use in nursing research. *Journal of Advanced Nursing* 33: 798–805

Further reading

Gibbs A (1997) *Focus Groups.* Guildford, Social Research Update, Issue 19, University of Surrey. *www.soc.surrey.ac.uk/sru/SRU19.html*

Dawson S, Manderson LA (1993) *A Manual for the Use of Focus Groups: methods for social research in disease.* Boston, MA, International Nutrition Foundation for developing countries (INFDC). *www.unu.edu/unupress/food2/UIN03E/uin03e00.htm*

24 Using Questionnaires

Tricia Murphy-Black

Key points

- Questionnaires are most commonly used in survey research but may feature in other research designs.
- Questionnaires form the basis of data collection by post, telephone or face-to-face.
- If questionnaires are designed for a specific study, the development and testing of validity and reliability is an important part of the preparation.
- When using existing scales, the validity and reliability have to be confirmed, and may need to be retested in different populations or conditions.

Purpose of questionnaires

Questionnaires are familiar: they may be used to evaluate a course, assess satisfaction with hospital care, or for market research. This familiarity might imply that using questionnaires is merely a process of writing a few questions, distributing them and then getting results. It is not quite so easy – the reasons for using a questionnaire, the type of people who will be asked to complete it and the wording and layout of the questionnaire have to be considered.

Questionnaires are research instruments. They are most commonly used in survey research but may be a feature of other research designs. They need to be designed for their purpose, which is to collect specific information that will provide answers to the research question. The data collected can only be as good as the questions asked. The most important stage is the preparation and design of the questionnaire itself. There are two ways of ensuring that a questionnaire will work within a survey.

- Use questionnaires that other researchers have developed and tested for validity and reliability, i.e. the questionnaire will measure what the study is investigating accurately and consistently.
- Use questionnaires that have been specifically designed and tested for the purpose.

Using previously-validated questionnaires

The advantages of using an established questionnaire are that the development work has been undertaken and there should be published information about the validity and reliability of the questionnaire with a specific population. However, the questionnaire will need to be tested for use with other populations. For example, the validity and reliability of a commonly used questionnaire, the General Health Questionnaire (GHQ) is well established. Nevertheless, its use in a non-English speaking country required that it was translated and the validity and reliability tested again before it could be used (Montazeri *et al.* 2003).

Questionnaires for specific purposes can be identified from research reports and some books provide details of different questionnaires (*see* further reading at the end of this chapter for examples). There are companies that supply questionnaires for a range of different patient groups (Jenkinson *et al.* 2003), e.g. the Picker Institute (*www.pickereurope.org/*). The advantage of using standardised questionnaires in different health care settings is that it allows for comparison across the sector. Disadvantages of 'off-the-shelf' questionnaires are that they may have copyright restrictions or charge a fee for use. The status of a questionnaire should be checked before it is used and permission sought, as appropriate, from the authors. It is important to recognise that a previously validated questionnaire may not be suitable for a specific project, in which case it is necessary to design a new questionnaire.

Designing a questionnaire

There are a number of sources of help in designing a questionnaire in textbooks, journals (*see* for example Meadows 2003; Boynton & Greenhalgh 2004) and the internet. Typing 'questionnaire design' in the Google search engine will result in thousands of sites, some commercial, some academic and some specifically for the NHS. While trying out a free account on QuestForm (*www.questform.co.uk*) is of limited value as it only allows five questions to be considered, it is a useful way to see how questions can be set out. Even with such templates for assistance, there comes a point where the questions have to be worked out.

The first decision to make is the type of questionnaire – will it be a postal questionnaire, used in a telephone interview or a face-to-face interview? The personal interaction that takes place in telephone or face-to-face interviews may allow for a slightly different approach in the wording but the main principles of questionnaire design are the same.

The next stage involves identifying the actual questions. The general principles laid out below apply to all types of questionnaire. Both of these stages (type and the wording) are strongly influenced by the nature of the project, the amount of funding, together with the time and people available. All these issues will interact with each other, and the initial plans may change considerably.

Designing a questionnaire involves deciding:

- *what* questions need to be asked: how much data is required to give the information needed to answer the research question
- *how* the questions should be asked: whether to use open or closed questions, fixed choice, or one of a variety of scales
- *when* questions should be asked: whether before or after an event of interest and the order within the questionnaire
- *where* the questions will be asked: whether in the street, at home, in hospital, alone, or in a group
- *why* the questions should be asked: whether these particular questions are more likely to get better answers than a different set of questions

Exploratory work is essential preparation of a questionnaire. This may involve reviewing the literature; group discussion with people similar to the proposed sample; testing ideas with experts or relevant individuals or groups (Riley & Peters 2000); or taking account of the special needs of particular groups (Hardyman & Tingle 1999).

When designing a questionnaire the following guidelines should be considered:

- The shorter the question, the better the respondents will like it.
- The larger the sample the more precise the results.
- The more relevant the topic to the respondent, and the more practical it is to answer, the better the response rate.

Content of questions

The content should be relevant to enable the respondents to answer the questions. The willingness to respond will be enhanced if the questions do not expose ignorance. The language needs to be pitched at the appropriate level for the population. Questions appropriate to health care professionals may not be suitable for patients. Piloting the questionnaire may reveal a better choice of words or phrases, appropriate to the group for which it is intended.

Length of questionnaire

Despite advice to keep questionnaires short, recent research examining the relationship between response rate and questionnaire length showed that responses were similar for short (4-page) and long (12-page) questionnaire groups (Jenkinson *et al.* 2003). However, a systematic review of methods influencing response rates for postal questionnaires reported that short questionnaires were more likely to be returned (Edwards *et al.* 2002). Questionnaires should only ask what is needed for this research project, despite the temptation to add questions that are interesting, but not necessarily relevant.

Wording

Each question should be specific, simple and straightforward. Questions should be kept short as long questions, with many different clauses, are difficult enough to follow when written but are even harder when they are spoken out loud in a face-to-face or telephone interview. Ambiguity, where a question could have different meanings, confuses the respondent and results in answers that are inconsistent. Vague words that could have a variety of meanings should be avoided. For example, 'regularly' could mean any of the following: once a day, once a month or once a year. In questionnaires concerning bowel habits or frequency of sexual intercourse, the interpretation of the questioner and the respondent might be very different. If asking 'how often?', phrase the question in the context of frequency within a time limit. For example:

How often do you shop in the city?
☐   once a month
☐   once a week
☐   every day

Never presume (e.g. State the number of children you have); either give options (e.g. How many children do you have? – this allows the respondent to say 'none') or use a filter (e.g. Please answer questions 3–5 if you have children or go to question 6 if you have none). Filter questions can also be used to funnel the replies from the general to the particular, for example:

• Have you read the Nursing and Midwifery Council Guidelines for records and recordkeeping?
• Have you been asked to comment?
• Have you given your views on this report?
• Please give your views below.

By using yes/no responses to the first three, it speeds up analysis and allows greater attention to be given to those who write out their answer to the final question.

Leading questions, which invite certain types of answers, should be avoided (e.g. Are you satisfied with hospital food?). Instead give the respondent a range of options (for example: Please indicate your view of the quality of hospital food: poor, reasonable, excellent). If looking for explanations of behaviour, it may be necessary to ask a number of questions to arrive at the desired answer. The first question asks about the behaviour:

How often do you exercise?
☐   every day
☐   twice a week
☐   once a week
☐   less than once a week?

Then the next question asks for reasons:

Please give three reasons for your response to the previous question.

Sometimes a hypothetical statement is useful to lead into a question about a difficult, sensitive or embarrassing subject. For instance the statement: 'Some men are unable to have an erection as often as they want' could lead to a question about impotence, offering a range of answers. By giving 'permission' to have the complaint, the respondents may feel they can answer the questions.

If the respondents are a homogenous group, such as nurses, it may not be necessary to define terms. For instance, most nurses in the UK will not need to be told that the length of the working week is 37.5 hours. If, however, the respondents are a heterogeneous group from varied backgrounds, and the purpose of the survey is very specific, it may be necessary to explain the terms. A number of definitions or explanations could be placed at the beginning of the questionnaire. If only one or two, then they can be included in a particular question.

The nature of the question and the type of response will guide the way the question is worded. For example, a factual question like 'Do you wear a watch?' will expect a 'yes' or 'no' answer and is unlikely to be influenced by other factors. The question 'How much do you spend on beer each week?' is different. The answer can be factual (the actual amount spent each week), wishful thinking (more than is spent to look generous), or less than is spent (to conceal heavy drinking). If the question is factual but about something that only occurs occasionally such as 'How much do you spend on liqueurs at Christmas?' there can be genuine problems with giving an accurate figure, especially if asked a few weeks or months later. Questions about smoking, drinking and sexual behaviour are commonly answered in the way the respondents think the questioner wants them to answer.

Types of questions

Different types of questions can be used.

Closed questions

Closed questions require a 'yes' or 'no' answer, for example, 'Have you been in hospital in the last year?' They may be used to direct those who say 'no' to skip several questions to reach the next relevant one. A series of closed questions reduces the time it takes to complete the questionnaire.

Forced choice

This is where the respondent has to choose between one of two categories, with the possible addition of 'don't know'. For example, 'Do you think nurses should take strike action?'

Multiple choice

Multiple choice or alternative statements specify whether the respondent is to choose one or more answers from a list. Unless the list is all-exclusive, it is worth adding, 'other, please specify' at the end. This approach can be used to ask straightforward questions where the respondent will fit into one category (for example, What is your age? under 21; between 21 and 64; over 65) or those which expect the respondent to choose one option (Who do you think should be the key worker for older frail people cared for in the community? District nurse, practice nurse, social worker, and general practitioner). The question might list different choices with the instruction, 'tick all that apply.'

Scales

There are a number of different scales that can be used in questionnaires. These may be little more than a closed question, expecting the respondents to 'agree' or 'disagree' with a statement or may give a range of options similar to multiple choice, some of which may have a weighting system for analysis. For example:

I was discharged from hospital:
- ☐ too soon
- ☐ at about the right time
- ☐ not soon enough

Ranking questions

Ranking questions ask the respondents to state their preference. This may be a list provided within the questionnaire, for example:

From the list of journals please rank them according to usefulness to your work; where 1 is the most useful and 5 is the least useful:

Nursing Times	☐
Nursing Standard	☐
Journal of Community Nursing	☐
Journal of Advanced Nursing	☐
British Journal of Nursing	☐

Alternatively respondents may be asked to provide their own list and then to rank them in order, for example:

Please give three reasons for choosing a professional journal and list below:

Reason for choosing journal	Rank order
1	☐
2	☐
3	☐

Considering the list given above, please rank according to importance to you, with 1 as most important and 3 as least important.

Likert scales

Likert scales, which have several different statements, ask respondents to choose one of five points between 'strongly agree' and 'strongly disagree' in relation to each statement.

Example:

	Strongly agree	Agree	Uncertain	Disagree	Strongly disagree
Job satisfaction is more important to nurses than a high salary	☐	☐	☐	☐	☐

This scaling method measures attitude with all items measuring the same dimension. Although this looks easy, it is important to follow the procedure set out by Likert. (The original description was published in 1932 however, details have been published more recently by Oppenheim 1993.) This involves developing a pool of statements that are subjected to different tests before their use in the questionnaire.

Pictorial scales

Pictorial scales use symbols such as faces, which range from sad (☹) to smiling (☺) and are similar to numerical rating scales. They can be used with children or those with literacy or visual problems.

Visual analogue scales

Visual analogue scales consist of a line, usually 10 cm long, and respondents are asked to indicate where their response lies by making a mark on the line. The ends have words to give the two extremes and the line may be numbered. Analysis is based on the distance that is measured from one end of the scale to the mark made by the respondent. This system is commonly used to assess pain but may be used for other health outcomes. For example:

Please draw a cross on the line below to indicate your reaction to aromatherapy

Not helpful   Very helpful

Open questions

Open questions such as 'How do you feel about the birth of your baby?' give respondents the freedom to answer in their own words. This can range from a single word or phrase, to extensive written text. In designing the questionnaire, it is essential to plan for such a variety of answers.

Validation of measurement scales

There are several ways of measuring health-related events, for example health outcomes, levels of pain, satisfaction with care, or changes in symptoms. Some studies use a range of different scales (*see* Box 24.1)

A questionnaire may consist of specifically designed questions for a particular study and/or measurement scales that have been used by others. (It should be noted that some authors of particular scales require that a specific format is used and this will need to be checked when getting permission to use the scale.)

There are two issues in the validation of measurement scales:

• Has the validity and reliability of this scale been established?

and if yes

• Will this measure be valid and reliable with the sample planned for this study?

The answer to the first question can be checked by identifying how the scale was developed and how it has been used. For example, the Nottingham Health Profile (NHP), a measure of well-being, was originally developed in 1986 (Hunt *et al.* 1986) and during the development phase was tested on two contrasting samples, a group of healthy mine rescue workers and a group of chronically sick people with osteoarthritis. Its validity was demonstrated by showing a difference between

---

Box 24.1   The use of different measurement scales.

Closs SJ, Barr B, Briggs M, Cash K, Seers K (2004) A comparison of five pain assessment scales for nursing home residents with varying degrees of cognitive impairment. *Journal of Pain and Symptom Management* 27: 196–205

In this study, 113 people with cognitive impairment living in nursing homes had their cognitive impairment measured using the Mini-Mental State Examination (MMSE). As the purpose of the study was to compare five different scales to assess pain, each resident was asked to complete one of the scales. These were a verbal rating scale, horizontal numeric rating scale, faces pictorial scale, colour analogue scale and a visual analogue scale. This meant that each resident only had to complete two scales – the MMSE and one of the pain assessments – but the study as a whole could compare the results from the different scales. The authors found that the verbal rating scale was the most successful as more than a third of those with severe cognitive impairment could complete it. It was necessary to give repeated explanations and this improved completion rates for all the scales. This study showed no difference in pain scores according to cognitive status.

the two groups. During the past 20 years it has been used in various research projects, for example, a study examining the changes in health outcome of older women experiencing sleep problems (Byles *et al.* 2003). In answering the second question, it is important to ascertain whether the scale has already been used on a similar sample to that of the proposed study, in which case it is possible to proceed with it. If, however, the scale has not been used with this particular group, then its validity and reliability needs to be established with the new group.

Validity and reliability

Questionnaires, whether they incorporate previously developed scales or are specifically designed for the purpose, should be tested for validity and reliability.

Validity

Validity refers to whether the questionnaire measures what it is intended to measure. It is difficult to assess and has many dimensions. While there are detailed and technical ways of demonstrating validity that are beyond the scope of this chapter the following general categories of validity can help structure its assessment.

Construct validity concerns the degree to which the questionnaire measures the construct it was designed to measure, for example whether a questionnaire intended to identify barriers to research utilisation actually achieves this objective. Increasing the number of different questions in a study will increase construct validity provided that the questions are measuring the same construct.

Content validity refers to the extent to which items on a questionnaire cover adequately the construct being studied, for example whether a questionnaire covers the full range of barriers to research utilisation. A related, but somewhat complex concept is *factorial validity*, which refers to the clustering of correlations of responses by groupings of items in the questionnaire. Factor analysis (a statistical procedure) can be used for this purpose. Nolan *et al.* (1999) undertook a factor analysis of the questionnaire used to examine barriers to research utilisation and were able to demonstrate how the questionnaire items could be grouped into four sets of barriers, i.e. those to do with the practitioner, the organisation, the quality of the research and how the research was communicated. The groupings should make sense to the researcher otherwise the questionnaire has poor factorial validity.

Criterion validity considers the extent to which items on a questionnaire actually measure the real-world conditions or events that they are intended to measure. This type of internal validity can be assessed by comparing questionnaire responses with objective measures of the condition to which they refer; for example comparing self-reported alcohol consumption with some objective physiological measure.

Reliability

Reliability refers to the extent to which a questionnaire would produce the same results if used repeatedly with the same group under the same conditions. Ideally, the reliability of a questionnaire would be determined by administering it several times to a large group of individuals, and analysing the results using statistical methods for measuring agreement. Normally this is not possible due to practical difficulties; changes in what is being measured over time in different individuals; and confounding effects such as individuals remembering their responses from previous applications of the questionnaire. To overcome these problems, statisticians have developed tests that can be applied to the single administration of a questionnaire to determine its reliability. The three main approaches to determining reliability are given below.

Retest method

A straightforward means to determine the reliability of a questionnaire is by the retest method in which the same questionnaire is given to the same people after a period of time. The reliability of the questionnaire can be estimated by examining the consistency of the responses between the two sets of data. If the same results are achieved on both occasions that the questionnaire is administered, then the reliability coefficient will be 1.00. Normally, the correlation of measurements across time will be less than perfect due to different experiences and attitudes that respondents have encountered from the time of the first test.

Split-halves method

To overcome the problems of administering a questionnaire on two occasions, statisticians developed the split-half halves method whereby the questionnaire items are split at random into halves and the score for an individual is calculated twice, once with one half of the items and once with the other half of the items. Tests with strong internal consistency show strong correlation between the scores calculated from the two halves. One drawback of the split-halves method is that the correlation between the two halves is dependent upon the method used to divide the items. The most common means is to assign the even numbered items to one half and the odd numbered items to the other half of the test.

Internal consistency method

This method provides an estimate of reliability following a single administration of the questionnaire. The most popular internal consistency reliability estimate is Cronbach's alpha. This statistical test is designed for use with questionnaires containing items that have no right answer, for example where respondents are asked to rate the degree to which they agree or disagree with a statement on a particular scale. An alpha coefficient of 0.8 or more is generally considered acceptable.

In addition to validity and reliability, a questionnaire should also be discriminating in that it is able to separate out important differences between the individuals being studied. The time and resource required to develop a valid, reliable and discriminating questionnaire should not be underestimated. If there is already a questionnaire that has been developed which fits the study purpose and has been validated with a population appropriate to the study then it should be used.

Box 24.2 provides an example of a study testing for reliability and validity.

Administering questionnaires

Before a questionnaire is administered a pilot study should be completed. This is a small-scale version of the main study undertaken to test the procedures and feasibility of study. It includes selecting a comparable sample to the main study, distributing the questionnaire, checking the returns, the analysis and the examination of the findings to see if the questionnaire provides the data expected.

Questionnaires can be administered by post, a face-to-face encounter or by telephone. A questionnaire handed out personally has the advantage that the respondent connects it with an individual or an organisation and this may improve the response rate (Edwards *et al.* 2002). Both postal and personally distributed questionnaires are self-administered, that is, the respondents are left to complete the answers themselves.

It is preferable for researchers to obtain the names of the people to whom they wish to send the questionnaire and then to distribute it themselves. Although some lists of names are in the public domain, for example the electoral register from which a random sample could be selected, in many instances permission has

---

Box 24.2 An example of a study testing for reliability and validity.

BenDebba M, Heller J, Ducker TB, Eisinger JM (2002) Cervical Spine Outcomes Questionnaire: its development and psychometric properties. *Spine* 27: 2116–2124

BenDebba *et al.* (2002) had developed a comprehensive, disease-specific questionnaire (The Cervical Spine Outcomes Questionnaire) for characterising complaints of neck pain and evaluating the outcomes of treatments for these complaints. This questionnaire was tested on 216 patients who underwent surgery for cervical spine disorders. They completed the questionnaire before treatment, and then at three and six months after treatment. The data were used to evaluate the reliability, validity, and responsiveness of the questionnaire. These authors showed that the Cervical Spine Outcomes Questionnaire had high test-retest reliability, good construct validity, and responsiveness to change after treatment.

to be sought to obtain the names and addresses of people to whom the question-naire is to be sent. For example, a list of nurses may need to be obtained from a nurse manager or the names of patients from a general practitioner. Release of personal information must comply with the Data Protection Act and this may be interpreted differently by different organisations. In some situations the organisa-tion in which the potential sample is based will release the names to the researcher. However, in other situations the organisation may require that they distribute the questionnaire on behalf of the researcher.

Response rates

Research studies that use a representative sample are dependent on a good response rate. A low response rate can have a significant impact on the usefulness of the findings. The generally accepted level of response to be aimed for is 80% but as shown in Table 24.1, this can vary considerably in published research.

Edwards *et al.* (2002) undertook a systematic review of randomised controlled trials of different strategies to influence response rates to postal questionnaires. Box 24.3 lists the strategies that will increase the likelihood of a good response.

Questionnaires are also less likely to be returned if they contain questions of a sensitive nature (Edwards *et al.* 2002). Detailed accounts of the issues of non-response are provided by Barriball and While (1999a;b).

Partial response

Partial response where some of the questions have been answered but others are left blank is irritating. It is worth checking the data carefully to see if there are any common patterns for non-completion. For instance, Clifford (1996) reported a relatively high level of non-response to the clinical component of a questionnaire to nurse teachers, which could be because they did not see this to be an important part of their role. In the general population, partial responses are more common in the elderly (Eaker *et al.* 998). Careful testing and piloting of the questionnaire can help to reduce partial response by checking whether the questions are understandable.

Table 24.1   Examples of variation in response rates.

Sample	Response (%)	Authors
Employees of geriatric homes and hospitals	80%	Tomasson *et al.* (2004)
Nurses, doctors and dentists in primary care	44%	Russell *et al.* (2004)
Nurse and midwife graduates	51%	Veeramah *et al.* (2004)
Mental health practitioners	53%	Skidmore *et al.* (2004)
Users/carers	14%	Skidmore *et al.* (2004)
Educationalists	33%	Skidmore *et al.* (2004)
Total sample	26%	Skidmore *et al.* (2004)

Box 24.3 Strategies to improve the response to postal questionnaires.

- monetary incentives: a better response can be obtained if the incentive is not conditional on the response
- short questionnaires
- using coloured paper
- questionnaires of interest to the participants
- contacting participants before sending the questionnaires
- personalised questionnaires and letters
- sending questionnaires by first-class post or recorded delivery
- using stamped return envelopes rather than business reply paid format
- follow up contact with non-respondents
- sending a second copy of the questionnaire to non-respondents
- originating from universities compared with commercial organisations

Source: Edwards *et al.* (2002)

Recall

One reason for partial response is poor recall. Any questions that ask respondents to remember events, behaviours or emotions are potentially subject to bias. Even something that focuses on a relatively recent event can be difficult to report accurately. Certain groups such as the elderly may have difficulty in remembering details (Worth & Tierney 1993) while critical life events may be easier to recall.

Non response

Are those who do not return postal questionnaires similar to or different from those who do return them? As there is always a danger of bias, this is an issue of considerable importance, yet it is not always reported. A meta-analysis of 210 studies showed that only 48% reported the response rate (Sitzia & Wood 1998). Some studies have demonstrated differences between responders and non-responders, which may be due to demographic characteristics, such as age or gender (Eaker *et al.* 1998).

Comparison between face-to-face and postal questionnaires

The strengths and weaknesses of face-to-face structured interviews and self-completion (usually postal) questionnaires are given in Box 17.3. Many of the issues to do with the design of a questionnaire are the same for a structured face-to-face interview schedule. There are similar concerns about the validity and reliability of questions in both methods of data collection as well as testing understanding of words used and the positioning of questions in the overall tool.

Questions for an interview schedule have to be written so they can be spoken. There can be visual aids, such as flash cards from which the respondent may choose items, which help comprehension. While there is greater flexibility for re-interpreting a question that a respondent does not understand when face to face, if there are a number of different interviewers, each one might explain a question in a slightly different way so that the respondents are not all answering the same question. Training all the interviewers collectively will help to prevent subtle changes in the presentation of questions.

Ethical issues associated with questionnaires

The ethical principles addressed in Chapter 3 apply to questionnaires as much as any other method of data collection. There are a number of issues to be considered in this context. Research participants have the right to know why they have been sent a questionnaire, what the study is about, why the information is being sought and what will be done with it. Their right to privacy should be addressed with regard to whether the questionnaire is anonymous; how the data will be handled, protected and reported. Such information should be included in a participant information sheet to accompany the postal questionnaire.

Participants also have the right to refuse to complete a questionnaire. Usually consent to participate in a survey is confirmed by return of a completed question-naire (rather than asking the respondent to complete a consent form). Written consent is often required for interview-based studies, especially those involving patients. Most of these issues need to be clarified for the respondent either in the letter accompanying the questionnaire or in an information sheet that goes with it. Sending a questionnaire through the post to a group of unknown people might result in distress for some of them. Where possible this should be anticipated and prevented by careful and thoughtful wording of the questions.

Conclusion

A questionnaire is a flexible and versatile method of collecting data. It can be used within a wide range of different research designs and has many advantages for both the novice and experienced researcher. There is much to learn about ques-tionnaire design and this chapter has just given an outline of some of the aspects to consider, which it is hoped will whet the appetite.

References

Barriball K, While A (1999a) Exploring variables underlying non-response in a survey of nurses and nurses' aides in practice. *Journal of Advanced Nursing* 4: 894–904

Barriball KL, While AE (1999b) Non-response in survey research: a methodological discussion and development of an explanatory model. *Journal of Advanced Nursing* 30:
677–686

BenDebba M, Heller J, Ducker TB, Eisinger JM (2002) Cervical Spine Outcomes Questionnaire:
its development and psychometric properties. *Spine* 27: 2116–2124

Boynton PM, Greenhalgh T (2004) Hands-on guide to questionnaire research 1: selecting,
designing and developing your questionnaire. *British Medical Journal* 328: 1312–1325

Byles JE, Mishra GD, Harris MA, Nair K (2003) The problems of sleep for older women:
changes in health outcomes. *Age and Ageing* 32: 154–163

Clifford C (1996) Collecting patients' views and perceptions of continence services: the
development of research instruments. *Journal of Advanced Nursing* 23: 603–611

Closs SJ, Barr B, Briggs M, Cash K, Seers K (2004) A comparison of five pain assessment
scales for nursing home residents with varying degrees of cognitive impairment. *Journal
of Pain and Symptom Management* 27: 196–205

Eaker S, Bergstrom R, Bergstrom A, Adami HO, Nyren O (1998) Response rate to mailed
epidemiologic questionnaires: a population-based randomized trial of variations in
design and mailing routines. *American Journal of Epidemiology* 147: 74–82

Edwards P, Roberts I, Clarke M, DiGuiseppi C, Pratap S, Wentz R, Kwan I (2002) Increasing
response rates to postal questionnaires: systematic review. *British Medical Journal* 324:
1183–1185

Hardyman R, Tingle A (1999) Studying the careers of nurse diplomats: the importance of
branch specific questionnaires. *Journal of Clinical Nursing* 8: 560–566

Hunt SM, McEwan J, McKenna SP (1986) *Measuring Health Status*. London, Croom Helm

Jenkinson C, Coulter A, Reeves R, Bruster S, Richards N (2003) Properties of the Picker
Patient Experience questionnaire in a randomized controlled trial of long versus short
form survey instruments. *Journal of Public Health Medicine* 25: 197–201

Meadows KA (2003) So you want to do research? 5: questionnaire design. *British Journal of
Community Nursing* 8: 562–570

Montazeri A, Harirchi AM, Shariati M, Garmaroudi G, Ebadi M, Fateh A (2003) The 12-item
General Health Questionnaire (GHQ-12): translation and validation study of the Iranian
version. *Health and Quality of Life Outcomes* 1: 1 66. *www.hqlo.com/content/1/1/66* 5apr05

Nolan M, Morgan L, Curran M, Clayton J, Gerrish K, Parker K (1999) Evidence-based care:
can we overcome the barriers? *British Journal of Nursing* 7: 1273–1278

Oppenheim AN (1993) *Questionnaire Design, Interviewing and Attitude Measurement*. London,
Pinter

Riley R, Peters G (2000) The current scope and future direction of perioperative nursing
practice in Victoria, Australia. *Journal of Advanced Nursing* 32: 544–553

Russell M, Lazenbatt A, Freeman R, Marcenes W (2004) Child physical abuse: health professionals' perceptions, diagnosis and responses. *British Journal of Community Nursing* 9:
332–338

Sitzia J, Wood N (1998) Response rate in patient satisfaction research: an analysis of 210
published studies. *International Journal of Quality Health Care* 10: 311–317

Skidmore D, Warne T, Stark S (2004) Mental health practice and the rhetoric-reality gap.
Journal of Psychiatric and Mental Health Nursing 11: 348–356

Tomasson K, Gunnarsdottir HK, Rafnsdottir GL, Helgadottir B (2004) Correlates of proba-
ble alcohol abuse among women working in nursing homes. *Scandinavian Journal of Public
Health* 32: 47–52

Veeramah V (2004) Utilization of research findings by graduate nurses and midwives.
Journal of Advanced Nursing 47: 183–191

Worth A, Tierney A (1993) Conducting research interviews with elderly people by telephone. *Journal of Advanced Nursing* 18: 1077–1084

Further reading

Bowling A (1991) *Measuring Health: a review of quality of life measurement scales.* 2nd edition. Milton Keynes, Open University Press

Bowling A (1997) *Research Methods in Health: investigating health and health services.* Buckingham, Open University Press

McDowell I, Newell C (1996) *Measuring Health: a guide to rating scales and questionnaires.* Oxford, Oxford University Press

Wall C, DeHaven M, Oeffinger K (2002) Survey methodology for the uninitiated. *The Journal of Family Practice* 51: 573

Website

www.ukmi.nhs.uk/Research/ResSkillsQDesign.asp – UK Medicines Information provides general guidance on questionnaire design

25 Using Observation

Hazel Watson and Rosemary Whyte

Key points

- The use of observation in research provides a first-hand account of behaviours or events, collected systematically for analysis and theory development.
- Depending on the theoretical approach of the research, observation may be anything from completely unstructured to highly structured, and observer roles may vary from complete observer to full participant.
- Participant observation is more commonly used within the qualitative paradigm, and requires immersion of the researcher in the field.
- Structured observation is more common in quantitative research, and requires the rigorous use of checklists and categories to record the observed data.

The purpose of observation

Observation is the use of human senses to gather information and develop an understanding of the world around us. It can involve using all of our senses, judging and interpreting what we perceive to enable us to make sense of the information. When providing clinical care for patients, nurses observe patients' physical condition while also observing for signs of pain or emotional and psychological distress.

In nursing research, observation is an active process by which data are collected about people, behaviours, interactions or events. The aim of data collection through observation is to gain detailed information that can contribute to understanding of the phenomena under study. Observational data provide a first-hand account of witnessed behaviours or events, collected through a systematic process that facilitates the development or testing of theories.

Observation can be used as the principal data collection method in both quantitative and qualitative studies. Whyte (2004) used observation in two ways, first by directly observing the ward setting where nurse-patient contact and interaction took place (Box 25.1). In addition, verbal exchanges between nurses and patients were captured through audiorecorded indirect observation.

Whyte's study provides an example of how observation can be used with a range of data collection methods in a qualitative study. The studies conducted by Booth et al. (2001) and Day et al. (2001) illustrate the use of observation within the context of quantitative research (Boxes 25.2 and 25.3).

Box 25.1   Using observation in qualitative research.

Whyte RE (2004) The provision of health education on smoking to patients in hospital: a critical evaluation of the role of diplomate nurses. Unpublished PhD thesis, Glasgow Caledonian University.

This study aimed to identify the extent to which nurses recognise and utilise opportunities to provide health education on smoking to patients in hospital. A qualitative case study, influenced by facets of ethnography, provided a critical evaluation of the role of 12 nurses in relation to health education on smoking. Data were collected through patient lifestyle questionnaires, tape-recorded nurse-patient interactions and interviews, observation, field notes, and examination of patients' nursing documentation. Triangulation of data enabled in-depth exploration of the nurses' health education interactions in acute wards and contributed to rigour in the study.

The findings indicated that smoking was part of nurses' health agenda, as evidenced by their recognition of opportunities to introduce the topic, although the content of their interactions was variable.

Box 25.2   Non-participant structured observation in quantitative research.

Booth J, Davidson I, Winstanley J, Waters K (2001) Observing washing and dressing of stroke patients: nursing and occupational therapists. What is the difference? *Journal of Advanced Nursing* 33: 98–105

This study used non-participant structured observation to compare the activities and interventions of qualified nurses with those of occupational therapists with stroke patients. Staff-patient interactions (n = 10) were observed by a single researcher. Twenty observation sessions in total were recorded manually during which time the activities, contacts and interactions were numerically coded and recorded at 20-second intervals on a standard proforma. Prior testing and use of the instrument ensured its reliability and validity. Statistical analysis showed that occupational therapists used 'prompting and instructing' commands more than nurses and used facilitation techniques significantly more (P = 0.0283). Nurses were significantly more likely to be engaged in 'supervision' interactions, spending 42.1% of their time performing this activity compared with 25.1% for occupational therapists. Reasons for the observed differences in the intervention styles used may be attributed to the approaches taken to assessment and treatment of stroke patients.

As a preliminary phase in research, observations can be used to identify routines, activities and happenings that occur within a setting to provide the basis for more focused observations during the main study. As the exploratory phase of a study of nurse-patient interactions, Whyte (2004) conducted non-participant

Box 25.3   Non-participant observation in experimental design.

Day T, Wainwright SP, Wilson-Barnett J (2001) An evaluation of a teaching intervention to improve the practice of endotracheal suctioning in intensive care units. *Journal of Clinical Nursing* 10: 682–696

This study investigated the relationships between knowledge and practice and evaluated the effectiveness of a research-based teaching programme on endotracheal suctioning. The study used a quasi-experimental design and was a randomised, controlled, single-blinded comparison of two research-based teaching programmes, with 16 intensive care nurses, using non-participant observation and a self-report questionnaire. Initial baseline data revealed a low level of knowledge for many participants, which was also reflected in practice, as suctioning was performed against many research-based recommendations. Following teaching, significant improvements were seen in both knowledge and practice. These were generally sustained four weeks later.

The study used non-participant observation to confirm that changes in knowledge were translated into improvements in practice.

observation to determine the organisation of nursing care in general hospital wards and to identify the times of nurse-patient contact (Box 25.1). The aim was to collect data about nursing activities in the wards to inform the development of data collection methods for the pilot and main studies.

Observation can be used to confirm or support data that have been collected through other methods such as questionnaire or interview (Box 25.3). Providing a record of behaviour or events as they occur can help to overcome sources of bias such as the effect of time on memory, or of participants giving socially acceptable answers. Instead, they provide a means of recording what people actually do as opposed to what they say that they do. When used in longitudinal studies, observation methods can uncover processes that evolve over time.

Observer roles

Depending on the theoretical approach of a study, the researcher may be a participant or a non-participant observer. In participant observation the researcher participates in the activities of those who are being observed, while in non-participant observation the researcher remains detached from those being observed. In a seminal paper, Gold (1969) identified four observational roles that researchers might adopt:

- *Complete participant* – the researcher participates fully in the activities of those being observed and attempts to act as one of the group. Observation may be conducted overtly or covertly.
- *Participant-as-observer* – the researcher participates in the activities of those who are being observed but the role is made explicit and observation is conducted overtly.

- *Observer-as-participant* – the researcher participates briefly with those being observed but spends most of the time observing behaviour/events.
- *Complete observer* – the researcher is chiefly concerned with observing behaviours and has no interaction with those being observed.

This may be seen as a continuum ranging from the researcher's complete participation with the work and activities of those being observed to complete detachment from them (Figure 25.1).

Where the researcher is a participant, irrespective of the extent of the participation, the research approach is generally qualitative, whereas in quantitative research the researcher assumes a non-participant role, i.e. that of complete observer.

The observer role may not be as rigid as Gold's typology would suggest and researchers may find their role changing during the course of observation. In their study of nursing practices in an intensive therapy unit (ITU), Turnock and Gibson (2001) experienced difficulty in maintaining non-participatory, detached roles as observers, especially in a unit where the staff knew them. As academic lecturers with previous experience of working in ITU, staff regarded them as 'quasi-insiders', sometimes asking them to 'watch' patients briefly while the nurses were engaged in other activities. At those times the complete observer role became 'observer-as-participant'.

Collecting observational data

Researchers who use observational methods may choose one of two forms of sampling, namely *event sampling*, or *time sampling*. Event sampling involves identifying specific events, such as used by Whyte (2004). The 'event' in her study was the provision of smoking-related information (Box 25.1). In time sampling, the researcher records on an activity sheet behaviours, which have previously been identified within a category system, at regular intervals throughout a specified period of time. Booth *et al.* (2001), for example, observed each participating patient every 20 seconds over a period of 1.5 hours (Box 25.2).

Observation data can be collected directly by the researcher 'on the spot' in the research setting, in which case observations are coded using an observation schedule. Alternatively, the activities to be observed can be videorecorded. This has the advantage that the researcher does not need to be present and is unconstrained by the need to code the data at the time that the observed phenomena are occurring. Events are recorded as they occur and analysis undertaken later.

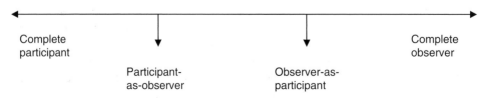

Figure 25.1   Observational roles (from Gold 1969).

Verbal interactions can be audiorecorded. This method of collecting observation data has been used successfully in studies of verbal exchanges during nurse-patient interactions to identify 'facilitating' and 'blocking' behaviours used by nurses (Macleod Clark 1982; Whyte 2004). When a range of behaviours is being observed, such as physical activity, non-verbal and verbal interactions, an activity checklist can be used simultaneously with audiotape recording, allowing the observer to concentrate on a limited range of phenomena at the time.

Participant observation

This form of observation, associated with the qualitative paradigm, is used in order to explore, understand and interpret a culture or group from an insider's or *emic* perspective. Participant observation has its origins in social anthropology where data are collected in the normal surroundings of the people or events being studied. For example, the anthropologists Mead (1935) and Malinowski (1922) studied the lives and traditions of groups of people in their social surroundings by immersing themselves in the cultures of the groups, sometimes for several years (*see* Chapter 14 for a more detailed account of the use of participant observation in ethnography).

Characteristics and purpose of participant observation

According to Gold's typology (1969) there are three roles the researcher might adopt as a participant observer, namely the complete participant, participant-as-observer, and observer-as-participant (*see* Figure 25.1).

As a complete participant, observation may be conducted covertly to ensure that those being observed are not aware of the researcher's purpose and do not change their behaviour. Covert observation has been used in sociological and anthropological studies, and to investigate sensitive topics to uncover and understand events or behaviours that would otherwise remain hidden (Mays and Pope 1995). In a study by Rosenhan (1973), eight participants were admitted to different psychiatric hospitals in America in order to observe the way in which psychiatric wards operated and the behaviour of staff towards psychiatric patients. The participants gained entry to the hospitals by claiming to 'hear voices'. Seven of the participants were diagnosed with schizophrenia and one with manic-depressive psychosis. Once admitted, the pseudo-patients stopped pretending to exhibit symptoms and reverted to 'normal' behaviour although the diagnoses of schizophrenia remained. Through covert participant observation the pseudo-patients recorded their experiences and those of other patients and demonstrated the powerlessness and depersonalisation that was the reality for psychiatric patients at that time. The data collected in the study could not have been obtained had the research been conducted overtly. However, the ethical issues associated with covert observation such as deception and observing participants without their knowledge and consent, make this a problematic role for nurse researchers.

In participant-as-observer and observer-as-participant the researcher's role is known and consent is obtained from the study participants. The openness of the role allows the researcher to ask group members to explain activities or events that have been observed. The amount of time the researcher spends in participation in each of these roles will depend on the data that are to be collected and the researcher may in fact switch between roles spending more time on participation or more time on observation as required (Waterman 1998).

Negotiating access and building rapport

As discussed in Chapter 10, those who wish to conduct research must obtain permission to access the study site. The process will require approval of the ethics committee and negotiation with nursing and medical personnel/gatekeepers before potential participants can be approached. Familiarity with aspects of nursing culture, and the language and traditions of hospitals and/or primary care will assist nurse researchers when entering a setting for the first time. The researcher may be considered an 'insider' and this can facilitate the exploration of practice processes and the understanding of the phenomenon being studied (Bonner and Tolhurst 2002). Nonetheless, this is only the first step and the researcher must spend time learning to integrate with people in the setting to gain their trust and acceptance.

Gerrish (1997) and Kennedy (1999) described their experiences of undertaking participant observation of district nurses (DNs) in practice. Both researchers had previously worked as DNs, which gave them credibility with the participants and enabled them to 'fit in' and gain access to the participants' roles. During 15 months of fieldwork Gerrish (1997), as *participant-as-observer*, involved herself in patient care where appropriate and developed a rapport with the DNs sufficient to be considered an honorary team member. Kennedy (1999) did not participate in patient care although she wore district nurse uniform when accompanying DNs on home visits. The focus of her *observer-as-participant* role was observing the work of the DNs. Through the rapport she had built up with the DNs, Kennedy helped them to overcome their anxiety about being observed. This may have helped to 'normalise' their behaviour and consequently enhanced the credibility of the observed data.

Negotiating access and building rapport with participants should be considered, not as a one-off event, but as a continuing process that requires patience and diplomacy to ensure that essential data are collected (Hammersley and Atkinson 1995; Robson 2002). Without the trust of participants, researchers may find they are not accepted and are unable to access the data they seek.

Working in the field and minimising disruption

Researchers conducting participant observation first enter the setting with a broad idea of what they want to observe and possibly a number of related questions.

The researcher's intention is to gain a 'feel' for the setting, the participants, how activities are conducted and the context in which they occur. Participation in the work and activities of a group, and a developing rapport with participants enables the researcher to refine the areas of observation, a process that Spradley (1980) referred to as 'forming a funnel'. This allows the observation to become more focused.

Researchers may spend long periods of time working alongside study participants in order to familiarise themselves with both the environment and the culture. This enables them to join in day-to-day activities and to share experiences with participants. Polit and Hungler (2003) call this 'getting backstage' to discover the reality of a group's experiences and behaviour, free from 'protective facades'. How well this is achieved is dependent on the trust and rapport that is developed between researcher and study participants.

Spending time in a site prior to data collection also enables participants to become familiar with the presence of the researcher and any audio or videorecording equipment that might be used. It is essential that the researchers' presence during data collection causes minimal disruption so that observed behaviours or events accurately reflect normality. While it is not possible to remove the effect of the researcher completely, it is important that researchers try to minimise the extent to which their presence is felt.

Recording observations – fieldnotes

Field notes are a record of the observations the researcher has made and should be recorded as soon as possible after observing an event to ensure accuracy. They may be written in a notebook used specifically for the purpose or may be recorded into a dictating machine. Whichever method is used, the security and confidentiality of the material is essential.

As a participant and an observer it may be difficult to record fieldnotes when and where they occur and the researcher may have to move out of an area to do so. It may also be useful to record fieldnotes in a place that is conducive to thinking about and interpreting observed data, away from an area that is particularly busy or noisy.

The way in which field notes are organised may be revised or refocused as observation progresses, or they may reflect themes that have been identified in the course of observation. The material constitutes collected data and, as the researcher attempts to make sense of observations and the contexts in which they occurred, the analytical process begins. An example of recorded field notes is presented in Box 25.4.

Most qualitative researchers keep a diary/journal record of their personal reflections during the periods of participant observation. In it they record their feelings, experiences and thoughts and acknowledge their position as a research instrument through which data pass.

Box 25.4   Fieldnotes.

Readiness to learn
Assessing readiness to learn is important for any chosen strategy for health education. Field notes made by Whyte (2004) during observation demonstrate a patient's lack of readiness not only to stop smoking but for information about smoking:

Case study 7
11:15 am: Nurse B (nurse participant) is working in the ward with a patient who is not in the study. I am in the ward dayroom with Sheila (patient participant).

Sheila is talking with three patients. They are all smoking and the talk is about smoking – ways of giving up, feeling like outcasts, problems caused by smoking. Sheila says she has spent a lot of money trying to give up and she wishes she hadn't bothered and just spent it on cigarettes instead. Doctors have been telling her for years that smoking is the cause of her heart trouble but she doesn't believe it as all of her family has had heart trouble and none of them smoke. She thinks it's in her genes and nothing to do with smoking, although she admits that she might be kidding herself. (observation and fieldnotes)

I don't think Sheila is ready to stop smoking.

2:00 pm: Nurse B and Sheila are sitting talking beside Sheila's bed. They appear quite relaxed.

Nurse B uses the opportunity to introduce the subject of smoking. Sheila's tone of voice becomes defensive when she is asked if she is a heavy smoker and she tries to change the subject. Nurse B talks about the harmful effects of smoking but Sheila eventually stops the conversation by saying '. . . nobody nags me to do anything about my smoking because they know what I've been through' (observation, field notes and taperecorded data)

Sheila is not ready to stop smoking – assessment of readiness would have identified that.

Researchers as participant observers must recognise the effect they might have on the study participants and the setting, and hence the data they collect. This process, called reflexivity, is defined by Schwandt (1997) as

'the process of critical self-reflection on one's biases, theoretical predispositions and preferences' (Schwandt 1997:136)

and contributes to the trustworthiness of the data.

Reflexivity should demonstrate that observed data is a reflection of the behaviour, events or activities of the study participants, while at the same time acknowledging the position of the researcher and how she/he may have affected the data.

Non-participant observation

In non-participant observation, the researcher assumes the role of complete observer and endeavours to have no influence on the phenomenon under observation. In quantitative research, a validated structured schedule is used for data collection, whereas in qualitative research, less structured forms of data collection are used. However, a systematic process to both the collection and analysis of data is equally important for both forms of research.

Recording unstructured observations

As outlined in Box 25.1, Whyte (2004) assumed a non-participant observer role in a qualitative study of the provision of smoking-related information, and used an unstructured approach to observation by audio-recording nurse-patient interactions. The audio-recordings were transcribed verbatim and the data were analysed qualitatively using a framework that was developed specifically for the study, based on literature on verbal communication and health education.

Observation methods using a structured method of data collection are appropriate for quantitative studies, collecting data about actions and behavioural interactions (Boxes 25.2 and 25.3).

Recording structured observations

In studies that use structured observation, the researcher is a non-participant observer who records the phenomena under examination using a framework for data collection. Such a framework is developed prior to commencement of the study. The researcher's aim is to devise a tool that will facilitate the systematic collection of data in a way that will, as far as possible, limit subjectivity and observer bias, enhancing validity and reliability. This involves a process which is similar to that followed when developing a questionnaire or structured interview schedule.

Category system

The first stage is to draw up a category system from which activity checklists and/or rating scales are developed for completion by the observer. A category system comprises a comprehensive list of the behaviours that are likely to arise within the situation under observation.

In developing the category system, the researcher needs to be clear about the phenomena that are to be observed. Expressing these as concise written statements is an important discipline in helping to ensure clarity. This also enables the researcher to identify subcategories for each category.

In observation research the categories often comprise the following:

- location
- time
- activity
- facial expression
- verbal interaction
- personnel

Each category has within it a range of attributes or subcategories that are amenable to observation (Box 25.5).

In designing observation schedules, it is important that the categories are mutually exclusive so that the observed phenomena can only be coded within one category (*see* the example of 'weeping' in Box 25.5).

When the category system has been developed, the next stage is to assess its face and content validity. This can be achieved by seeking the views of a panel of individuals who have expertise in the topic of the investigation. When testing for face validity, the individuals are asked to comment on the appropriateness of the categories and the clarity of the wording. Assessing the content validity involves asking for views of the appropriateness of each item of the category system and whether, in their view, it is sufficiently complete or whether additional behaviours should be recorded.

Activity checklist

Activity checklists are developed from the sub-category systems. These can be simple lists that require to be coded, as shown in Figure 25.2. Alternatively they can be more complex. Using a numerical coding scheme to rate the activity can

---

Box 25.5   Category system for structured observation.

Location
Bed, bedside, dayroom, treatment room, bathroom

Time
Starting time, finishing time

Activity
Sleeping, eating, walking, reading, watching television

Facial expression
Natural repose, smiling, laughing, grimacing, weeping*

Verbal interaction
The nature of the interaction – e.g. question, explanation, reassurance, humorous exchange
   The tone of voice – e.g. soft, harsh

Personnel
Patient, nurse, doctor, occupational therapist, family member

*Note that the word 'weeping' is used rather than 'crying', which could be interpreted as 'crying out' as, for example in pain or anger. The careful use of descriptive words is crucial in avoiding ambiguity and subsequent errors in coding.

Patient	Sleeping	Eating	Walking	Reading	Watching TV
1		✓			
2	✓				
3	✓				
4			✓		
5					✓

Figure 25.2 A simple activity checklist.

Box 25.6 An activity checklist used in structured observation.

Walking
1. Unable to walk, even with maximum assistance.
2. Constant assistance of one or two persons is required during ambulation.
3. Assistance is required with reaching aids and/or their manipulation. One person is required to offer assistance/support.
4. The patient is independent in walking up to 50 yards/metres, or may require supervision for confidence or safety.
5. The patient must be able to assume the standing position, sit down and use necessary walking aids correctly. The patient must be able to walk 50 yards/metres without help or supervision.

---

provide a more qualitative level of observation, as indicated in Box 25.6 where 'Walking' is rated using the criteria given for ambulation in the Modified Barthel Index (Shah *et al.* 1989).

The next stage in the process is to establish the reliability of the schedule. Reliability in observational methods refers to the consistency with which categories of observation are identified and recorded when the same behaviours are observed and recorded, either by different observers, or by the same observer on different occasions. There are therefore two aspects of reliability that ought to be tested during the development of the schedule. These are the *inter-observer* reliability, i.e. the level of reliability of the schedule when used by more than one observer, and its *intra-observer* reliability, i.e. the level of reliability of the schedule when used by the same observer on more than one occasion.

If more than one observer is used to collect data on the same phenomena, it is important that they are trained in using the observation schedule and that the *inter-observer* reliability is evaluated. This involves each observer collecting and recording data on the same situation at the same time and using statistical procedures to analyse the results. The Kappa statistic is a measure of agreement based on the proportion of subjects who give the same responses (Armitage and Berry 1994). The value of Kappa can range from zero, which indicates no agreement, to 1.0 for perfect agreement. A value that exceeds 0.75 represents excellent agreement; values less than 0.4 indicate poor agreement. *Intra-observer* reliability can be assessed using the same statistical procedure but in this case the data are collected and recorded on the same behaviours on different occasions by only one observer. It may be difficult to ensure that the same behaviours can be observed on separate occasions. This can be overcome by using a videotape recording of the activity and making recordings during a series of showings.

The observation schedule can be used in conjunction with a diagram of the physical environment and fieldnotes can be made to provide a verbal description to place the quantitative recordings in context.

Advantages and disadvantages of observation

Observational methods have the advantage that they can uncover and describe practice and behaviours as they actually happen, rather than as self-reported activities. Observation also allows the researcher to access the context in which study participants are operating. This can help to explain the phenomena that are observed. Unlike studies that rely on self-report data, real-time observational data is not subject to the effects of recall, or to misinterpretation by the participant. They are therefore inherently more reliable. Observation can offer verification of self-report data and contribute to the reliability, validity, trustworthiness and rigour of a study.

Using a structured observation schedule helps to minimise observer bias in that the data that are collected are predetermined, as is the coding scheme. An advantage of using a previously validated observation schedule is that it allows researchers to replicate the work of others in different settings or with different populations. Since structured observation offers a means of collecting quantitative data, this method of data collection can be incorporated into descriptive or cross-sectional surveys or experiments. Designing a schedule provides other researchers with a tool with which to conduct replication studies.

Structured observation schedules undoubtedly have advantages in terms of reliability and validity. However, highly structured systems for coding and recording behaviour may prevent the capture of complex activities that occur spontaneously. Use of a rating scheme can have the effect of 'pigeonholing' observed behaviours such that inappropriate judgements are made about events under examination.

While useful in helping us to understand *what* people do, structured observation, offers little insight into *why* they do it. Underlying meanings that are ascribed to behaviours remain inaccessible when structured observation is used as the primary and sole source of data. Participant observation, on the other hand, is intrinsically more flexible.

Participant observation allows the researcher to reflect the reality of events as they occur and can be used to provide in-depth descriptions of behaviours, events and activities. Analysis of observations contributes to explanations of behaviours, events, and activities in their natural contexts. The opportunity for the researcher to assume a participant role facilitates the development of trust between researcher and those being observed. This may help to break down barriers and lead to enhanced understanding of the subtleties of complex behaviour and dynamic interpersonal interaction. Participant observation offers a means of studying the art of nursing, whereas structured observation can be used to investigate its science. For any form of observation study, however, it has to be remembered that events that are observed represent only a 'snapshot' of the overall activity.

Throughout participant observation the researcher has two roles – as both nurse and researcher. This dual role has the potential to be a source of conflict. There is a risk that researchers may become immersed in the culture and fail to maintain sufficient distance between themselves, the culture and the participants, thereby losing their research perspective and threatening the credibility of the data.

One of the strongest criticisms that can be levelled at observation methods is that the presence of the observer, be that a person or a camera, may influence the very behaviours that are the focus of the study. Patton (1990) has argued that prolonged exposure to observation reduces the likelihood of behaviour resulting from the 'observer effect'. However, this contention is problematic since one cannot know what the behaviour would have been had the subjects not been observed.

Observational methods of data collection are relatively time-consuming as the researcher needs to be present during the period of direct observation, or when conducting or viewing videorecordings.

Issues of validity and reliability

As has been seen, observation can be used in both qualitative and quantitative studies. In qualitative studies, the terms used to encompass the concepts of validity and reliability have been described as 'trustworthiness' or 'rigour' (see Chapter 27).

In structured observation, the terms 'reliability' and 'validity' are pertinent. The use of a carefully designed tool for recording the observations is important. Using a structured observation schedule helps to minimise observer bias in that the data that are collected are predetermined, as is the coding scheme. All personnel who are involved as observers need to undergo training in using the schedule and in coding and recording the data to ensure consistency and inter-observer reliability of the study. Careful piloting can help to identify problems such as observer bias so that corrective action can be taken before the main study is conducted.

The trustworthiness or validity of an observation study can be affected if the observer misconstrues certain phenomena, misinterprets their importance, or is temporarily distracted or tired. Some behaviours may be outside the range of the observer's field of vision or may not be captured, being outwith the observation period. Actions may be misinterpreted because the observer is not sufficiently knowledgeable about the topic of the study, or the observer may be influenced by a preconception of the situation that is observed.

The presence of the observer can also influence the behaviour of those being observed and hence the trustworthiness and validity of the data. The likelihood of this increases when a researcher conducts an observation study within his or her own workplace (Mulhall 2003).

Ethical issues associated with observation

There are key principles that govern the ethics of nursing research. Adherence to these principles ensures that practitioners involved in undertaking research respect the autonomy and personhood of all participants.

Covert observation

In studies where covert observation is used researchers should ensure that disclosure is made and de-briefing provided for each participant when their participation in the study is completed. However, as indicated earlier in this chapter covert observation is problematic for nurses and health care professionals. As a general principle covert observation is not considered ethical because the autonomy of the individuals who are being observed, their right to information about the study and their right to consent are breached. In cases where covert observation is considered, alternative, more open ways of addressing the problem should be sought.

Overt observation

The researcher should plan the study such that all individuals who may be present during any period of observation are given full information about the study in advance so that they can decide whether or not to take part. This may, however, prove difficult if, during the observation, an unanticipated event occurs which necessitates the presence of another individual or group of people. In this instance, the researcher may be required to seek consent retrospectively.

A further dilemma concerns what constitutes 'full information'. It could be argued that failure to provide full information diminishes the autonomy of the individual to make an informed decision regarding consent to participate. On the other hand, by providing full details of the phenomena to be observed, the researcher may risk influencing the participant's behaviour, thereby diminishing the validity of the findings of the study. As it is unethical to undertake research that is rendered less valid by the information that is given, it may be necessary to reach a compromise.

The principle of non-maleficence requires that the research does not cause harm. The researcher may come across an incident where s/he feels the need to intervene in clinical care, perhaps because of a sense of the need to 'help out' when clinical colleagues are overstretched, or where he or she observes inappropriate practice. This poses problems on at least two fronts. First, such a distraction will prevent the continuous observation of the focus of the study. Second, it raises ethical issues concerning the professional clinical role of the nurse researcher. The Code of Professional Conduct for Nurses and Midwives (NMC 2002) is clear in stating the necessity for intervention if patient care or safety is compromised. In situations that do not involve patients, researchers may need to discuss what has been observed with members of staff or colleagues. In such cases the researcher's role as a participant observer may be changed to such an extent that the study can no longer continue.

Conclusion

Recording and analysing observed events and activities as they actually occur in naturalistic settings can enhance a study's scope to provide reliable and valid findings. This method of data collection is appropriate for either qualitative or quantitative studies and, depending on the nature of the study, the researcher's role may involve participation to varying degrees. Importantly, when using observation the researcher must consider the ethical issues associated with this method of data collection.

References

Armitage P, Berry G (1994) *Statistical Methods in Medical Research*. Oxford, Blackwell

Bonner A, Tolhurst G (2002) Insider-outsider perspectives of participant observation. *Journal of Advanced Nursing* 9: 7–19

Booth J, Davidson I, Winstanley J, Waters K (2001) Observing washing and dressing of stroke patients: nursing and occupational therapists. What is the difference? *Journal of Advanced Nursing* 33: 98–105

Day T, Wainwright SP, Wilson-Barnett J (2001) An evaluation of a teaching intervention to improve the practice of endotracheal suctioning in intensive care units. *Journal of Clinical Nursing* 10: 682–696

Gerrish K (1997) Being a 'marginal native': dilemmas of the participant observer. *Nurse Researcher* 5: 25–34

Gold R (1969) Roles in sociological field observation. In McCall, G, Simmons, J (eds) *Issues in Participant Observation: a text and reader*. London, Addison-Wesley

Hammersley M, Atkinson P (1995) *Ethnography: principles in practice*, 2nd edition. London, Routledge

Kennedy C (1999) Participant observation as a research tool in a practice-based profession. *Nurse Researcher* 7: 56–65

Macleod Clark J (1982) *Nurse-patient verbal interaction: an analysis of recorded conversations on selected surgical wards*, London, University of London

Malinowski B (1922) *Argonauts of the Western Pacific*. London, Routledge & Kegan Paul

Mays N, Pope C (1995) Qualitative research: observational methods in health care settings. *British Medical Journal* 311: 182–184

Mead M (1935) *Sex and Temperament in Three Primitive Societies*. New York, Morrow

Mulhall A (2003) In the field: notes on observation in qualitative research. *Journal of Advanced Nursing* 41: 306–313

Nursing and Midwifery Council (2002). *Code of Professional Conduct*. London, NMC

Patton M (1990) *Qualitative Evaluation and Research Methods*. Newbury Park, Sage

Polit DE, Hungler B (2003) *Essentials of Nursing Research: methods, appraisal and utilisation*, 5th edition. Philadelphia, Lippincott

Robson C (2002) *Real World Research*, 2nd edition. Oxford, Blackwell

Rosenhan D (1973) On being sane in insane places. *Science* 179: 250–258

Schwandt T (1997) *Qualitative Inquiry: a dictionary of terms*. London, Sage

Shah S, Vanclay F, Cooper B (1989) Improving the sensitivity of the Barthel Index for stroke rehabilitation. *Journal of Clinical Epidemiology* 42: 703–709

Spradley JP (1980) *Participant Observation*. New York, Holt, Rinehart and Winston

Turnock C, Gibson V (2001) Validity in action research: a discussion on theoretical and practice issues encountered while using observation to collect data. *Journal of Advanced Nursing* 36: 471–477

Waterman, H (1998) Data collection in qualitative research. In Roe B, Webb C (eds) *Research and Development in Clinical Nursing Practice*. London, Whurr

Whyte RE (2004) The Provision of Health Education on Smoking to Patients in Hospital: a critical evaluation of the role of diplomate nurses. Unpublished PhD Thesis, Glasgow Caledonian University

Website

www.trentfocus.org.uk/Resources/observations_research_project.htm

26 Physiological Measurement

Mark Johnson and S José Closs

Key points

- Accurate measurement of physiological variables is essential in many kinds of research as well as in clinical practice.
- Objectivity is important in such measurement, though some clinical measures such as pain have to use self-report.
- Physiological variables have a range of different characteristics, and need to be measured with accurate and appropriate instruments.
- Assessment of validity and reliability of physiological measurement is important.
- Specific ethical issues arise in the use of physiological measurement, particularly relating to the use of tissue samples.

Introduction

Although much of the research undertaken by nurses uses methods from the social and psychological sciences, some involves physiological measurements. This is particularly true for those employed as research nurses on clinical trials, who are frequently asked to collect large amounts of physiological data. It is important for such nurses to understand the impact of accurate and precise measurement on the validity of the entire research study. They may also need to be aware of the ethical implications of storage and processing of such data.

Human physiology can be defined as the science of body processes, i.e. how body parts function (Tortora & Grabowski 2003). Physiological processes can be studied at different levels such as molecular, cellular, tissue, organ, system and organism although these levels overlap. Furthermore, physiological processes may be reflected indirectly in psychological and other outcomes.

In clinical practice, health care professionals assess physiological processes in a variety of ways. Sometimes physiological processes are assessed by watching (observation), touching (palpation) and listening (auscultation) to the body and its parts. Sometimes physiological processes are assessed by taking samples and specimens of living tissue to check its composition and/or characteristics. Sometimes physiological processes are assessed by monitoring ongoing activity of body parts using instruments like the electrocardiogram (ECG), which monitors the heart. In any research project it is important to be clear about what is to be measured, why it is to be measured and how best this can be achieved.

In this chapter we aim to clarify what is involved in the measurement of physiological phenomena and their psychological concomitants for research purposes. This includes the breadth of type of measurements that may be made; the selection and use of measurement instruments; measurement procedures; the interpretation of measurements; and a brief mention of ethical issues.

What is measurement?

One definition of measurement is

> 'the operationalisation of abstract constructs into concrete variables [through the] formal assignment of numbers to objects according to well-defined rules' (Powers & Knapp 1995:99).

In the context of this chapter, we can consider measurement to be the process of assigning numbers to physiological phenomena.

Clinical nurses take physiological measurements to provide answers (or clues to answers) to questions concerning health status. In nursing practice, for example, the questions may be about infection (Is the temperature above normal?) or diabetes (Is there any glucose in their urine?). Nurse researchers take measurements to provide answers to research rather than clinical questions. By using numbers to represent physiological and psychological processes practitioners and researchers can:

- describe a phenomenon or process
- compare a given physiological or psychological measurement with established values for health and illness
- explore associations between physiological and non-physiological items
- examine the effect of an intervention (Box 26.1)
- examine how an intervention works (Box 26.2)

When taking physiological measurements it is important that the overall procedure reduces as much measurement error as possible. This necessitates the use of reliable, carefully calibrated instruments, with an appropriate level of sensitivity and specificity, at an appropriate time (or time intervals) and to be able to understand what the measurement means in the context of the question.

Types of measurement

Measurements made in clinical practice that are commonly used in research are mostly physiological or psychological in nature. These may produce continuous, discrete or categorical data (*see* Chapter 28), but measurement may also be conceptualised as objective or subjective.

Box 26.1 Examining the effect of an intervention.

Johnson MI, Tabasam G (2003) An investigation into the analgesic effects of interferential currents and transcutaneous electrical nerve stimulation on experimentally induced ischaemic pain in otherwise pain-free volunteers. *Physical Therapy* 83: 208–223

The aim of this study was to compare the analgesic effects of Interferential Current Therapy (IFT) and Transcutaneous Electrical Nerve Stimulation (TENS) on experimentally induced ischaemic pain in 30 pain-free healthy participants using a modified version of the submaximal-effort tourniquet technique. A single-blind, sham-controlled, parallel-group method was used and the primary outcome measure was the change in the self-report of pain intensity during one of three possible interventions: (1) IFT, (2) TENS, or (3) sham electrotherapy using a dummy stimulator. Unpaired t-tests showed that IFT and TENS reduced pain intensity when compared with sham electrotherapy but that there were no statistically significant differences between IFT and TENS. In conclusion, IFT and TENS reduced experimentally-induced ischemic pain in healthy participants to a greater extent than sham electrotherapy but there were no differences in the magnitude of pain relief between IFT and TENS.

Box 26.2 Reasons for undertaking physiological measurement.

Reason	Example
To describe a phenomenon or process	What is the time course for a leg ulcer to heal? Area and depth of wound could be measured regularly over time until healing is complete.
To compare a given measurement with a standard	Does the body weight of adult female prisoners differ from population norms? If adult female prisoners had significantly lower body weight than women in the general population, this might mean either that the adult female prisoners had different eating and exercise habits (?anorexia) or that the diet provided in prison was less fattening than that eaten by the general population of comparable women. Or there may be other, less obvious reasons for the difference.
To explore associations between measurable items	Are post-operative infection rates associated with the duration of surgery, the grade of surgeon undertaking the operation, the type of dressing used, the grade of nurse undertaking the wound re-dressing and/or the frequency of changing the dressing? Multivariate statistical procedures could be used to identify whether any of these factors were associated with infection rates, and whether some were more strongly associated than others.
To examine the effect of an intervention	Does aromatherapy using lavender oil have a calming effect on women about to undergo breast lump biopsy? Two groups of patients could be used – intervention (receiving aromatherapy) and control (no aromatherapy). Comparisons of heart rate and blood pressure could be used as indicators of calmness. Self-report of feelings of calmness would add validity.

Measured values (data) are often said to lie on a continuum from 'objective' to 'subjective'. Objectivity is related to things happening outside oneself and not necessarily constrained by our human senses, for instance we cannot see microwaves but know that they exist because we can detect and measure their existence using instruments. Objective data are obtained through measurements such as physical examination, laboratory tests, height and weight. Subjectivity is personal; it arises from our own experience and is not perceptible to others. Subjective data are obtained from patients or family and friends' reports of their feelings or perceptions about health, such as morale, fear, anxiety and pain. For example, the level of someone's morale can only be described by the person experiencing it, not by someone observing the person. An observer has no means of confirming that the person's report of their morale is a true reflection of their actual morale, since the patient could be deceiving the observer that their morale is good, when in fact it is not (and *vice versa*).

Objectivity

Absolute objectivity does not exist and is a myth now generally rejected. True objectivity is elusive because all measurements incur a certain degree of error, due in the main either to the measurement instrument, changes in the environment, fluctuations in the phenomenon being measured, or the person taking the measurement.

Instruments that take 'objective' measurements have the potential to be more reliable (reproducible) because they are less susceptible to errors in human judgement. For example, if researchers weighed patients by simply lifting them up and estimating, there would be substantial variation in the answers from researchers with different levels of strength and fitness. However, if weighing scales were used they would give very similar measurement values, even if different models of scales were used, providing they were correctly calibrated. This is because weighing scales are fit for purpose and are detached from a judgement based on a researcher's viewpoint or past experience. The scales improve the 'objectivity' of the measurement because they are 'impartial' or 'neutral' to the measurement process, i.e. they do not have an 'opinion' of what the answer should be. However, all instruments are imperfect and prone to error because they are designed and used by humans.

Subjectivity

Measurements of psychosocial attributes such as health status, quality of life, coping and stress rely heavily on a patient's self-report. A researcher has no means of confirming the authenticity of a self-report so researchers may also measure physiological processes to substantiate measurements of psychosocial attributes. An example of this might be an obese middle-aged man complaining of extreme fatigue and daytime sleepiness. Tiredness and satisfaction with sleep are measured by self-report – only the sleeper knows how satisfied he is. However, sleep itself can be monitored by electroencephalogram and be shown to be very disturbed – if respiratory rate is also monitored it might be shown that the man suffers from sleep apnoea, waking many times during the night because of the inability to breathe.

One clinical phenomenon commonly experienced by patients and less commonly monitored by nurses is pain. The experience of pain is entirely subjective, and can only be meaningfully assessed using self-report. Researchers have developed a variety of approaches to the identification and quantification of the experience of pain. Different approaches should be selected for different conditions, types of pain, patient groups and so on. For example, intensity of pain can be measured with a visual analogue scale – usually a 10 cm long horizontal line with anchors such as 'no pain' and 'worst possible pain' at opposite ends. The patient then indicates the point on the line which best represents how he or she feels (as used in the example in Box 26.1). While this approach is sensitive to small changes, it is not appropriate for use with some groups, such as older people and in particular those who have cognitive impairments, since conceptually it is difficult for some to grasp (Box 26.3). A simple verbal rating scale, where the person selects from a list of descriptions such as 'no pain, mild pain, moderate pain, severe pain or excruciating pain' is a simpler and more widely usable approach.

It must be remembered that an objective measure cannot replace a subjective one, e.g. increased cortisol levels cannot be used to 'prove' that someone is in pain. Therefore, objective and subjective measures have crucial and sometimes complementary roles in gathering knowledge.

Box 26.3   Comparison of pain assessment scales.

Closs SJ, Barr B, Briggs M, Cash K, Seers K (2004) A comparison of five pain assessment scales for nursing home residents with varying degrees of cognitive impairment. *Journal of Pain and Symptom Management* 27: 3 196–205.

The aim of this study undertaken in the north of England was to compare five different pain assessment scales for use with people with different levels of cognitive impairment residing in nursing homes. The verbal rating scale (VRS), horizontal numeric rating scale (NRS), faces pictorial scale (FS), colour analogue scale (CAS) and mechanical visual analogue scale (MVAS) were presented in random order to 113 residents. Cognitive impairment was assessed using the Mini-Mental State Examination (MMSE). The use of the VRS was the most successful with this group, completed by 80.5% overall, and 36% of those with severe cognitive impairment. The MVAS was the least successful. Repeated explanation improved completion rates for all the scales. Consistency between scores on the five scales was good for those with none to moderate cognitive impairment and poor for those severely impaired. This study showed no difference in pain scores according to cognitive status.

Making physiological measurements

When making physiological measurements it is necessary to:

- identify clearly the characteristics of the physiological variable to be measured
- select an appropriate instrument that can measure the physiological variable
- set up a measurement procedure that measures the physiological variable and minimises measurement error

Characteristics of physiological variables

Understanding the characteristics of physiological variables is necessary when setting up a measurement procedure. Some examples of physiological attributes and the instruments suitable for measuring them are shown in Box 26.4.

Physiological processes are dynamic and will fluctuate over time. Some occur within very short periods of time, e.g. the action potential of a nerve impulse takes milliseconds; some processes fluctuate rhythmically, e.g. breathing, heart beat and menstruation; while others fluctuate in an irregular (but not chaotic) fashion, e.g. the generation of nerve impulses. The measurement of many physiological functions therefore needs to be timed carefully and sometimes repeatedly, such as the blood glucose of someone with diabetes. Other attributes, such as height, can be considered to be stable, since their rate of change is so slow.

Selecting a measurement instrument

Measuring instruments generate numbers that are related to the object or phenomenon being measured (i.e. the measured variable). It is the researcher's responsibility to ensure that they have selected an instrument that is related specifically to the physiological variable under study, i.e. is fit for purpose. This requires information about the range of instruments at their disposal and a basic understanding of how the different instruments take their measurements. There is a wide range of instrumentation available to capture information about physiological processes (*see* Box 26.4).

Types of instrument

Our human senses can be used to quantify physiological processes by simply listening, observing, smelling or touching the patient. Paper-based instruments can be used to quantify a researcher's observation, such as a score for the patient's ability to undertake a range of activities of daily living, or to record patients' self-reports of experiences such as pain (e.g. using a verbal rating scale, VRS) or depression (e.g. using the Hospital Anxiety and Depression Scale, HADS).

Box 26.4   Examples of measuring instruments.

Measuring the physical quantity of a physiological variable

Physiological characteristic	Measuring instrument
Weight	Weighing scales, e.g. mechanical, electronic
Body temperature	Thermometers, e.g. electronic, mercury, infrared
Electrical conductivity of the heart	Electrocardiogram (ECG)
Rate of peak expiratory flow	Peak flow meter
Proteinuria/haematuria	Dipstick/urinalysis
Brain structure	Computed tomography (CT) scanner
	Magnetic resonance imaging (MRI) scanner
Selected blood tests including ammonia (plasma), bilirubin, high and low density lipoprotein cholesterol, creatine phosphokinase (CKP), protein, haemoglobin	Laboratory analysis
Area of bruising or wound	Trace outline of bruise/wound and measure total surface area

Measuring a physiological variable by a researcher's observation

Physiological characteristic	Measuring instrument
Neurological development	Bayley scales of infant development
	Motor development index
	Mental development index
Functional ability	Barthel index (Mahoney & Barthel 1965)

Measuring the self report of a patient's own experience

Physiological characteristic	Measuring instrument
Pain intensity	0–10 cm numeric rating scale (NRS)
Pain quality	McGill pain questionnaire (Melzack 1975)
Depression	Hospital anxiety and depression scale (HADS) (Zigmond & Snaith 1983)
	Beck Depression Inventory (BDI) (Beck et al. 1961)
Morale	The Philadelphia Geriatric Center morale scale (PGCMS) (Lawton 1975)
Self-esteem	Coopersmith self-esteem inventory (Coopersmith 1981a;b)

Adapted from Burns and Grove (1993); Fulbrook (1993)

Instruments can be used to aid measurements using our senses, e.g. a watch to record time when palpating the radial pulse to measure heart rate or a thermometer to confirm our sense that a patient feels hot, and quantify temperature.

Many physiological processes cannot be detected without the aid of instruments. For example, it is not possible to measure ketone bodies (which indicate diabetes mellitus) without instruments to test urine samples. Some instruments measure body structure, such as X-rays and magnetic resonance imagers (MRI);

while others measure function, such as an electroencephalogram (EEG) measuring the electrical activity of the brain. Some measure activity in real time, such as an electrocardiogram (ECG); while others measure physiological processes *post hoc* (after the event), e.g. by taking a specimen or sample for testing.

How instruments work

When instruments quantify a variable and derive a number they do so in a series of operational steps. Often physiological instruments operate by detecting a physical characteristic of the physiological process and converting it in to a signal that can be quantified and displayed (e.g. weighing scales). The researcher is responsible for checking that the components within the instrument are functioning correctly and that the final reading is accurate. Ideally, measuring instruments should not change in their properties during use, since this would introduce error in the measurement obtained. For example, a ruler should not expand between measurements and a clock should not run at a variable speed.

Nowadays, computers are used to speed up the processing, analysis and display of physiological data. However, the more technologically impressive an instrument is, the harder it is for the end user to be confident about its accuracy, precision, and reliability.

Operating a measurement instrument

When using instruments there are certain procedures that will enhance the validity and reliability of measurements taken.

Safe and effective operation

It is crucial that instruments are in good working order. Most instruments come with guidelines for operation, technical specifications and sometimes contraindications for their use. These should always be read carefully before use. The performance of the instrument should be checked in the environment in which it will be used and against the technical specifications provided by the manufacturer.

Calibrating instruments against a standard

Physiological instruments often need to be calibrated against standardised norms, and in some cases this needs to be done prior to each occasion they are used. This ensures, for example, a 1 kg weight is measured as 1 kg by a set of measurement scales, or an oxygen meter can accurately measure a mixture of gas with a known content of oxygen. Manufacturers will calibrate instruments before they leave the factory but it is worth checking the performance of new instruments against the technical specifications whenever possible.

Choice of range and setting the scale ends

In some instruments you have to choose the range and the sensitivity of the measurement scale and this will affect the precision of the measurement. Many instruments also have a limit to their range so it is important that the physiological variable does not fall outside of the measurement limits of the instrument (*see* Figure 26.1). This may result in some or all of the data being lost. If the scale is too sensitive it may also produce data that is unnecessary or meaningless, e.g. measuring height to ten decimal places. Some instruments have a 'gain' (amplifier) setting that enables the size of a display to be increased or decreased, e.g. with ECG recordings.

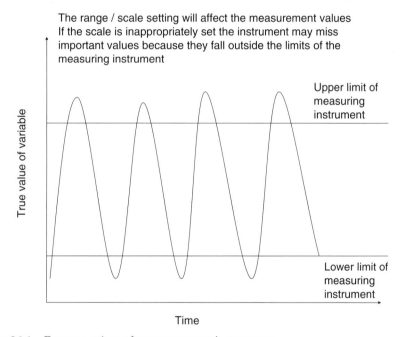

Figure 26.1   Range setting of measurement instrument.

Instrument 'drift' and 'stabilisation' during measurements

Drift is a gradual change in a reading of an instrument when a measured variable is known to remain stable, i.e. changes in the measurement are not caused by the measured variable changing (*see* Figure 26.2).

Drift affects the reliability of readings and may be caused by an instrument being faulty or intrinsically unstable or the environment progressively changing. Some instrumentation needs time to stabilise its measurement or 'warm up', e.g. a thermometer needs time to equilibrate with the patient's temperature otherwise the measurement will be lower than the true temperature (*see* Figure 26.3).

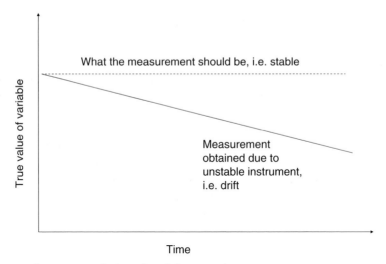

Figure 26.2 Instrument drift and stabilisation during measurement.

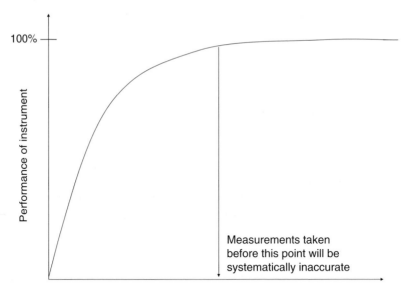

Figure 26.3 Time taken to stabilise measurement.

Measurement procedures

Devising a measurement procedure or protocol takes much thought and is critical to the quality of a research study. It is important to consider the following aspects of data collection.

Collection procedures of specimens and samples

Physiological measurements can be taken using specimens of living tissue or samples of body fluids obtained from the patient and measured at a later time, usually in a laboratory. Such measurements are termed *in vitro*. Specimens and samples taken from a patient may need to be sterile if contaminants from the environment affect the tissue and/or interfere with the performance of the measurement instrument. Biological samples also deteriorate over time so the integrity of the specimen may depend on the delay between collection and measurement. To reduce contamination and deterioration, collection procedures may involve storing specimens in ice or freezing them in liquid nitrogen. It is also important that a sufficient quantity of a sample is obtained. Too large a sample may affect the donor's health and too small a sample may be unable to meet the operational requirements of the instrumentation.

The physiological context in which the measurement is taken

Physiological measurements can be made directly from the patient so that a value is obtained from living tissue within the person. Such measurements are termed *in vivo*. Some *in vivo* measurements are affected by the site of the measurement, e.g. blood pressure differs according to where in the circulatory system the measurement is taken, i.e. systemic, pulmonary, arterial or venous. Sometimes body site does not affect the measurement, e.g. pulse can be taken from the brachial, radial or carotid artery.

Some measurements can be taken at a single (discrete) time point, e.g. height or weight if the measures are to be used to describe the characteristics of a study population. The duration of the measurement may simply be the time it takes the measuring scales to stabilise when a person stands on them. Some measurements are taken continuously over the entire duration of an experiment as is the case in sleep experiments when electroencephalographic (EEG) data are collected over the entire night of sleep to determine a participant's sleep pattern. Commonly, measurements of physiological processes are taken intermittently.

Timing of measurements

The time interval between physiological measurements, sometimes called the sampling rate, can be critical. Intrinsic body rhythms have a profound influence on many physiological variables. Many hormones, such as cortisol and melatonin have clearly-defined fluctuations, while in women oestrogen and progesterone have approximate monthly rhythms. Body temperature fluctuates predictably during the day, increasing during the morning, dipping a little after lunch and then continuing to increase until the early evening when it starts to decrease until the early hours of the morning. Measurements of body temperature taken in the afternoon would therefore be systematically higher than those taken early in the morning. If very accurate changes in body temperature are required in a research study, these normal variations need to be taken into consideration (Figure 26.4).

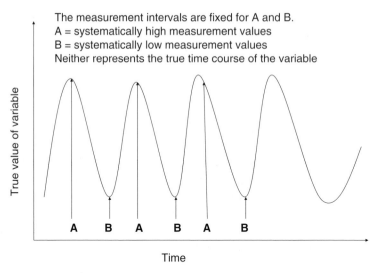

Figure 26.4   Timing of measurements.

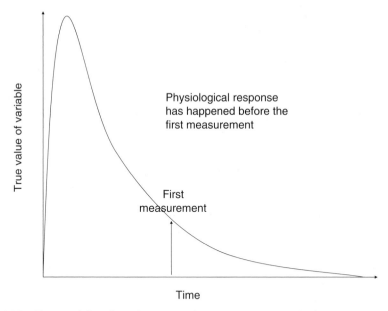

Figure 26.5   Error arising from inappropriate measurement timing.

If the time interval between measurements is too small, unmanageably large amounts of data may be obtained. It would be impractical to measure healing of an ulcer on a minute-by-minute basis, for example. The time course of healing could be achieved adequately by measuring on a weekly basis. However, the duration between measurements should not be so large as to miss any changes (Figure 26.5). This is particularly important in studies that are measuring the time course of a physiological process or a response to an intervention. Monitoring of the effect of consuming confectionery on insulin levels would miss meaningful changes in insulin levels if measurements were taken only once a day. The interval between measurements ultimately depends on whether it was important to establish changes in a physiological attribute every few seconds, minutes, hours, days or weeks.

Within and between subject variation

The characteristics of a physiological process can vary within an individual over time as seen above. This is termed *within* subject variation. The characteristics of a physiological process can also vary between individuals because of differences such as age, gender, diet and environment. This is termed *between* subject variation. Measurements are often repeated to establish the extent of this variation, because it will give an indication of the similarity of the measurements within and between individuals. This is especially important when measurements are being used to generalise to a wider context as it provides an estimate of the reliability of the research finding.

Researchers design experiments that are able to measure the physiological variable against this 'background noise' of within and between subject variation. Some factors that contribute to physiological variation between patients cannot be changed, such as age and gender. The researcher may match or standardise the age and gender of patients between experimental groups to reduce the influence of these factors. Alternatively, they may randomly allocate patients to experimental groups so that the effect of age and gender cancels out between the groups. Researchers may standardise room temperature, time of day, and consumption of substances like alcohol or caffeine prior to measurements so that all participants are exposed to similar conditions when the measurement is taken.

Interpreting physiological measurements

Several factors need to be considered when interpreting physiological measurements, including the validity and reliability of the measurement as well as the spread of the measurements and their normal range.

Validity and reliability depend on the accuracy of the measurements made. Errors are the difference between reality and what was measured and are due to the instrument, the environment or the researcher. Measurement errors can be systematic, affecting the validity of measurement, or random, affecting the reliability of the measurement.

Validity

Validity is the extent to which the instrument and procedure actually measure what they claim to measure. This is also referred to as *internal* validity. *External* validity refers to the generalisability of research findings to the wider population of interest.

The internal validity of the interpretation of a measurement is compromised whenever some kind of systematic error is introduced into the measurement

procedure, such as an investigator choosing an inappropriate instrument or consistently misreading an appropriate instrument. For example, heart rate cannot
measure sympathetic nervous system activity because heart rate is controlled by
sympathetic and parasympathetic nerves and it would not be possible to determine which nerve was influencing heart rate.

Reliability

Reliability is a generic term that reflects a measure's consistency and reproduc-
ibility. It is influenced by random errors, sometimes called artefacts, which affect
the consistency of the measurement. When considering physiological measurements, test-retest reliability and inter-rater reliability are important.

Test-retest reliability

Test-retest reliability is concerned with the stability of a measuring instrument and
is compromised by instrument 'drift'. A researcher may need to take steps to
assess the test-retest reliability of any instrument they might be using prior to
starting a study. Statistical tests would be undertaken in order to ensure that the
correlations between repeated measures were at acceptable levels.

Inter-rater reliability

It is important that different people can repeat a measurement accurately, particularly when large research studies demand that many different data collectors are
involved. For example, when taking an aural temperature, one person might position the probe exactly as the manufacturers instruct, while another might routinely
place it too far away from the heat source, producing a lower temperature than
when placed correctly. This might be a fault either of the person not paying careful
attention to the technique required to obtain an accurate reading, or it might be an
instrumental fault, where the construction of the probe is such that it is impossible
for the user to know whether it is in the required position or not. Therefore it is
important to determine inter-rater reliability. This can be done by two or more
people (raters) undertaking and recording a measurement at a given time. Statistical
techniques can then be used to assess the degree of agreement between raters.

Normal range of measurements

The physiological context is central to any measurement, e.g. the importance of
knowing the sex of a person from whom a blood sample had been taken for the
identification of oestrogen levels. Obviously normal levels would be very different
in men and women. Physiological measurements are usually norm referenced,
i.e. compared against large sets of measurements taken from healthy people. It is
then possible to compare a measurement taken with what you would expect. For
example, if an accurate measurement of resting blood pressure was 140/100 mmHg,
the inference for someone aged 50 years may be that it is 'normal' whereas it might
be considered to be 'high' for a teenager. The norm depends on many factors
including age, gender and lifestyle and the researcher must be aware of the extent

of normal physiological variations that may contribute to the measured values. Many data sets are available which provide a basis for the interpretation of individual and pooled measurements.

Ethical issues

Ethics related to informed consent to participate in research are discussed elsewhere in this book (*see* Chapters 3 and 10). For this kind of clinical physiological research, informed consent is required concerning all measurement procedures, as well as ensuring that the person is aware of how any tissue samples will be used; and consent is also required for the storage and potential future use of samples (Medical Research Council (MRC) 2001).

Researchers should be aware of cultural and/or religious beliefs concerning the body before approaching potential participants. Obviously, any measurements being made, particularly any that involve invasive procedures (such as taking blood samples), need to be explained fully and carefully to the participant. Foreseeable harm as a result of the measurement or other use of tissue should be minimised and the patient should be made aware of all known risks and follow-up support put in place to deal with this. Harm may be physiological and/or psychological, if for example the measurement is potentially embarrassing (e.g. involves the collection of urine).

Participants need to be aware that they can withdraw consent at any time and that they can request the destruction of specimens. In intervention studies the patient needs to know whether there is a potential for receiving a placebo and that no conventional treatment will be withheld. Written information describing any procedures should be provided, and potential subjects should have a minimum of 24 hours to consider whether or not they wish to take part.

The patient needs to know how any samples or specimens will be handled, and how long they will be kept before they are destroyed. It is usual for the principal investigator (PI) to have day-to-day responsibility for the management of tissue samples, while the PI's host institution (university, hospital, etc) usually has formal responsibility for the custodianship of such material.

It is possible that a physiological measurement undertaken as part of a research study might indicate some kind of ill-health or abnormality in the research subject. In such cases, the best interest of the patient has to be the priority, even if as a result they need to withdraw from the study. Further information about research ethics can be obtained from the COREC website, (*www.corec.org.uk/*) and the MRC Ethics Series (e.g. MRC 2001).

Conclusion

Nurse researchers may use physiological measurements to answer a range of research questions, producing descriptive, associative and causal results. The quality of the results depends on the quality of the measurement and as has been discussed here, this depends on understanding what needs to be measured; selecting appropriate instruments; using instruments properly; and careful interpretation of the findings.

References

Beck AT, Ward CH, Mendelson M, Mock J, Erbaugh J (1961) Inventory for measuring depression. *Archives of General Psychiatry* 4: 561–571

Burns N, Grove SK (1993) Measurement strategies in nursing (Chapter 14). In Burns N, Grove SK (eds) *The Practice of Nursing Research*. conduct, critique and utilisation, 2nd edition. Philapdelphia, WB Saunders, 357–359

Closs SJ, Barr B, Briggs M, Cash K, Seers K (2004) A comparison of five pain assessment scales for nursing home residents with varying degrees of cognitive impairment. *Journal of Pain and Symptom Management* 27: 196–205

Coopersmith S (1981a) *The Antecedents of Self-Esteem*. Palo Alto, Consulting Psychologists Press

Coopersmith S (1981b) *Self-Esteem Inventories*. Palo Alto, Consulting Psychologists Press

Fulbrook P (2000) Physiological measurement (Chapter 28) In Cormack DFS (ed) *The Research Process in Nursing*, 4th edition. Oxford, Blackwell pp337–351

Johnson MI, Tabasam G (2003) An investigation into the analgesic effects of interferential currents and transcutaneous electrical nerve stimulation on experimentally induced ischemic pain in otherwise pain-free volunteers. *Physical Therapy* 83: 208–223

Lawton MP (1975) The Philadelphia Geriatric Center Morale Scale: a revision. *Journal of Gerontology* 30: 85–89

Mahoney FI, Barthel DW (1965) Functional evaluation: the Barthel Index. *Maryland State Medical Journal* 14: 61–65

Medical Research Council (2001) *Human tissue and biological samples for use in research: operational and ethical guidelines*. MRC Ethics Series, London, MRC

Melzack R (1975) The McGill Pain Questionnaire: major properties and scoring methods. *Pain* 1: 277–299

Powers BA, Knapp TR (1995) *A Dictionary of Nursing Theory and Research*, 2nd edition. London, Sage

Tortora GJ, Grabowski SR (2003) *Principles of Anatomy and Physiology*, 10th edition. New York, John Wiley

Zigmond AS, Snaith RP (1983) The hospital anxiety and depression scale. *Acta Psychiatrica Scandinavica* 67: 361–370

Further reading

Bland JM, Altman DG (1986) Statistical methods for assessing agreement between two methods of clinical measurement. *The Lancet* 1: 307–310

Willard HH, Merritt LL, Dean JA, Settle FA (1988) *Instrumental Methods of Analysis*. Belmont, Wadsworth pp30–31

Section 5
Making Sense of Data

Section 5 is short, but the processes it describes are of critical importance in any research study. Without analysis of data, it would be impossible to convey with any clarity or precision what exactly the research has discovered. It is also the stage in the research process that is often most taxing and confusing, as the researcher wades through a mass of statistical or narrative data, and wonders how to bring order out of the seeming chaos.

Chapter 27 tackles qualitative data analysis. This is a huge subject, and the serious student is referred to major texts on the subject (e.g. Miles and Huberman 1994, *see* references for Chapter 27). However a clear overview of the broad principles of analysis is presented here, with the aim of getting the novice researcher started, and able to make a choice between the major methods such as narrative analysis, framework analysis, and grounded theory. The chapter builds upon earlier chapters in Section 3 (Chapters 13–15), and the reader is encouraged to use the four chapters in parallel.

Chapters 28 and 29 are designed to be read together, as they are written by the same authors and use a consistent worked example throughout. Chapter 28, however, may be sufficient for some readers who want only to be able to describe and present quantitative data in a basic way. For those wishing to test hypotheses or analyse relationships, Chapter 29 takes the reader further into statistical analysis and provides some basic methods of making inferences from data. Again, as with Chapter 27, there is much more to statistical analysis than can be presented here, and these chapters include recommendations for further reading.

27 Qualitative Analysis

Judith Lathlean

Key points

- There are a number of different approaches to qualitative analysis, depending on the research design and nature of the data.
- Qualitative data analysis is usually ongoing and iterative throughout the research process; as such it can inform the research design as well as provide an interpretation of the findings.
- The validity of the analysis, triangulation and reflexivity are all important concepts when undertaking qualitative analysis.
- Different frameworks and software packages exist to assist in the practical process of qualitative data analysis.

Introduction

For the qualitative researcher in nursing, the process of analysing data is not linear or even predictable. Qualitative research studies do not follow the traditional route of hypothesising or identifying a research problem, doing a literature review to clarify what is already known about that proposition or problem, collecting some data and only then analysing these data. Indeed, the actual analytical process can start at the very beginning and inform all the aspects and stages of the research. Furthermore, there is no one 'right' way of doing the analysis and no standard recipe for success. It depends as much on what one wants to achieve as the view of what would lead to the production of a rich account and a deep understanding about the phenomena being studied.

Despite the relative lack of prescription, much has been written about qualitative data analysis and there is general agreement that there are some helpful principles to consider, as well as some tried and tested schematic approaches and practical aids. This chapter explores these principles and discusses several more popular methods of analysis in some detail. It also looks at the practicalities of qualitative data handling and analysis including the growing use of software packages.

Principles of qualitative analysis

Objectivity or subjectivity?

In thinking about the nature of qualitative research, the discussions have fre-quently been presented as dichotomous choices. Are objective or subjective data being generated and are the analysis processes lending themselves to objective or subjective descriptions? Is the aim for replication (that is, if a finding holds true in one setting, does it also hold true in another comparable setting?) or for authen-ticity (is this an authentic and credible portrait of what is being examined)? Is the aim to study representative samples or is there more interest in purposively selected samples? Is the ability to generalise conclusively being sought or is it accepted that all situations are unique, and therefore only tentative theoretical generalisations are possible? In reality these distinctions are not clear-cut, although the qualitative analyst will tend to lean more towards the right-hand position in these dichotomies.

Building theory

Qualitative researchers almost invariably agree that theory (or theorisation) should be the primary goal of research. Nevertheless, they frequently reject the formula-tion of theories in advance of their fieldwork, considering this to be unduly con-straining. The process of developing and testing theory is often said to proceed in tandem with data collection, and the main methods of analysis, such as analytic induction and grounded theory, offer fruitful strategies for theory building. So, for example, in analytic induction the analyst tries to formulate generalisations that hold true across all of his or her data, and when adopting a grounded theory approach, the theory is inductively derived from the study of the phenomenon it represents.

Eisenhardt (1989) provides a useful description of how to build theories from case study research. In doing so she draws on grounded theory building and the analytical methods described by Miles and Huberman (1994). Her logical step-by-step approach to developing theory includes tips on entering the field, analysing within-case data, searching for cross-case patterns, shaping hypotheses, compar-ing emergent concepts and theory with the existing literature and reaching closure (the point when the analyst ceases to add cases and stops going back and forth between theory and data).

Concurrent data collection and analysis

It is common in qualitative research for data that are analysed early on in research to inform the rest of the data collection, the research design and sometimes even the actual research questions. This is illustrated by a study I undertook of the implementation and development of lecturer practitioner roles in nursing (Lathlean 1997). At the outset, I had anticipated using an action research approach where I tried to find out 'how' these new roles should be developed and what processes were necessary to enhance their effectiveness. Following initial data collection and analysis, it quickly became obvious that the prime question was not to do with 'how' but rather 'what' i.e. 'what is the nature and reality of the job of lecturer practitioner?' So I chose an ethnographic research design with a number of different stages, each being thoroughly analysed before proceeding to the next one.

Another reason for analysing data as a study progresses is to identify when the data have reached 'theoretical' saturation (*see* Chapter 13).

Validation by respondents or researchers

In qualitative research the distinction is sometimes made between internal validity (the extent to which research findings represent reality) and external validity (the extent to which abstractions and concepts are applicable across groups). The qualitative analyst has strategies that can be used to ensure or at least facilitate both. These include giving the original data (e.g. an interview transcript) to the interviewee and asking them to clarify the meaning of their responses. Participant observation (which is common in ethnographic studies) allows data to be collected over a prolonged period and this is accompanied by continual data analysis. In this way constructs can be refined and checked out with participants. A crucial test of qualitative research accounts is whether those people whose beliefs and behaviour are supposedly presented in the accounts actually recognise the validity of the accounts. However, it is necessary to be cautious about the process of respondent validation, since it can not be assumed that any actor is a privileged commentator on his or her actions, in the sense that the intentions, motives and beliefs involved are accompanied by a *guarantee* of truth.

Triangulation

Data-source triangulation involves the comparison of data relating to a phenomenon that have been derived, for example, from separate phases of the field-work, or from the accounts of various participants including the researcher. The claim is that if different kinds of data lead to the same conclusion, this increases confidence in the conclusions. This approach has been supported by a number of authors, but it should not be confused with 'method triangulation'. This is where, for example, the results of interviews are compared with the researcher's observations or with data from very structured questionnaires relating to the same phenomenon. This can be problematic, since it assumes that there is a single 'reality' that is waiting to be discovered, a suggestion that is anathema to most qualitative researchers.

In my research on lecturer practitioners, the presentation of my accounts of their lives to the participants was a way of 'validating' those accounts and a form of triangulation (Lathlean 1997). The accounts generated at the three different stages were compared and contrasted for each participant as well as being examined for consistency across cases. However, I needed to be careful to distinguish between differences that occurred as a result of the way the data had been collected (for example, the interviews may have thrown up different points about the experiences of the lecturer practitioners than I gleaned in my role as observer), and differences that were the result of real disparities in their lives at separate points in time.

Following on from my three-year longitudinal study, I surveyed the perspectives of all lecturer practitioners who were in post in one health authority at that time, using a structured questionnaire. Conducting this separate study could have been construed as a form of triangulation on the grounds that the intention was to achieve a fuller and more penetrating understanding of the lecturer practitioners. But I had to be cautious about interpreting the results. A match or mismatch between the perceptions of the participants in the survey and the 'reality' of the lecturer practitioners as observed in the ethnographic study did not necessarily confirm or put into question the validity of either study. Rather it could simply mean that there were differences between the lives of lecturer practitioners and other people's understandings of those lives.

Reflexivity

Qualitative research stresses the importance of reflexivity whereby the researcher recognises that he or she has a social identity and background that has an impact on the research process. Reflexivity is especially relevant in nursing research because often the researcher is also a nurse. In such circumstances the researcher needs to think carefully – to reflect – on the impact that being a member of the same professional group as study participants may have on all aspects of the research process, especially interpretation of research findings. So, for example, in a qualitative study that was undertaken of community mental health nurses' experience of taking part in a clinical trial of treatment for patients with common mental health problems (*see* Kendrick *et al.* 2005), the researcher (Lucy Simons) – a nurse herself – had to make a conscious effort to 'reflexively bracket' her experience (Ahern 1999), so that it did not unduly bias the process of the research nor the interpretations she drew. Simons' use of narrative analysis in her study, with its emphasis on the nurses' talk itself and the *way* they told their stories, was also helpful in this respect.

Examples of methods of analysis

Two particular general strategies for analysis are frequently cited – analytic induction and grounded theory. In addition there are other approaches that are especially suited to more open-ended forms of textual data such as discourse, conversation and narrative analysis. Finally, since policy and applied research is increasingly important in nursing, analytical methods such as the 'Framework' approach have been developed.

Analytic induction

Analytic induction is a process of analysing data where the researcher tries to find explanations by carrying on with the data collection until no cases (referred to as deviant or negative cases) are found that are inconsistent with a hypothetical explanation of a phenomenon. The process of analytic induction is illustrated in Box 27.1.

From this brief description it can be seen that the analytic induction method shares attributes of 'positivism' or a 'realist' stance in research, for example, the setting up of a 'hypothesis' and the confirmation or refutation of that hypothesis. However, it is based on a case study research design, whereby cases are not selected to be representative and therefore theoretical rather than statistical generalisation occurs. Furthermore, the final explanations that result from analytic induction may specify the conditions that are *sufficient* for a phenomenon to occur, but rarely those that are *necessary*. So, for example, studies have shown that certain people in particular circumstances become drug or alcohol dependant but analytic induction will not shed light on why other people with the same characteristics in similar circumstances do *not* become addicted. Also, in analytic induction, there are no hard and fast rules as to how many cases need to be investigated before the absence of negative cases and the validity of the hypothesis can be confirmed.

Grounded theory

For a detailed discussion of grounded theory, *see* Chapter 13. However, it is referred to briefly here since it is one of the most widely cited approaches to the analysis of qualitative data. While there is some disagreement about the precise nature of the grounded theory approach, most consider that there are usually four aspects in the analytical process: theoretical sampling, coding, theoretical saturation and constant comparison (Box 27.2).

Some researchers claim to be using a grounded theory methodology when what they really mean is that they are employing some of the stages or principles of

---

Box 27.1   Steps in analytic induction.

1. Set up a definition of a problem.
2. Provide a hypothetical explanation of the problem.
3. Investigate a number of cases.
    a. Find that these cases are in line with the hypothesis – hypothesis is confirmed.
    b. Find cases that deviate from hypothesis.
        i.   Reformulate hypothesis and go back to 3 *or*
4. Redefine hypothetical explanation to exclude deviant cases and end data collection.

Box 27.2   Key aspects in a grounded theory approach to analysis.

Theoretical sampling – this is

'the process of data collection for generating theory whereby the analyst jointly collects, codes and analyses his (sic) data and decides what data to collect next and where to find them, in order to develop his theory as it emerges' (Glaser & Strauss 1967)

Coding – this is where data are broken down into component parts and names are given to the parts.

Theoretical saturation – this refers to the point when no further coding is necessary because no new instances are required to confirm a category, and/or when no new data collection is required as there is sufficient confidence about the nature of the emerging concepts.

Constant comparison – this is the process whereby the data and the subsequent conceptualisations from it are compared to ensure that there is a good fit. This happens throughout data analysis.

analysis such as theoretical saturation or constant comparison. This is not necessarily a problem but, in these instances, it needs to be recognised that only parts of the approach are being adopted.

Analysing narrative

The most common approaches to analysing narrative are conversation analysis, discourse analysis and narrative analysis. Conversation analysis is based on an attempt to describe people's methods for producing orderly social interaction and has a relatively long history. It is concerned with the sequential organisation of talk – how talk overlaps and the lengths of pauses in a conversation are key attributes. Silverman (1998) says that is important in conversation analysis to try to identify sequences of related talk, to examine how speakers take on certain roles or identities through their talk, such as 'client–professional', and to look for particular outcomes in talk such as laughter and then work back from there to see how it was produced. For an introduction to conversation analysis, see Heritage (2004).

Discourse analysis is very similar to conversation analysis in that it seeks to analyse the activities present in talk. However, unlike conversation analysis, discourse analysis possesses the following three features: it is concerned with a far broader range of activities such as gender relations or social control; it does not always use analysis of ordinary conversation as a baseline for understanding talk in organisational settings and it works with far less precise transcripts than conversation analysis.

A good example of the use of discourse analysis is to be found in the study of violent behaviour in an acute mental health setting by Benson *et al.* (2003) (Box 27.3). In this study, discourse analysis was found to be illuminative because of 'its capacity to reveal constructions of the self, the other and the world, and the ways in which actors understand social actions and interactions' (Benson *et al.* 2003:918). In this respect, the authors are referring to the work of Potter and Wetherell (1995), which is a good reference source for discourse analysis, as is Potter (2004).

Narrative analysis stems from the idea that in research, as in life, stories are told and these are then taken as the object of investigation. In research interviews, as long as the questions are not too focused and require more than 'yes' or 'no' answers, the respondent will often reply at length and sometimes organises these 'turns' into quite substantial stories. Traditional approaches to qualitative analysis tend to fragment these 'blocks' of text, in order to thematise and eventually to draw interpretations and generalisations. The narrative analyst is not only interested in the content of the story but in asking the question 'why was the story told *that* way?' A helpful description of the theory behind narrative analysis as well as the practicalities of doing it is given by Riessman (2002).

Narrative methods can also be combined with other forms of qualitative analysis. In the aforementioned study by Simons on the experiences of community mental health nurses within a treatment trial involving people suffering from

---

Box 27.3   Example of a study using discourse analysis.

Benson A, Secker J, Balfe L, Lipsedge M, Robinson S, Walker J (2003) Discourses of blame: accounting for aggression and violence on an acute mental health inpatient unit. *Social Science and Medicine* 57: 917–926

This study was based on 16 semi-structured interviews in one mental health unit, and aimed to address the paucity of research on how all involved in such a setting understand the attributed meaning to violent or aggressive situations, and how these attributions justified individual perceptions, reactions and actions. Although the analysis was based on only two incidents involving one client (the other clients being unwilling or unable to give retrospective accounts), it clearly demonstrates how discourse analytic techniques can be used to examine client accounts and those of staff members engaged in the incidents. The findings reveal that participants discussed key themes in terms of dilemmas: e.g. whether the violent or aggressive behaviour was 'mad' or 'bad'; predictable or unpredictable; and had resulted from a personality disorder or mental illness. It also indicated that discourses of staff and clients were remarkably similar and had at their core the attribution of blame.

common mental health problems, first of all a thematic analysis of the interviews with the nurses was carried out. This identified a main theme that related to the nurses' goal to be agents of change (e.g. through practical means, by improvements in patients' symptoms, by facilitating self-efficacy among patients and through sustained change). It also emerged, though, that with trial patients the ability to be agents of change could be constrained by the treatment-centred approach required by the trial protocol. In turn, the narrative analysis portrayed *how* change did or did not happen and *why*, through the way in which the nurses constructed their stories about their experiences. Thus in looking at how the nurses used language to produce their accounts of nurse-patient encounters, this gave deeper insights into the perceptions of their role and function – both in the trial and in their everyday professional practice.

Framework analysis

Ritchie and Spencer (1994) developed 'Framework' as a method of data analysis particularly suited to policy and applied research. It involves a number of distinct though interconnected stages (*see* Box 27.4). An example of a project in health care where Framework analysis was used is a study by Elkington *et al.* (2004) (*see* Box 27.5). A worked example of how codes are attached and how a coding framework is developed when adopting this strategy is given in Box 27.6.

Box 27.4   Five key stages of data analysis in the 'Framework' approach.

Familiarisation – immersion in the data (e.g. listening to tapes, reading transcripts, studying notes, etc.) to get an initial feel for the key ideas and recurrent themes.

Identifying a thematic framework – the process of identifying key issues, concepts and themes and the setting up of an index or framework. This can be used for sifting and sorting data including *a priori* issues (used to inform the focus of the research and the data collection guides), emergent themes raised by respondents and analytical themes that are evident through recurring patterns in the data.

Indexing – the process of systematically applying the index or framework to the text form of the data, by annotating the text with codes in the margin.

Charting – data are 'lifted' from their original context and rearranged according to themes in chart form. There may be separate charts for each major subject or theme and they will contain data from several different respondents. This process involves considerable synthesis and abstraction.

Mapping and interpretation – the charts are used to define concepts, map the range and nature of phenomena, create typologies, and find associations between themes in order to provide explanations for the findings. This process is guided by the original research questions as well as themes and relationships emerging from the data.

Box 27.5   Example of a study using the Framework approach to analysis.

Elkington H, White P, Addington-Hall J, Higgs R, Pettinari C (2004) The last years of life of COPD: a qualitative study of symptoms and services. *Respiratory Medicine* 98: 439–445

This study set out to assess the symptoms experienced and their impact on patients' lives in the last year of chronic obstructive pulmonary disease (COPD), and to assess patients' access to and contact with health services. The Framework approach was used for the qualitative analysis of in-depth issues with 25 carers of COPD patients who had died in the preceding 3–10 months. Five phases of the approach are described: familiarisation, identification of a thematic framework, indexing, charting and mapping and interpretation. The paper presents two key areas to emerge from this process – the first relating to the symptoms experienced and their impact on patients' lives and the second relating to patients' contact with health services in the community.

Box 27.6   Example of analysis using the Framework approach.

As part of a study of out-of-hours health services (Lattimer *et al.* 2005) a postal survey of patient satisfaction with the services was undertaken, resulting in both quantitative and qualitative data. The qualitative data were in the form of open-ended comments which were analysed using the Framework approach. First, extracts from 3 comments related to the telephone contact are presented with codes attached. Second an excerpt is given from the coding frame and third, the chart shows how these can be compared across different sites.

Comment A: I was quite happy with phone service; I'd seen notices about it in the doctor's surgery and I read about it in the local paper; but there was one small aspect that I found irritating and it could be improved – different people asking the same questions *(balanced – 1.1)*

generally satisfied (2.1)

well advertised (2.1.1)

repeated questioning (2.2.1)

Comment B: Can't fault [the phone service]; got to speak to nurse immediately which was good *(all positive – 1.3)*

put straight through to nurse/doctor (2.1.7)

Comment C: Didn't realise that I'd have to phone GP and NHS Direct as well; so I was not pleased and then the operator spoke so fast I couldn't take it in *(all negative – 1.2)*

ringing doctor and then NHS (2.1.10)
person spoke too fast

(Continues)

Extract from coding framework (with examples of codes)
Balance of comments overall: 1
- Balanced comments   1.1
- All negative comments   1.2
- All positive comments   1.3

Theme: Ease of access over the phone: 2
- Positive   2.1
  General
    Well-advertised   2.1.1
    Good recommendation of other services   2.1.2
    Continuity of information between services   2.1.3 etc.
    Waiting time
    Put straight through to nurse/doctor   2.1.7 etc.

- Negative   2.2
  Questioning
    Repetitive questioning   2.2.1
    Repetitive questioning causing delay   2.2.2
    Perceived irrelevant questioning   2.2.3 etc.
    Clarity of process
    Ringing doctor and then NHSD   2.2.10
    Emergency doctors with no access to information   2.2.11 etc.
    Communication problems
    Person spoke too fast   2.2.19
    Difficulty communicating with call handler   2.2.20 etc.

Extract from chart comparing responses across sites

	Code	Site 1		Site 2		Site 3	
		n	%	n	%	n	%
Balance of comments	1						
• Mixed comments	1.1	47	29.4	31	26.1	30	29.1
• All negative comments	1.2	47	29.4	35	29.4	27	26.2
• All positive comments	1.3	66	41.2	53	44.5	46	44.7
All comments coded		160		119		103	
Returned questionnaires		332		274		249	
Theme: Ease of access over the phone	2						
Positive	2.1	23	35.9	9	25.0	7	35.0
Negative	2.2	41	64.1	27	75.0	13	65.0
Total		64	40.0	36	30.3	20	19.4

Practicalities

Recording and transcribing data

In order to be able to analyse data from interviews, a verbatim record of the interview should be gained. By far the best approach is to tape (or video) record the interaction and then to transcribe the tape. Some researchers use a transcription service, but wherever possible it is better for the interviewer to do this him or herself, since it is a good opportunity to start the process of 'immersion' in the data. The extent to which every single word is extracted, and every pause and emphasis is noted, will depend on the particular approach to analysis. So, for example, if thematic analysis is chosen, then pauses are not essential to record, whereas with discourse and narrative analyses, there are conventions that must be followed in preparing the transcript (see for example the narrative analysis in Box 27.3). Transcription is a very lengthy process, with a 60-minute interview needing several hours for transcription.

Fieldnotes in observation can follow a structure, according to the purpose of the observation, or they can be more free-flowing. If a structure is used, this can form the basis for the analysis. On the other hand, a predetermined structure may be unduly constraining. Sometimes it is a good idea to take a few notes during an interview as well, even when it is being tape-recorded. This can be helpful both as prompts for further questioning in a relatively unstructured or semi-structured interview and as a back-up, should the tape recorder fail, or the tape run out.

Doing qualitative analysis

The most usual way of condensing or grouping data is to attach codes to it. These codes may have been decided upon in an *a priori* way or they may emerge as the fieldwork unfolds. Different approaches to analysis use the word 'code' to mean slightly different things so the best plan when following one particular type of analysis is to be clear about what constitutes a 'code' in that approach. All the forms of analysis refer to the development of themes and categories, but the way in which they are derived or they emerge is again related to the analytical method.

A thematic analysis process is illustrated by an ongoing study of prisoners' views of a telepsychiatry service, conducted by Sarah Leonard. She undertook 20 taperecorded semi-structured interviews with prisoners after they had participated in an experimental telepsychiatry initiative. The questioning focused on the experience of the prisoners being assessed in terms of their mental health by a videorecorded link with a remote psychiatrist in a setting far from the prison. While their feelings about the experience of assessment using this process were central to the interview, the prisoners also talked graphically about their lives in prison.

These interviews were analysed using the stages outlined by Cresswell (1998). First, each interview was transcribed by the researcher herself and the transcription was then shared with the interviewee. This was to check out with them her understanding of the language they used – which tended to rely quite heavily on prison 'jargon' – rather than to 'validate' the transcripts. She then imported the text of the transcripts into a software package, NUD*IST (*see* section below). The second stage involved familiarisation with the range, depth and diversity of the data by listening to the tapes, reading the transcripts several times, and reflecting on each interview. During this 'immersion' in the data, 'memos' – consisting of initial impressions, key ideas and recurring themes – were written in the margins of the transcript. The next stage entailed description, the identification of codes and the clustering of similar ones under theme headings. Examples relating to the prisoners' life in prison included: 'lack of structure and meaningful activity', 'routines and lack of change' 'rigid system', and 'predictability'. Finally, the data clustered under these themes were again scrutinised and presented within a framework of main headings. Thus the aforementioned became sub-themes under the main heading of 'factors that help or hinder adaptation' to prison life. Verbatim comments were used to provide evidence of the participants' experience.

Examples of analyses

As referred to previously, different types of analytical approaches require the transcribed data to be presented in particular ways. Two contrasting examples are given to illustrate this – a narrative analysis (*see* Box 27.7) and a piece of analysis using the 'Framework' approach (*see* Box 27.6). It should be noted that while these are quite different strategies, for example, the narrative analysis requires the data to be presented with every single utterance, repetition and pause and with lines identified, whereas the Framework analysis works on chunks of verbatim quotes with undue repetition left out, there are still similarities. Thus the analyst in both works from the transcripts, identifying key concepts and producing an analytical framework, which can then be used to compare across other cases.

Analysing qualitative data is never easy, despite the impression given by many published studies that the results flow effortlessly from an obvious process, and it is often not possible to stick slavishly to one particular approach. A helpful sourcebook of methods, which is as much for the novice as for the more experienced researcher, is that of Miles and Huberman (1994). They define analysis as 'consisting of three concurrent flows of activity: data reduction, data display, and conclusion drawing/verification' (1994:10). Data reduction refers to the process of selecting, focusing, simplifying, abstracting and transforming the data found in fieldnotes and transcriptions and it occurs throughout the project – not just at the end of a data collection period.

The second type of activity is data display, which can mean the presentation of extended quantity of text – or at the very least copious snippets of verbatim quotes. Miles and Huberman provide examples of different types of display such as charts, graphs, matrices and networks that can work well to begin to show relationships and connections. The third 'stream' of activity is that of conclusion

Box 27.7 Example of narrative analysis.

This example is from Lucy Simons' qualitative study of community mental health nurses' experiences of treating patients with common mental health problems within a randomised trial (Kendrick *et al.* 2005). It is in three parts: first a story described by Len about his experience, presented using the conventions of narrative analysis, see Reismann (2002); second, the detailed analysis of this story and third, the template that this story is placed in so that it can be compared and contrasted with the other narratives in the study.

The story: 'Len, the most rewarding of all'	Line No.
Erm (1) but I think actually one of the most rewarding ones was	*105*
the e:r (,) um was a relatively young guy (.) who worked in a local Bank	*106*
who um (1) lived I think with his sister so a single guy um (.) and um	*107*
who actually not only told me that his problems were resolved by the end	*108*
but actually said you know how he now understood about tackling his	*109*
future problems you know in view of you know (.) that he not only not	*110*
only resolved his current problems but had learnt had learnt a way of	*111*
tackling (.) um how he perceives things in the future you know um which I	*112*
I find that (.) actually the most rewarding of all um (.) erm: you know	*113*
because hopefully you know not only has it resolved during the time	*114*
that I saw him but he will be able to do it himself next time, which is	*115*
what of course was said on the on the course itself but um (.) he	*116*
actually he actually came out with that himself and when he when he did	*117*
it um you know that was quite encouraging.	*118*
I think like	*508*
I said it was great when that guy said to me you know that he got	*509*
something he got something (.) for himself for the future he could use	*510*
you know and how to perceive things differently if you know I think that	*511*
was ur extremely good.	*512*

The detailed analysis of the story

Narrative characters and how Len wants them to be known

Len provided an introduction to the patient at the start of this narrative. He is constructed as a single young man who held a respectable job and lived with his sister (lines 106–107). Within this narrative Len hardly features and little is learnt about his character. This narrative featured some time into the interview and Len had already made identity claims earlier on.

Social positioning

The patient has the most dominant social position in this narrative in that all the actions that take place are attributed to him. The patient's actions are related to what he tells Len about the outcome of the encounter – that his problems were resolved (line 108) and that he had learnt to manage better in the future (lines 109–110). These ideas were then repeated twice (lines 110–112, 114–115). The patient had also offered this information to Len without prompting (line 117). When Len returned to the narrative much later in the interview the actions taken were still the patients' actions of telling Len that he had learnt for the future (lines 509–510).

In contrast Len did not attribute any actions to himself during the narrative. He described how he felt about the encounter: it was 'rewarding' (line 105), which he found 'quite encouraging' (line 118) and 'extremely good' (line 512), but it was not clear what actions Len had

(Continues)

actually taken to help bring about the problem resolution and the skills that the patient told him he had acquired. Len was the passive recipient in this narrative, as the patient told him what the outcome of the encounter was and even where Len refers to the problem-solving training course he frames this as what was said to him rather than what he learnt (line 116).

Although the patient was the most active and agentic character in the narrative the activity attributed to him is about telling Len the result of the treatment encounter. The problems were described as being 'resolved' (lines 108, 111, 114) by the end of the encounter without any clear idea who or what was responsible for this outcome.

Other narrative/discursive devices

Repetition

Len repeated the main idea of the narrative on three occasions throughout the whole narrative but rather than build on or add detail to the idea at each repetition he simply restated what happened.

Analytical framework

Who are the characters in the story? Are they dominant or subordinate? Type of story? What action takes place?	*Patient* (dominant): young, single guy *Len* (subordinate): on receiving end of action Change achieved and possibly successful PST* *Patient:* 108: told Len problems were resolved 109: told Len understood how to tackle problems 111: had resolved current problems 117: identified learning from the encounter 509: told Len what he had got from the encounter *Len:* none
Does the patient achieve change? Social positioning of characters:	Yes, problems resolved *Patient:* 108: problems resolved (no action taken) 110–112: resolved problems (taken action) and learnt how to in future 114: resolved during the time (no action) 115: future action indicated *Len:* 108, 117, 509: informed by patient 118, 512; encouraged by events of this encounter
Other narrative devices used:	Repetition Main idea returned to much later in interview
Blame (if no change achieved)	n/a

*(*Problem-solving technique used to treat patients randomised to this intervention)*

drawing and verification. This process does in fact start in the data collection stage when the researcher begins to note possible patterns, explanations and propositions. However, 'final' conclusions may not be apparent until the data collection is completed. Then the conclusions need to be 'tested' and 'verified' lest the analyst is left with an interesting story of what happened but one of unknown truth and utility.

Using computer software for qualitative data analysis

In the pre-computer age, most researchers took multiple copies of transcripts of interviews and field notes and wrote codes or categories alongside the text, usually in the margin. The use of different coloured highlighters was very popular to identify different types of code or category or to mark particularly apt or illustrative quotations. The next step was often to cut up the copies according to the different codes and place the pieces of text in piles, either over several desks and tables, or on the floor. Problems occurred when one part of the text could relate to more than one code, hence the need for multiple copies, or when there were

Box 27.8 The advantages and disadvantages of analysing qualitative data using software packages.

Advantages
- enables medium to large amounts of qualitative data to be stored in a single place, organised and cross-referenced
- allows quick and easy access to material and retrieval of data
- provides a comprehensive approach in that all data need to be considered and included
- encourages consistent coding and categorisation of data.
- allows more sophisticated analysis using algorithms to identify co-occurring codes

Disadvantages
- there are an increasing number to choose between; deciding on the best one for a purpose may require external advice
- it takes time, especially for novice researchers, to develop proficiency in their use
- some packages are relatively inflexible and impose a particular structure on the data
- making changes can be difficult after they have been completed
- they may persuade researchers that they can manage much larger amounts of data and increase the 'power' of their study, but qualitative studies are not designed to be statistically generalisable (Pope *et al.* 2000)

Adapted from Cresswell (1998)

hundreds of codes or one simply ran out of space! Wordprocessing was a major step forward. The data could be typed and then later scanned into a document and manipulated through the 'copy' and 'paste' facility. However, it is still a cumbersome and laborious process, with large amounts of data, and cross-referencing is still problematic.

The use of dedicated software packages for qualitative data is the next logical step. The advantages and disadvantages are summarised in Box 27.8.

QSR NUD*IST (or Non-numerical, Unstructured Data Indexing, Searching and Theorising) (and more recently NVivo which has come out of the same stable) alongside ATLAS.ti, are perhaps the most widely used of the packages. NUD*IST can be used to generate theory – it was initially developed for grounded theory – yet it is not rigidly tied in to a particular method of analysis. A detailed description of the use of NUD*IST or other packages is beyond the scope of this chapter. The reader is directed to Robson (2002) who provides an accessible overview of the NUD*IST approach, and then relates its application to different types of research such as ethnography, case studies and grounded theory.

Above all, software packages can help with the process of analysing data, but they are not shortcuts to rigorous analysis and they still require the researcher to make decisions about categorisation. As such they are tools to facilitate the analytical process but many would say that they are no substitute for immersing oneself in the data, and really getting a feel for the nature of the data and the inter-relationships between different aspects. In essence, they are geared more to medium-sized to larger projects where there are reasonable amounts of data, Conversely, where the beginning researcher has perhaps a few short interviews, they can provide learning opportunities for use in future projects.

Conclusion

In conclusion, qualitative data analysis in nursing research is a complex, creative process, which is ongoing, interactive, inductive and reflexive. It occurs throughout the study from the initial conception of the idea to the production of the final report or account. While it can be quite different from the processes used to analyse quantitative data, nevertheless it still needs to be rigorous, systematic and transparent.

References

Ahern KJ (1999) Ten tips for reflexive bracketing. *Qualitative Health Research* 9: 407–411

Benson A, Secker J, Balfe E, Lipsedge M, Robinson S, Walker J (2003) Discourses of blame: accounting for aggression and violence on an acute mental health inpatient unit. *Social Science and Medicine* 57: 917–926

Cresswell JW (1998) *Qualitative Inquiry and Research Design: choosing among five traditions.* Thousand Oaks, Sage

Eisenhardt K (1989) Building theories from case study research. *Academy of Management Review* 14:4 532–550. Reprinted in Huberman AM, Miles MB (eds) (2002) *The Qualitative Researcher's Companion*. Thousand Oaks, Sage pp5–35

Elkington H, White P, Addington-Hall J, Higgs R, Pettinari C (2004) The last years of life of COPD: a qualitative study of symptoms and services. *Respiratory Medicine* 98: 439–445

Glaser B, Strauss AL (1967) *The Discovery of Grounded Theory*. Chicago, Aldine

Heritage J (2004) Conversation analysis and institutional talk: analysing data. In Silverman D (ed) *Qualitative Research: theory, method and practice*. London, Sage pp161–182

Kendrick T, Simons L, Mynors-Wallis L, Gray A, Lathlean J, Pickering R, Harris S, Rivero-Arias O, Gerard K, Thompson C (2005) A trial of problem-solving by community mental health nurses for anxiety, depression and life difficulties among general practice patients. The CPN-GP study. *Health Technology Assessment Monograph* September, 9(37): 1–104

Lathlean J (1997) *Lecturer Practitioners in Action*. Oxford, Butterworth-Heinemann

Lattimer V, Turnbull J, Burgess A, Surridge H, Gerard K, Lathlean J, Smith H, George S, (2005) Effect of introduction of integrated out-of-hours care in England: observational study. *British Medical Journal* 331: 81–84

Miles M B, Huberman AM (1994) *Qualitative Data Analysis: an expanded sourcebook*, 2nd edition. Thousand Oaks, Sage

Pope C, Ziebland S, Mays N (2000) Qualitative research in healthcare: analysing qualitative data. *British Medical Journal* 320: 114–116

Potter J, Wetherell M (1995) Discourse analysis. In Smith JA, Harre R and Van Langenhove (eds) *Rethinking Methods in Psychology*. London, Sage pp80–92

Potter J (2004) Discourse analysis as a way of analysing naturally occurring talk. In Silverman D (ed) *Qualitative Research: theory, method and practice*. 2nd edition. London, Sage pp144–160

Reissman CK (2002) Narrative analysis. In Huberman AM, Miles MB (eds) *The Qualitative Researcher's Companion*. Thousand Oaks, Sage pp217–270

Ritchie J, Spencer L (1994) Qualitative data analysis for applied policy research. In Bryman A, Burgess R (eds) *Analysing Qualitative Data*. London, Routledge. Reprinted in Huberman AM, Miles MB (eds) (2002) *The Qualitative Researcher's Companion*. Thousand Oaks, Sage pp305–331

Robson C (2002) *Real World Research*, 2nd edition. Oxford, Blackwell

Silverman D (1998) *Harvey Sacks and Conversation Analysis* (Polity Key Contemporary Thinkers Series). Cambridge, Polity Press

Further reading

Bryman A, Burgess R (eds) (1994) *Analysing Qualitative Data*. London, Routledge

Huberman AM, Miles MB (eds) (2002) *The Qualitative Researcher's Companion*. Thousand Oaks, Sage

Miles MB, Huberman AM (1994) *Qualitative Data Analysis: an expanded sourcebook*, 2nd edition. Thousand Oaks, Sage

28 Descriptive Analysis of Quantitative Data

Jenny Freeman and Stephen Walters

Key points

- Different types of quantitative data need to be handled, presented and described in appropriate ways.
- Data checking and cleaning are essential first steps in recording and entering data for analysis.
- Charts, tables and graphs are commonly used to display data, but attention needs to be paid to presentation.
- Summary statistics such as means, medians and standard deviation are used to describe quantitative data.

Introduction

The prospect of collecting and analysing quantitative data can be daunting, especially the first time. However, it need not be and the purpose of this and the next chapter is to demystify the process and introduce some basic statistical ideas, so that when preparing to conduct a study the tools with which to proceed are available. This chapter describes the basic data types encountered in quantitative analysis, together with some simple ways of describing and displaying them. The following chapter introduces the concept of hypothesis testing and describes some basic methods for testing hypotheses. In order to provide continuity, data from the same study will be used throughout both chapters to illustrate key concepts. This study is described in Box 28.1, but briefly, it is a randomised controlled trial (*see* Chapter 16) of standard care versus specialist community leg ulcer clinics for treatment of venous leg ulcers. Patients were assessed at entry to the study, after three months and one year, and outcome measures included healing rates, health-related quality of life, satisfaction with the service and treatment cost.

Data types

In order to collect and analyse data as part of the research process it is necessary to understand the different types of data there are. Figure 28.1 shows a basic hierarchy of data types. Data are either *quantitative* or *categorical*. Quantitative variables can be either discrete or continuous. *Discrete* data are also known as

Box 28.1   Case study of a randomised controlled trial.

Morrell CJ, Walters SJ, Dixon S. Collin s KA, Brereton LML, Peters J, Brooker CGD (1998) Cost effectiveness of community leg ulcer clinics: randomised controlled trial. *British Medical Journal* 316: 1487–1491

This study comprised a randomised controlled trial looking at the cost effectiveness of community leg ulcer clinics. 233 patients with venous leg ulcers were randomly allocated to either usual care at home by district nursing team (control group, n = 113) or weekly treatment with four layer bandaging in a specialist leg ulcer clinic (intervention group, n = 120). In addition to looking at the relative costs for each group, other outcomes included time to complete ulcer healing, patient health status, recurrence of ulcers, satisfaction with care and use of services.

At the end of 12 months the mean time (in weeks) that each patient was free from ulcers during follow up was 20.1 and 14.2 in the clinic and control groups, respectively. On average, patients in the clinic group had 5.9 more ulcer-free weeks (95% confidence interval 1.2 to 10.6 weeks) than the control patients. Mean total NHS costs were £877.60 per year for the clinic group and £863.09 for the control group (P = 0.89). The researchers concluded that the community-based leg ulcer clinics with trained nurses using four-layer bandaging is more effective than traditional home-based treatment and this benefit is achieved at a small additional cost.

Health status or health-related quality of life (HRQoL) was measured at three-time points, recruitment or baseline, three months and six months follow-up using the Short-Form (SF)-36. The SF-36 is a 36 item self-completed questionnaire that measures HRQoL on eight dimensions, including general health, on a 0 (poor) to 100 (good health) scale (Brazier *et al.* 1992).

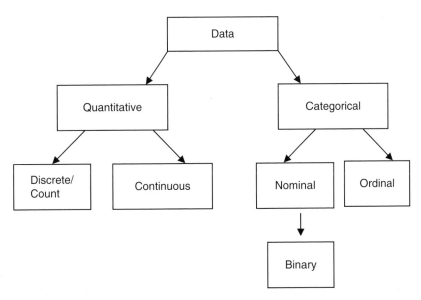

Figure 28.1   Types of data.

count data and occur when the data can only take whole numbers, such as the number of children in a family or the number of visits to a GP in a year. *Continuous* data are data that can be measured and they can take any value on the scale on which they are measured. They are limited only by the scale of measurement and examples include height, weight, and blood pressure.

Data are described as *categorical* when they can be categorised into distinct groups, such as ethnic group or disease severity. Although categorical data may be coded numerically, for example gender may be coded 1 for male and 2 for female, these codes have no intrinsic numerical value; it would be nonsense to calculate an average gender. Categorical data can be divided into either *nominal* or *ordinal*. Nominal data have no natural ordering and examples include eye colour, marital status and area of residence. *Binary* data is a special subcategory of nominal data, where there are only two possible values, for example (male/female, yes/no, treated/not treated). Ordinal data occurs when there can be said to be a natural ordering of the data values, such as better/same/worse, grades of breast cancer or social class.

Recording data

When collecting data either *forms* or *questionnaires* may be used. Forms are used to record factual information such as a subject's age, ethnic group or blood pressure. They are often completed by the study investigator(s) and thus need to be clearly laid out and familiar to all investigators. Although questionnaires may ask about basic demographic information they are generally used to measure more personal, subjective attributes such as attitudes and opinions, or levels of pain. When designing the layout of questionnaires it is usual for the data to be recorded in a series of boxes, as this will aid data entry.

In addition to collecting data using forms and questionnaires, a *data coding sheet* may be useful. This document is a link between the data collected on paper and the data stored on a computer as it contains information about how the individual variables are to be named, labelled and coded in the chosen computer package or spreadsheet. It should also have details of any special codes that are to be used for data that are missing or not applicable. It is a common convention when coding data to reserve 9, 99, 999, etc as codes for missing data. Table 28.1 is an example of a data coding sheet.

Use of spreadsheets and statistical packages

Once the data have been collected and the questionnaires and forms completed, the information recorded can then be input directly onto the computer ready for analysis. Two of the most commonly used packages for data storage and basic statistical analysis are Excel and SPSS (Statistical Package for the Social Sciences). Both are Windows packages with easy-to-follow pull-down menus. Excel is a

Table 28.1 Example of data coding sheet.

Variable	Label	Values	
ID	Patient ID number		
Age	Age (years)	999	missing
Sex	Sex	0	Male
		1	Female
		9	Missing
Hgt	Height (metres)	999	missing
Wgt	Weight (kg)	999	missing
BMI	Body mass index	999	Missing
Group	Study group	1	Clinic
		2	Control
Folup12	Patient available for follow-up at 12 months	1	Responder
		2	Died
		3	Referred elsewhere
		4	Moved away
		6	Hospital
		7	Nursing home
		8	Non-responder
			Etc...

spreadsheet with some statistical functions. It also has good facilities for producing graphs. However, if more than the most basic statistical analyses are planned, it is better to use SPSS as this has more comprehensive and flexible statistical analysis and data management facilities. Data can be entered into either package and, most usefully, it is possible to transport files and data between the two, should this be necessary. SPSS will read Excel files, while it is possible to save SPSS files as Excel files.

As stated previously, all data should be coded numerically when being entered into the computer, unless it is free text. Free text is data that is entered as a string of words. For example, in the leg ulcer trial, patients were asked to comment on their satisfaction with the services and their replies would have been entered into a single variable as a string of words. In SPSS it is possible to label both variables and the individual values of a categorical variable to ensure that all output is appropriately labelled and readily understandable.

Data entry and data storage

When entering data on to the computer either into a spreadsheet or a statistical package, it is conventional for each column to represent a different variable, and each row to represent the data for an individual subject. For categorical variables, the different categories should be input as distinct numerical values. This is because the standard statistical packages can have problems handling non-numerical data; they are not able to test for a difference between the two groups 'male' and 'female'; they would, however, be able to test for a difference between groups 1 and 2. Figure 28.2 shows the data view window of SPSS for the leg ulcer trial data (*see* Box 28.1).

Each row contains the data for a particular patient, identified by their (unique) patient identification number (PATID) and each column contains the data for a particular variable; for example the first column contains patient ID number (PATID), the second column contains information on patient follow-up status at three months (FOLUP3M) and so on. Although the latest version of SPSS (v13) at the time of writing will allow variable names longer than eight characters, in general, statistical packages including older versions of SPSS restrict the length of variable names to eight characters. Thus the data coding form can be useful in linking the variable names on the computer to a longer more informative label.

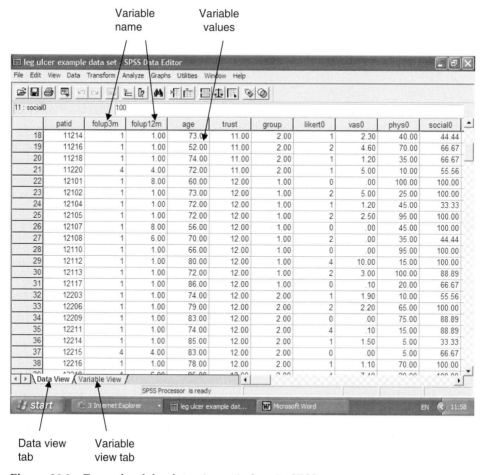

Figure 28.2 Example of the data view window in SPSS.

Data checking

Errors in recorded data are common. Errors can be made when measurements are taken (data collection), when the data are originally recorded, when they are transcribed from the original source (such as from hospital notes), or when being typed into a computer (data transfer). It is not always possible to know what is correct and so attention must be restricted to making sure that the recorded values are plausible. The data should be scrutinised for potential errors and omissions, and if possible these should be corrected, either by checking the original questionnaire or re-measuring the variable. This process is known as *data checking* (or *data cleaning*). Since the data will be analysed on a computer, this checking should take place after the data have been entered on the computer.

Initial checks should be made that the values are logical and that there are no missing or clearly implausible values. For categorical variables this can be as basic as tabulating the values (i.e. calculating the frequency for each value and putting these into a table) and checking that they are all possible. If for example, sex can only take the numerical values 1 (male), 2 (female) and 9 (missing) then any values outside these three are clearly wrong.

For continuous measurements, it should be possible to specify lower and upper limits on what is reasonable for the variable concerned. For example, for age, limits of 0 and 100 may be used. Age values above 100 should be checked since although these are possible they are unlikely. Equally if adults are being studied, values below 18 should be checked. Values that lie away from the main body of the data are known as *outliers*. They may be genuine observations from individuals with extreme values of the measurement, or they may be erroneous. As with all error checking, once outliers have been checked, they should only be changed if they are known to be wrong and values remaining outside a prespecified range must be left as they are, or recorded as 'missing'. Values should never be removed from the data set simply because they are higher or lower than would be expected, although the presence of these outlying values may influence the choice of statistical technique used (as outlined in the following chapter).

One method for ensuring that few errors occur in data entry is to enter the data twice and compare the two datasets. This technique is known as double entry and any values that are not the same can be checked against the original source. The disadvantage of this approach is that it can be expensive and time consuming, particularly for large datasets. However, this must be balanced against the fact that the errors that can occur in data entry will have been minimised. It is important to note that this method should never be used as a substitute for the logical and range checking described above once the data have been entered.

A by-product of data cleaning is that any missing observations will be identified. As stated earlier it is usual to use codes such as 9, 99, 999 or 99.9, according to the nature of the variable, although some computer programs, such as SPSS, allow a full stop (.) to indicate a missing observation. If a numeric value is used in SPSS, it is essential to identify the value as a 'user-defined' missing value before analysing the data. It is easy to forget that one or two values are missing, perhaps coded as 999, when carrying out an analysis and the effects on the subsequent analysis can be severe.

As a final point, it is worth considering why the data are missing. In particular, is there a reason related to the nature of the study? If this is the case it can have serious implications for the generalisability of the study results. Frequently, however, values are missing essentially at random for reasons not related to the study. As with impossible values, it may be possible to check with the original source of the information that missing observations are really missing.

Presenting data in charts

As a first step to any analysis it is useful to plot the data and examine it visually. This will show any extreme observations (outliers) together with any interesting patterns. In addition to being a useful preliminary step to analysis, information can also be displayed pictorially when summarising the data and reporting results. Figures are useful as they can be read quickly, and help particularly when presenting information to an audience. However, when using figures for presentation purposes care must be taken to ensure that they are not misleading. A figure should have a title explaining what is displayed and axes should be clearly labelled. A fundamental principle for both figures and tables is that they should maximise the amount of information presented for the minimum amount of ink used (Tufte 1983). Gridlines should be kept to a minimum as they act as a distraction and can interrupt the flow of information. All the figures and tables covered in the following sections were drawn using data from the leg ulcer trial as described in Box 28.1.

Basic charts for categorical data

Categorical data may be displayed using either a *bar chart* or a *pie chart*. Figure 28.3 shows a bar chart of marital status for the leg ulcer patients. Along the horizontal axis are the different marital status categories while on the vertical axis is percentage. Each bar represents the percentage of the total population in that category. For example, examining Figure 28.3, it can be seen that the percentage of participants who were married was about 45%.

Figure 28.4 shows the same data displayed as a pie chart. Generally pie charts are to be avoided, as they can be difficult to interpret particularly when the number of categories becomes greater than five. In addition, unless the percentages in the individual categories are displayed (as here) it can be much more difficult to estimate them from a pie chart than from a bar chart. For both chart types it is important to include the number of observations on which it is based, particularly when comparing more than one chart. And finally, neither of these charts should be displayed as three-dimensional as these are especially difficult to read and interpret (Huff 1991).

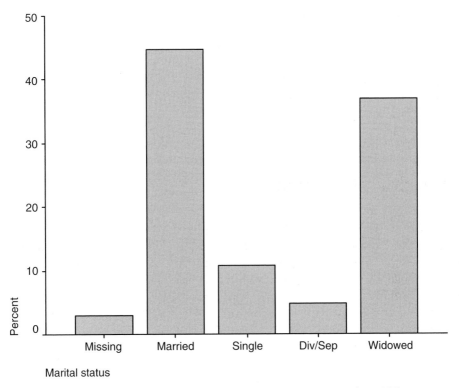

Marital status

Figure 28.3   Bar chart of marital status for the leg ulcer patients (n = 233).

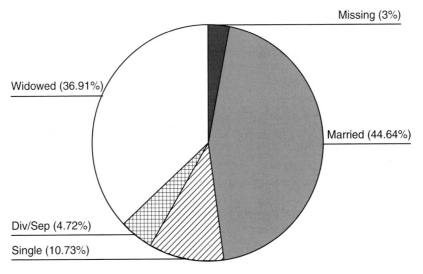

Figure 28.4   Pie chart of marital status (n = 233).

Basic charts for quantitative data

There are several charts that can be used for quantitative data. *Dot plots* are one of the simplest ways of displaying all the data. Figure 28.5 shows a dot plot of the heights for the leg ulcer patients, by sex. Each dot represents the value for an individual and is plotted along a vertical axis, which in this case, represents height in metres. Data for several groups can be plotted alongside each other for comparison; for example, data for men and women are plotted separately in Figure 28.5 and the differences in height between men and women can clearly be seen.

The most common method for displaying continuous data is a *histogram*. In order to construct a histogram the data range is divided into several non-overlapping equally sized categories and the number of observations falling into each category counted. The categories are then displayed on the horizontal axis and the frequencies displayed on the vertical axis, as in Figure 28.6.

The way that data are distributed can be examined using a histogram. Occasionally they display the percentages in each category on the vertical axis rather than the frequencies and it is important that if this is done, the total number of observations that the percentages are based upon is included in the chart. For the leg ulcer data there are a total of 233 observations and it is convention to write

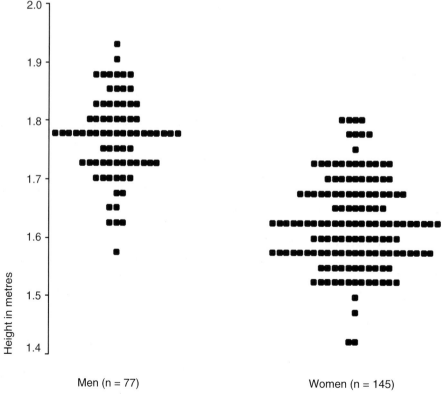

Figure 28.5   Dot plot of height, for leg ulcer patients.

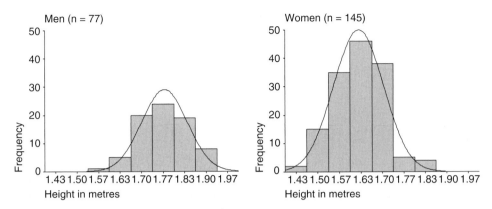

Figure 28.6   Histograms for height for men & women.

this as 'n = 233'. The choice of number of categories is important: too few categories and much important information is lost, too many and any patterns are
obscured by too much detail. Usually between 5 and 15 categories will be enough
to gain an idea of the distribution of the data. One useful feature of a histogram
is that it makes it possible to see whether the distribution of the data is approximately *normal*. The histogram of normally distributed data will have a classic 'bell'
shape, with a peak in the middle and symmetrical tails, such as that in Figure 28.6
for the height of men and women, displayed here with a theoretical normal
distribution curve. The *normal distribution* (sometimes known as the Gaussian
distribution) is one of the fundamental distributions of statistics, and its
properties underpin many of the methods explored in the following chapter.

Another extremely useful method of plotting continuous data is a *box-and-
whisker* or *box plot*. Box plots can be particularly useful for comparing the distribution of the data across several groups. The box contains the middle 50% of the
data, with the lowest 25% of the data lying below it and the highest 25% of the
data lying above it. In fact the upper and lower edges represent a particular quantity called the interquartile range (described later, *see* Box 28.3). The median is
shown by the horizontal line across the box (this is described later, *see* Box 28.2,
but briefly it is the value such that half of the observations lie below this value
and half lie above it). The whiskers extend to the largest and smallest values
excluding the outlying values. The outlying values are those values more than
1.5 box lengths from the upper or lower edges, and are represented as the dots
outside the whiskers. Figure 28.7 shows box plots of the heights of the men and
women in the leg ulcer trial. The gender differences in height are immediately
obvious from this plot and this illustrates the main advantage of the box plot over
histograms when looking at multiple groups. Differences in the distributions
of data between groups are much easier to spot with box plots than with
histograms.

The association between two continuous variables can be examined visually by
constructing a *scatterplot*. The values of one variable are plotted on the horizontal
axis (sometimes known as the X-axis) and the values of another are plotted on the

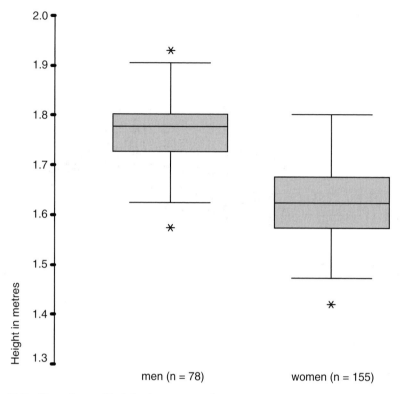

Figure 28.7   Box plots of height for men and women.

vertical axis (Y-axis). If it is known (or suspected) that the value of one variable (independent) influences the value of the other variable (dependent), it is usual to plot the independent variable on the horizontal axis and the dependent variable on the vertical axis (the reason for this will be explained in the following chapter). Figure 28.8 shows the scatterplot of weight against height and each dot represents the height and weight values for an individual. As height determines weight, to an extent, and not the other way around, it is plotted on the horizontal axis, although the variables could legitimately be plotted the other way around!

Describing data

Describing categorical data

A first step to analysing categorical data is to count the number of observations in each category and express them as percentages of the total sample size. For example, as part of the leg ulcer trial the participants were asked about their marital status. There were five categories, as displayed in Table 28.2.

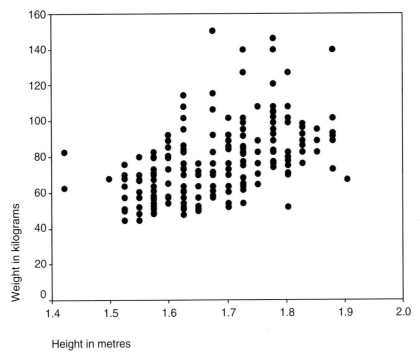

Figure 28.8   Scatterplot of height and weight (n = 215).

The first column shows category names, while the second shows the number of individuals in each category together with its percentage contribution to the total. In addition to tabulating each variable separately, it might be of interest to compare two categorical variables at the same time and in this case the data can be *cross-tabulated*. Table 28.3 shows the distribution of marital status by study group; in this case it can be said that marital status has been cross-tabulated with study group. Table 28.3 is an example of a contingency table with five rows (representing marital status) and two columns (representing treatment group). This table suggests that the distribution of marital status is broadly similar between the two study groups and in the following chapter this will be formally tested.

Describing quantitative data

As it can be difficult to make sense of a large set of numbers, an initial approach would be to calculate summary measures, to describe the *location* (a measure of the 'middle value') and the *spread* (a measure of the dispersion of the values) of each variable. These are of great interest, particularly if a comparison between groups is to be made or the results of the study are to be generalised to a larger group, and so it is necessary to find reliable ways of determining their values.

Table 28.2   Marital status for the leg ulcer trial patients (n = 233).

Marital status	n	%
Single	25	(10.7)
Married	104	(44.6)
Divorced/separated	11	(4.7)
Widowed	86	(36.9)
Missing	7	(3.0)

Table 28.3   Marital status for the leg ulcer trial patients, by study group.

Marital status	Control group		Clinic group	
	n	(%)	n	%
Single	11	(9.7)	14	(11.7)
Married	50	(44.2)	54	(45.0)
Divorced/separated	4	(3.5)	7	(5.8)
Widowed	45	(39.8)	41	(34.2)
Missing	3	(2.7)	4	(3.3)

Measures of location

There are several commonly used measures of location, as summarised in Box 28.2. The simplest is the *mode*. This is simply the most common observation and is the highest bar of the histogram. Looking at the histograms (Figure 28.6) for height, 1.77 m is the modal height for men as this is the height category with the highest bar on the histogram and 1.63 m is the modal category for women. However, the mode is rarely used since its value depends upon the accuracy of the measurement. If, for example the age bands were 10 years wide rather than 5 years, the mode would change to 1.82 m. In addition, it can be difficult to determine if there is more than one distinct peak such as that for height for all patients (Figure 28.9). In this case the presence of two peaks is a reflection of the differing distribution of height between men and women.

Two other more useful and commonly calculated measures are the *median* and the *mean*. The median is the middle observation, when the data are arranged in order of increasing value. It is the value that divides the data into two equal halves. If there is an even number of observations, the median is calculated as the average of the two middle observations. For example, if there are 11 observations the median is simply the sixth observation, but if there are 10 observations the median is the (fifth + sixth observation)/2. The median is not sensitive to the behaviour of outlying data, thus if the smallest value was even smaller, or the largest value even bigger it would have no impact on the value of the median.

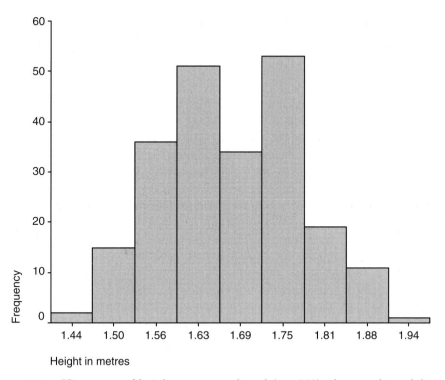

Height in metres

Figure 28.9   Histogram of height, sexes combined (n = 222), showing bimodality of height, when the data for men and women are combined.

Box 28.2   Measures of location.

Mode   Most common observation

Median   Middle observation, when the data are arranged in order of increasing value. If there is an even number of observations the median is calculated as the average of the middle two observations

Mean   Sum of all observations
Number of observations

For example, consider the ages (in years) of five patients recruited to the leg ulcer trial: 82, 72, 81, 85 and 58.

The most common observation is: 82 or 72 or 81 or 85 or 58. Unfortunately, multiple modes exist in this example, so there is no unique **mode**.

The five ages in ascending order are: 58, 72, 81, 82, and 85. The **median** is the middle or third value of the ranked or ordered ages i.e. 81 years.

The **mean** is: 82 + 72 + 81 + 85 + 58 = 378 divided by the number of observations, 5, i.e. 75.6 years.

Generally the most useful measure of the central value of a set of data is the *mean*. It is calculated as the sum of all observations divided by the total number of observations. Each observation makes a contribution to the mean value and thus it is sensitive to the behaviour of outlying data; as the largest value increases this causes the mean value to increase and conversely, as the value of the smallest observation becomes smaller the value of the mean decreases.

Both the mean and median can be useful, but they can give very different impressions when the distribution of the data is *skewed*, because of the relative contributions (or lack of, in the case of the median) of the extreme values. Skewed data are data that are not symmetrical. This is best illustrated by examining the shape of the histogram for age (Figure 28.10).

There are few observations at lower ages, while the majority of observations are clustered at the older ages. This is described as being negatively skewed, as there is a long left-hand tail at lower values. Data that have a long right-hand tail of higher values, but where the majority of observations are clustered at lower values, are called positively skewed. The weight data in Figure 28.11 are an example of positively skewed data. There are no firm rules about which to use, but when the distribution is not skew it is usual to use the mean. However, if data are skew then it is better to use the median, as this is not influenced by the extreme values and may not be as misleading as the mean.

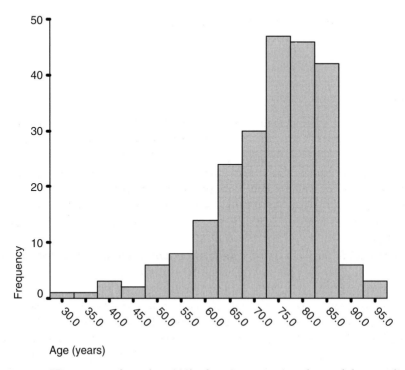

Age (years)

Figure 28.10 Histogram of age (n = 233), showing negative skew of the age distribution for this sample (long tail of younger ages & clustering of values at older ages).

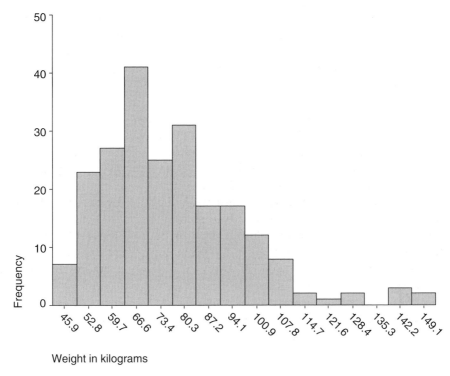

Weight in kilograms

Figure 28.11 Histogram of weight in kilograms (n = 218), showing positive skew of the weight.

Measures of spread

In addition to finding measures to describe the location of a dataset, it is also necessary to be able to describe its spread. Just as with the measures of location, there are both simple and more complex possibilities (as summarised in Box 28.3). The simplest is the *range* of the data, from the smallest to the largest observation. The range of age for the leg ulcer patients is 32 to 97 years (or 65 years as a single number). The advantage of the range is that it is easily calculated, but its drawback is that it is vulnerable to *outliers*, extremely large and extremely small observations.

A more useful measure is to take the median value as discussed above and further divide the two data halves into halves again. These values are called the quartiles and the difference between the bottom (or 25th percentile) and top quartile (or 75th percentile) is the *interquartile range* (IQR). This is the observation below which the bottom 25% of the data lie and the observation above which the top 25% lie. The middle 50% of the data lie between these limits. Unlike the range it is not as sensitive to the extreme values. The IQR for the age of the patients involved in the leg ulcer trial is 67 to 82 years or 15 years. Strictly speaking the range and IQR are single numbers but frequently the two values, minimum and

---

Box 28.3 Measures of spread.

Range   Minimum observation to the maximum observation

Interquartile range   Observation below which the bottom 25% of data lie and the obser-
                             vation above which the top 25% of data lie. If the value falls between
                             two observations, e.g. if 25th centile falls between 5th and 6th
                             observations then the value is calculated as the average of the two
                             observations (this is the same principle as for the median)

Standard deviation $\sqrt{\dfrac{\sum\limits_{i=1}^{n}(x_i-\bar{x})^2}{n-1}}$ where $\bar{x}$ is the sample mean, x_i is the ith observa-

                             tion, n is the sample size and the notation $\sum\limits_{i=1}^{n}$ represents the

                             addition or summing up of all the squared deviations from the
                             sample mean from the first ($I = 1$) to the last (n^{th}) observation.

*For example, consider the ages (in years) of five patients recruited to the leg ulcer trial: 82,
72, 81, 85 and 58.*

The **range** of the data is from 58 to 85 years or 27 years.

The five ages in ascending order are: 58, 72, 81, 82, and 85. The bottom 25% of data,
falls somewhere between the 1st and 2nd ordered observations, i.e. 58 and 72, so we can
take the average of these two observations $58 + 72 = 130/2 = 65.0$. The top 25% of data fall
somewhere between the 4th and 5th ordered observations, i.e. 82 and 85. So the 75th percentile is the average of the two observations $82 + 85 = 167/2 = 83.5$. Hence the **interquartile
range** is 65.0 to 83.5 years or 18.5 years.

The **standard deviation** is calculated by first working out the squared deviation of each
observation from the sample mean of 75.6 years i.e. $(82 - 75.6)^2 + (72 - 75.6)^2 + (81 - 75.6)^2$
$+ (85 - 75.6)^2 + (58 - 75.6)^2 = 481.2$ years^2.

This result is divided by the number in the sample minus one (i.e. $5 - 1 = 4$)
i.e. $481.2/4 = 120.30$ years^2. Finally, we take the square root of this number to give us a
standard deviation of 10.97 years.

---

maximum, or the 25% and 75% percentiles respectively, are reported as this can
be more informative.

However, the most common measure of the spread of the data is the standard
deviation (Box 28.3). It provides a summary of the differences of each observation
from the mean value. The standard deviation has units on the same scale as the
original measurement (e.g. metres if height is being measured).

As with the measures of location, when deciding which measure of spread to
present it is necessary to know whether the data are skewed or not and this will
also have a bearing on how the data will be analysed subsequently, as will be seen
in the following chapter. When the distribution is not skew it is usual to use the
standard deviation. However, if data are skew then it is better to use the range or
interquartile range.

Presenting data and results in tables

Some basic charts for displaying data have been described earlier in this chapter. As stated, plotting data can be a useful first stage to any analysis, as this will show extreme observations together with any interesting patterns. Charts are useful as they can be read quickly, and are particularly helpful when presenting information to an audience such as in a seminar or conference presentation. Although there are no hard and fast rules about when to use a chart and when to use a table, when presenting the results in a report or a paper it is often best to use tables so that the reader can scrutinise the numbers directly. Tables can be useful for displaying information about many variables at once, while charts can be useful for showing multiple observations on groups or individuals (such as a dot plot or a histogram). As with charts, there are a few basic rules of good presentation.

- Numerical precision should be consistent throughout and summary statistics such as means and standard deviations should not have more than one extra decimal place compared to the raw data. Spurious precision should be avoided, although when certain measures are to be used for further calculations or when presenting the results of analyses greater precision may be necessary.
- Gridlines can be used to separate labels and summary measures from the main body of the data in a table. However, their use should be kept to a minimum, particularly vertical gridlines, as they can interrupt eye movements, and thus the flow of information. Elsewhere white space can be used to separate data, for example, different variables from each other.
- The information in tables is easier to comprehend if the columns (rather than the rows) contain like information, such as means and standard deviations, as it is easier to scan down a column than across a row.
- Tables should be clearly labelled and a brief summary of the contents of a table should always be given in words, either as part of the title or in the main body of the text.

When summarising categorical data, both frequencies and percentages can be used, but if percentages are reported it is important that the denominator (i.e. total number of observations) is given.

For summarising numerical data, the mean and standard deviation may be used, or, if the data have a skewed distribution, the median and range. As with categorical data, the number of observations should be stated.

Conclusion

This chapter has looked at the different types of data encountered in quantitative analysis, together with ways of displaying these different data types. Basic summary measures of both location and spread have been discussed and advice given on the best way of presenting these statistics. In the next chapter some basic approaches to the analysis of these types of data will be examined.

References

Brazier JE, Harper R, Jones NMB, O'Cathain A, Thomas KJ, Usherwood T, Westlake L (1992) Validating the SF-36 health survey questionnaire: new outcome measure for primary care. *British Medical Journal* 305: 160–164

Huff D (1991) *How to Lie With Statistics.* London, Penguin Books

Morrell CJ, Walters SJ, Dixon S, Collins KA, Brereton LML, Peters J, Brooker CGD (1998) Cost effectiveness of community leg ulcer clinics: randomised controlled trial. *British Medical Journal* 316: 1487–1491

Tufte ER (1983) *The Visual Display of Quantitative Information.* Connecticut, Graphics Press

Further reading

Altman DG (1991) *Practical Statistics for Medical Research.* London, Chapman & Hall

Altman DG, Machin D, Bryant TN, Gardner MJ (2000) *Statistics with Confidence: confidence intervals and statistical guidelines,* 2nd edition. London, BMJ Publishing

Bland M (2000) *An Introduction to Medical Statistics.* Oxford, Oxford Medical Publications

Campbell MJ, Machin D, Walters SJ (2006) *Medical Statistics: a commonsense approach.* 4th edition. Chichester, Wiley

Field A (2000) *Discovering Statistics Using SPSS for Windows.* London, Sage

Freeman JV, Walters SJ, Campbell MC (in press 2006) *How to Display Data.* Oxford, Blackwell

Hart A (2001) *Making Sense of Statistics in Healthcare.* Oxford, Radcliffe Medical Press

Kinnear PR, Gray CD (2004) *SPSS for Windows Made Simple,* Release 12, Hove, Psychology Press

Petrie A, Sabin C (2000) *Medical Statistics at a Glance.* Oxford, Blackwell Science

Swinscow TDV, Campbell MJ (2002) *Statistics at Square One,* 10th edition. London, BMJ Publishing

Websites

www.sghms.ac.uk/depts/phs/guide/guide.htm#brief – statistics guide for research grant applicants

www.statsoftinc.com/textbook/stathome.html – an electronic statistics textbook offering training in the understanding and application of statistics

www-users.york.ac.uk/%7Emb55/pubs/pbstnote.htm – statistics notes in the British Medical Journal

members.aol.com/johnp71/javastat.html – convenient, accessible, multiplatform statistical software package and links to online statistics books, tutorials, downloadable software, and related resources

www.bettycjung.net/ – information for public health and healthcare researchers

peltiertech.com/Excel/Charts/statscharts.html#BoxWhisker – Excel charts, biostatistics charting and graphing data, charting data, Excel charting tutorials, charts for statistics, box-and-whisker plots

www.coventry.ac.uk/discuss/ – Statistics tutorial DISCUSS (Discovering Important Statistical Concepts Using Spread Sheets) provides web-based interactive spreadsheets, designed for teaching elementary statistics

29 Examining Relationships in Quantitative Data

Jenny Freeman and Stephen Walters

Key points

- There are two basic approaches to statistical analysis: hypothesis testing using P values, and estimation using confidence intervals.
- Appropriate statistical methods for analysing relationships in quantitative data include tests for differences between groups, and tests for relationships between variables.
- Choice of the correct statistical test for the purpose of the study, the nature of the research question, and the type of data collected, is crucially important.

Introduction

The previous chapter looked at the different types of data encountered in quantitative analysis, together with ways of displaying them. Basic summary measures of both location and spread were discussed and advice given on the best ways of presenting these statistics. This chapter will examine the two basic approaches to statistical analysis: *hypothesis testing* (using P values) and *estimation* (using confidence intervals) and consider some elementary approaches to analysing the types of data outlined in the previous chapter, including the use of statistical techniques for investigating differences between groups. Example outputs from the Statistical Package for the Social Sciences (SPSS) will be shown, but formulae and mathematical detail will be kept to a minimum, and the interested reader is referred to the more advanced texts, as listed at the end of Chapter 28 and this chapter. As with the previous chapter, all the example analyses will be based upon data from the leg ulcer trial as outlined in Box 28.1 of Chapter 28.

Statistical analysis

It is rarely possible to obtain information on an entire population and usually data are collected on a sample of individuals from the population of interest. The main aim of statistical analysis is to use the information from the sample to draw conclusions (*make inferences*) about the population of interest. For example, the leg ulcer trial (Box 28.1) was conducted as it was not possible to study all individuals with venous leg ulcers. Instead, a sample of individuals with venous leg ulcers in the Trent Region was studied in order to estimate the potential cost effectiveness of specialist clinics compared to standard care. The two main approaches to statistical analysis, hypothesis testing and estimation, are outlined in the following section.

Hypothesis testing (using P values)

Before examining the different techniques available for analysing data it is first essential to understand the process of hypothesis testing and its key principles, such as what a P value is and what is meant by the phrase 'statistical significance'. Figure 29.1 describes the steps in the process of hypothesis testing. At the outset it is important to have a clear research question and know what the outcome variable to be compared is.

Once the research question has been stated, the null and alternative hypotheses can be formulated. The null hypothesis (H_0) assumes that there is no difference in the outcome of interest between the study groups. The study or alternative hypothesis (H_1) states that there is a difference between the study groups. In general, the direction of the difference (for example: that treatment A is better than treatment B) is not specified. For the leg ulcer trial, the research question of interest is:

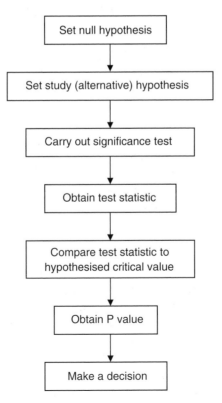

Figure 29.1   Hypothesis testing: the main steps.

For patients with leg ulcers, does specialist treatment at a leg ulcer clinic affect the number of ulcer-free weeks over the 12-month follow-up compared to district nursing care at home?

The null hypothesis, H_o, is:

There is no difference in ulcer-free weeks between the control (home) and intervention (clinic) group.

and the alternative hypothesis, H_1, is:

There is a difference in ulcer-free weeks between the control and intervention groups.

Having set the null and alternative hypotheses the next stage is to carry out a significance test. This is done by first calculating a *test statistic* using the study data. This test statistic is then used to obtain a *P value*. For the comparison above, patients in the clinic group had, on average, 5.9 more ulcer-free weeks after 12 months than the control (home) group and the P value associated with this difference was 0.014. The final and most crucial stage of hypothesis testing is to make a decision, based upon the P value. In order to do this it is necessary to understand first what a P value is and what it is not, and then understand how to use it to make a decision about whether to reject or not reject the null hypothesis.

So what does a P value mean? *A P value is the probability of obtaining the study results (or results more extreme) if the null hypothesis is true.* Common misinterpretations of the P value are that it is either the probability of the data having arisen by chance or the probability that the observed effect is not a real one. The distinction between these incorrect definitions and the true definition is the absence of the phrase 'when the null hypothesis is true'. The omission of 'when the null hypothesis is true' leads to the incorrect belief that it is possible to evaluate the probability of the observed effect being a real one. The observed effect in the sample is genuine, but what is true in the population is not known. All that can be known with a P value is, if there truly is no difference in the population, how likely is the result obtained (from the study data).

It is important to remember that a P value is a probability and its value can vary between 0 and 1. A 'small' P value, say close to zero, indicates that the results obtained are unlikely when the null hypothesis is true and the null hypothesis is rejected. Alternatively, if the P value is 'large', then the results obtained are likely when the null hypothesis is true and the null hypothesis is not rejected. *But how small is small?* Conventionally the cut-off value or *significance level* for declaring that a particular result is *statistically significant* is set at 0.05 (or 5%). Thus if the P value is less than this value the null hypothesis (of no difference) is rejected and the result is said to be statistically significant at the 5% or 0.05 level (Box 29.1). For the example above, of the difference in the number of ulcer-free weeks, the P value is 0.014. As this is less than the cut-off value of 0.05 there is said to be a

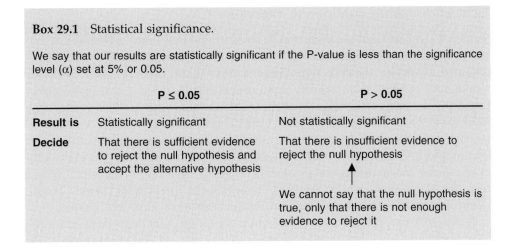

Box 29.1 Statistical significance.

We say that our results are statistically significant if the P-value is less than the significance level (α) set at 5% or 0.05.

	P ≤ 0.05	**P > 0.05**
Result is	Statistically significant	Not statistically significant
Decide	That there is sufficient evidence to reject the null hypothesis and accept the alternative hypothesis	That there is insufficient evidence to reject the null hypothesis
		We cannot say that the null hypothesis is true, only that there is not enough evidence to reject it

Table 29.1 Making a decision.

		The null hypothesis is actually:	
		False	**True**
Decide to:	Reject the null hypothesis	Correct	Type I error (α) (false positive error)
	Not reject the null hypothesis	Type II error (β) (false negative error)	Correct

statistically significant difference in the number of ulcer-free weeks between the two groups at the 5% level.

Though the decision to reject or not reject the null hypothesis may seem clear-cut, it is possible that a mistake may be made, as can be seen from the shaded cells of Table 29.1.

Whatever is decided, this decision may correctly reflect what is true in the population: the null hypothesis is rejected, when it is in fact false or the null hypothesis is not rejected, when in fact it is true. Alternatively, it may not reflect what is true in the population: the null hypothesis is rejected, when it is in fact true (*false positive* or *Type I error*, α); or the null hypothesis is not rejected, when in fact it is false (*false negative*, *Type II error*, β).

The probability that a study will be able to detect a difference, of a given size, if one truly exists is called the *power* of the study and is the probability of rejecting the null hypothesis when it is actually false. It is usually expressed in percentages, so for a study that has 80% power, there is a likelihood of 80% of being able to detect a difference, of a given size, if there genuinely is a difference in the population.

Estimation (using confidence intervals)

Statistical significance does not necessarily mean the result obtained is clinically signifi-cant or of any practical importance. A P value will only indicate how likely the results obtained are when the null hypothesis is true. It can only be used to decide whether the results are statistically significant or not, it does not give any informa-tion about the likely effect size. Much more information, such as whether the result is likely to be of clinical importance, can be gained by calculating a *confidence interval*. A confidence interval may be calculated for any estimated quantity (from the sample data), such as the mean, median, proportion, or even a difference, for example the mean difference in ulcer-free weeks between two groups. It is a measure of the precision (accuracy) with which the quantity of interest is esti-mated (in this case the mean difference in the number of ulcer-free weeks).

Technically, the 95% confidence interval is the range of values within which the true population quantity would fall 95% of the time if the study were to be repeated many times. Crudely speaking, the confidence interval gives a range of plausible values for the quantity estimated; although not strictly correct, it is usually interpreted as the range of values within which there is 95% certainty that the true value in the population lies. For the leg ulcer example above, the quantity estimated was the mean difference in the number of ulcer-free weeks between the groups, 5.9 weeks (*see* Figure 29.3, explained fully below). The 95% confidence interval for this difference was 1.2 to 10.5 weeks.

Thus, while the best available estimate of the mean difference was 5.9 weeks, it could be as low as 1.2 weeks or as high as 10.5 weeks, with 95% certainty. The P value associated with this difference was 0.014 and in the previous section it was concluded that this difference was statistically significant at the 5% level. While the P value will give an indication of whether the result obtained is statistically significant, it gives no other information. The confidence interval is more informa-tive as it gives a range of plausible values for the estimated quantity. Provided this range *does not* include the value for no difference (in this case 0) it can be concluded that there is a difference between the groups being compared.

Choosing the statistical method

What type of statistical analysis depends on the answer to five key questions (Box 29.2) and given answers to these, an appropriate approach to the statistical analy-sis of the data collected can be decided upon. The type of statistical analysis depends fundamentally on what the main purpose of the study is. In particular, what is the main question to be answered? The data type for the outcome variable will also govern how it is to be analysed, as an analysis appropriate to continuous data would be completely inappropriate for binary data. In addition to what type of data the outcome variable is, its distribution is also important, as is the summary measure to be used. Highly skewed data require a different analysis compared to data that are *normally* distributed.

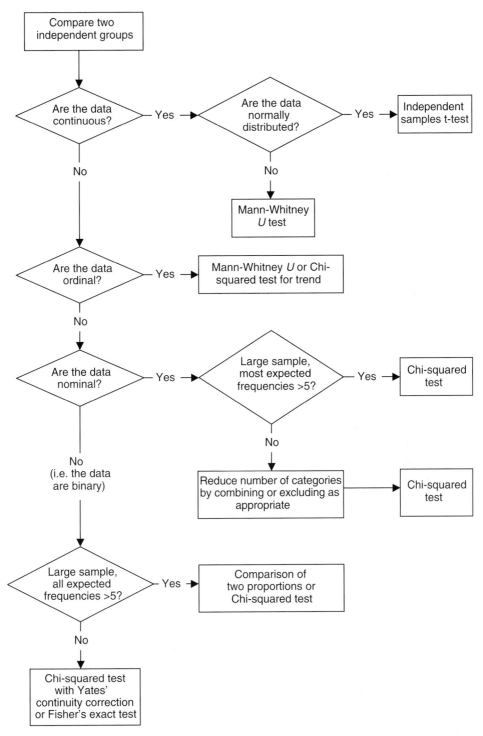

Figure 29.2 Statistical methods for comparing two independent groups or samples.

Group Statistics

	Group	N	Mean	Std. Deviation	Std. Error Mean
Leg ulcer free time (weeks)	Clinic	120	20.0821	18.49067	1.68796
	Home	113	14.2035	17.56148	1.65204

As the standard deviations for the two groups are similar, results from the 'Equal variance assumed' row in the table below can be used.

Independent Samples Test

		Levene's Test for Equality of Variances		t-test for Equality of Means					95% Confidence Interval of the Difference	
		F	Sig.	t	df	Sig. (2-tailed)	Mean Difference	Std. Error Difference	Lower	Upper
Leg ulcer free time (weeks)	Equal variances assumed	1.632	.203	2.485	231	.014	5.87860	2.36555	1.21779	10.53942
	Equal variances not assumed			2.489	230.982	.014	5.87860	2.36188	1.22503	10.53218

The P value is 0.014. Thus the results are unlikely when the null hypothesis (that there is no difference between the groups) is true. The result is said to be *statistically significant* because the P value is less than the significance level (α) set at 5% or 0.05 and there is sufficient evidence to reject the null hypothesis and accept the alternative hypothesis that there is a difference in mean ulcer free weeks between the clinic and control groups.

Figure 29.3   SPSS output from the independent samples *t*-test.

Box 29.2   Five key questions to ask.

- What are the aims and objectives?
- What is the hypothesis to be tested?
- What type of data is the outcome data?
- How is the outcome data distributed?
- What is the summary measure for the outcome data?

The choice of method of analysis for a problem depends on the comparison to be made and the data to be used. This chapter outlines the methods appropriate for the three most common problems in statistical inference as outlined in Box 29.3. Before beginning any analysis it is important to examine the data, using the techniques described in Chapter 28; adequate description of the data should precede and complement the formal statistical analysis. For most studies and for randomised controlled trials (RCTs) in particular, it is good practice to produce a table or tables that describe the initial or baseline characteristics of the sample.

Comparison of two independent groups

Before comparing two independent groups it is important to decide what type of data the outcome is and how it is distributed, as this will determine the most appropriate analysis. This section describes, for different types of data, the statisti-

Box 29.3   Three most common problems in statistical inference.

- Comparison of independent groups, e.g. groups of patients given different treatments.
- Comparison of the response for paired observations, e.g. in a crossover trial, or for matched pairs of subjects.
- Investigation of the relationship between two variables measured on the same sample of subjects.

Box 29.4   The assumptions underlying the use of the independent samples *t*-test.

- The groups are independent.
- The variables of interest are continuous.
- The data in both groups have similar standard deviations.
- The data is normally distributed in both groups.

cal methods available for comparing two independent groups, as outlined in Figure 29.2.

Independent samples t-*test for continuous outcome data*

The independent samples *t*-test is used to test for a difference in the mean value of a continuous variable between two groups. For example, one of the main questions of interest in the leg ulcer trial was whether there was a difference in the number of ulcer-free weeks between the control and the clinic groups. As the number of ulcer-free weeks is continuous data and there are two independent groups, assuming the data are normally distributed in each of the two groups, then the most appropriate summary measure for the data is the sample mean and the best comparative summary measure is the difference in the mean number of ulcer-free weeks between the two groups.

When conducting any statistical analysis, it is important to check that the assumptions that underpin the chosen method are valid. The assumptions underlying the two-sample *t*-test are outlined in Box 29.4.

The assumption of normality can be checked by plotting two histograms, one for each sample; these do not need to be perfect, just roughly symmetrical. The two standard deviations should also be calculated and as a rule of thumb, one should be no more than twice the other.

Figure 29.3 shows the SPSS output for comparing ulcer-free weeks between the two groups using two independent samples *t*-test. It can be seen that there is a significant difference between the groups; *the 95% confidence interval for the difference* suggests that that patients in the clinic group have between 1.21 and 10.53

more ulcer-free weeks than patients in the control group and the best estimate is a mean difference of 5.87 more ulcer-free weeks.

Mann–Whitney U test

There are several possible approaches when at least one of the requirements for the *t*-test is not met. The data may be transformed (e.g. the logarithm transformation can be useful, particularly when the variances are not equal) or a *non-parametric method* can be used. Non-parametric or distribution-free methods do not involve distributional assumptions, i.e. making assumptions about the manner in which the data are distributed (for example that the data are normally distributed). An important point to note is that it is the test that is parametric or non-parametric, not the data.

When the assumptions underlying the *t*-test are not met, then the non-parametric equivalent, the Mann–Whitney *U* test, may be used. While the independent samples *t*-test is specifically a test of the null hypothesis that the groups have the same mean value, the Mann–Whitney *U* test is a more general test of the null hypothesis that the distribution of the outcome variable in the two groups is the same; it is possible for the outcome data in the two groups to have similar measures of central tendency or location, such as mean and medians, but different distributions. The Mann–Whitney *U* test requires all the observations to be ranked as if they were from a single sample. From this the statistic *U* is calculated; it is the number of all possible pairs of observations comprising one from each sample for which the value in the first group precedes a value in the second group. This test statistic is then used to obtain a P value.

Examining the output from the Mann–Whitney *U* test in SPSS (Figure 29.4) there is sufficient evidence to *reject the null hypothesis* and accept the alternative hypoth-

NPAR TESTS

Mann-Whitney Test

Ranks

	Group	N	Mean Rank	Sum of Ranks
Leg ulcer free time (weeks)	Clinic	120	126.87	15224.00
	Home	113	106.52	12037.00
	Total	233		

Test Statistics[a]

	Leg ulcer free time (weeks)
Mann-Whitney U	5596.000
Wilcoxon W	12037.000
Z	-2.388
Asymp. Sig. (2-tailed)	.017

a. Grouping Variable: Group

P value: probability of observing the test statistic under the null hypothesis. As the value of 0.017 is less than the significance level (α) set at 0.05 or 5% this means that the result obtained is unlikely when the null hypothesis is true and it is said to be statistically significant. Thus there is sufficient evidence to reject the null hypothesis and accept the alternative hypothesis that there is a difference in ulcer free weeks between the clinic and control groups.

Figure 29.4   SPSS output from the Mann–Whitney *U* test.

esis that there is a difference in ulcer-free weeks between the clinic and control (home) groups.

In the majority of cases it is reasonable to treat *discrete data*, such as number of children in a family or number of visits to the GP in a year, as if they were continuous, at least as far as the statistical analysis goes. Ideally there should be a large number of different possible values, but in practice this is not always necessary. However, where ordered categories are numbered such as stage of disease or social class, the temptation to treat these numbers as statistically meaningful must be resisted. For example, it is not sensible to calculate the average social class or stage of cancer, and in such cases the data should be treated in statistical analyses as if they are ordered categories.

Comparing more than two groups

The methods outlined above can be extended to more than two groups. For the independent samples *t*-test, the analogous method for more than two groups is called the *analysis of variance (ANOVA)* and the assumptions underlying it are similar. The non-parametric equivalent for the method of ANOVA when there are more than two groups is called the *Kruskall–Wallis test*. A fuller explanation of these methods is beyond the scope of this chapter and the interested reader is referred to the more advanced statistical textbooks listed at the end of this chapter and Chapter 28.

Chi-squared test for categorical outcome data

Sometimes when comparing two independent groups the outcome is categorical rather than continuous, for example in the leg ulcer trial it was of interest to know whether there was a difference between the groups in the proportions with healed ulcers at 12 weeks. With two independent groups (clinic and control) and a binary (ulcer healed *vs* not healed) rather than a continuous outcome, the data can be cross-tabulated as in Table 29.2. This is an example of a 2×2 contingency table with 2 rows (for treatment) and 2 columns (for outcome) i.e. 4 cells in total. The most appropriate summary measure is simply the proportion in the sample whose leg ulcer has healed at 12 weeks and the best comparative summary measure is the difference in proportions healed between the two groups. The most appropriate hypothesis test, assuming a large sample and all expected frequencies >5, is the *chi-squared test*.

Table 29.2 Cross-tabulation of treatment group *vs* ulcer status at 12 weeks.

Treatment	Outcome: leg ulcer healed at 12 weeks					
	Not healed		Healed		Total	
Clinic	98	(81.7%)	22	(18.3%)	120	(100%)
Control	96	(85.0%)	17	(15.0%)	113	(100%)
Total	194		39		233	

The null hypothesis is that the two classifications (*e.g. group and ulcer healed status at 12 weeks*) are unrelated in the relevant population (*leg ulcer patients*). More generally the null hypothesis, H_0, for a contingency table is that there is no association between the row and column variables in the table, i.e. they are independent. The general alternative hypothesis, H_1, is that there is an association between the row and column variables in the contingency table, i.e. they are not independent or unrelated. For the chi-squared test to be valid two key assumptions need to be met, as outlined in Box 29.5. If these are not met, Fisher's exact test can be used for 2×2 tables.

Figure 29.5 shows the results of analysing Table 29.2 in SPSS. The P value of 0.620 indicates that there is little evidence of a difference in leg ulcer healing rates at 12 weeks between the clinic and control groups.

Box 29.5   Guidelines for the chi-squared test to be valid.

- At least 80% of cells should have expected frequencies greater than 5.
- All cells should have expected frequencies greater than 1.

Two groups of paired observations

When there is more than one group of observations, it is vital to distinguish the case where the data are paired from that where the groups are independent. Paired data may arise when the same individuals are studied more than once, usually in different circumstances, or when individuals are paired as in a case-control study. For example, as part of the leg ulcer trial, data were collected on health related quality of life (HRQoL) at baseline, 3 months and 12 months follow-up. Methods of analysis for paired samples are summarised in Figure 29.6.

Paired t-test

HRQoL at baseline and 3 months are both continuous variables and the data are paired as measurements are made on the same individuals at baseline and 3 months; therefore, interest is in the mean of the differences not the difference between the two means. If we assume that the paired differences are normally distributed, then the most appropriate summary measure for the data is the sample mean, at each time point, and the best comparative summary measure is the mean of the paired difference in HRQoL between baseline and 3 months. Given the null hypothesis (H_0) that there is no difference (or change) in mean HRQoL at baseline and 3 months follow-up in patients whose leg ulcer had healed by 3 months, the most appropriate test is the paired *t*-test.

There were 36 patients with a healed leg ulcer at 3 months. Examining the SPSS output for the comparison of HRQoL for these 36 patients at baseline and 3 months shows that the result is statistically significant (Figure 29.7). *The 95% confidence interval of the difference* suggests that we are 95% confident that HRQoL has

CROSSTABS

Case Processing Summary

	Cases					
	Valid		Missing		Total	
	N	Percent	N	Percent	N	Percent
Leg ulcer healed at 12 weeks * Group	233	100.0%	0	.0%	233	100.0%

Leg ulcer healed at 12 weeks * Group Crosstabulation

			Group		Total
			Clinic	Home	
Leg ulcer healed at 12 weeks	Not healed	Count	98	96	194
		% within Group	81.7%	85.0%	83.3%
	Healed	Count	22	17	39
		% within Group	18.3%	15.0%	16.7%
Total		Count	120	113	233
		% within Group	100.0%	100.0%	100.0%

Chi-Square Tests

	Value	df	Asymp. Sig. (2-sided)	Exact Sig. (2-sided)	Exact Sig. (1-sided)
Pearson Chi-Square	.452[b]	1	.502		
Continuity Correction[a]	.247	1	.620		
Likelihood Ratio	.453	1	.501		
Fisher's Exact Test				.599	.310
Linear-by-Linear Association	.450	1	.502		
N of Valid Cases	233				

a. Computed only for a 2x2 table

b. 0 cells (.0%) have expected count less than 5. The minimum expected count is 18.91.

To improve the approximation for a 2 x 2 table, Yates' correction for continuity is sometimes applied. Altman (1991) recommends the use of Yates' correction for all chi-squared tests on 2 x 2 tables. In a 2 x 2 table when expected cell counts are less than 5, or any are less than 1 even Yates' correction does not work and thus Fisher's exact test is used. When comparing frequencies amongst groups that have an ordering (e.g. group by pain score), any difference among the groups would be expected to be related to the ordering and the Mantel-Haenszel test for linear association or trend can be carried out. Although the Mantel-Haenszel statistic is displayed, it should not be used for purely nominal data, like we have here.

This suggests that the chi-squared test is valid as all the expected counts are greater than 5.

The P value of 0.62 indicates that the results obtained are likely if the null hypothesis (of no association between the rows and columns of the contingency table above) is true. Thus there is insufficient evidence to reject the null hypothesis and the results are said to be not statistically significant.

Figure 29.5   SPSS output for Crosstabs procedure and Chi-squared test.

changed by between 1.74 and 12.93 points between baseline and 3 months and the best estimate is a mean change of 7.33 points. In fact, HRQoL has declined over time from a mean of 66.3 at baseline to a mean of 58.9 at 3 months follow-up!

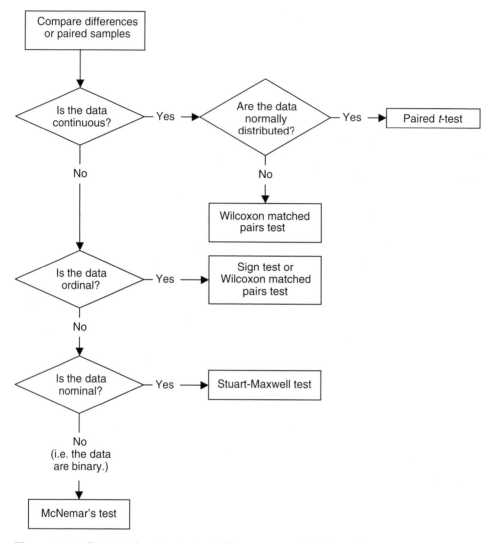

Figure 29.6   Statistical methods for differences or paired samples.

The assumptions underlying the use of the paired *t*-test are outlined in Box 29.6. If these are not met a non-parametric alternative, the *Wilcoxon signed rank sum test*, can be used.

The relationship between two continuous variables

Many statistical analyses are undertaken to examine the relationship between two continuous variables within a group of subjects (Table 29.3).

Paired Samples Statistics

	Mean	N	Std. Deviation	Std. Error Mean
Health related quality of life: baseline	66.2778	36	18.83251	3.13875
Health related quality of life: 3 months	58.9444	36	21.95052	3.65842

Paired Samples Correlations

	N	Correlation	Sig.
Health related quality of life: baseline Health related quality of life: 3 months	36	.681	.000

Paired Samples Test

	Paired Differences					t	df	Sig. (2-tailed)
	Mean	Std. Deviation	Std. Error Mean	95% Confidence Interval of the Difference				
				Lower	Upper			
Health related quality of life: baseline Health related quality of life: 3 months	7.333	16.53222	2.75537	1.7396	12.9270	2.661	35	.012

The P value is 0.012, indicating that the results obtained are unlikely when the null hypothesis is true. The result is statistically significant because the P value is less than the significance level (α) set at 0.05 or 5% and there is sufficient evidence to reject the null hypothesis. The alternative hypothesis, that there is a difference or change in mean HRQoL between baseline and 3 months follow-up in patients whose leg ulcer had healed by 3 months, is accepted.

Figure 29.7   SPSS output for paired *t*-test.

Box 29.6   The assumptions underlying the use of the paired *t*-test.

- The paired differences are plausibly normally distributed (it is not essential for the original observations to be normally distributed).
- The paired differences are independent of each other.

Two of the main purposes of such analyses are:

- to assess whether the two variables are associated. There is no distinction between the two variables and no causation is implied, simply *association*
- to enable the value of one variable to be predicted from any known value of the other variable. One variable is regarded as a *response* to the other *predictor* variable and the value of the predictor variable is used to *predict* what the response would be.

Table 29.3   Statistical methods for relationships between two variables measured on the same sample of subjects.

	Continuous, normal	Continuous, non-normal	Ordinal	Nominal	Binary
Continuous	Regression Correlation: (Pearson's r)	Regression Rank correlation: (Spearman's r_s)	Rank correlation: (Spearman's r_s)	One-way analysis of variance	Independent samples t-test
Continuous, non-normal		Regression Rank correlation: (Spearman's r_s)	Rank correlation: (Spearman's r_s)	Kruskall–Wallis test	Mann–Whitney U test
Ordinal			Rank correlation (Spearman's r_s)	Kruskall–Wallis test	Mann–Whitney U test Chi-squared test for trend
Nominal				Chi-squared test	Chi-squared test
Binary					Chi-squared test Fisher's exact test

For the first of these, the statistical method for assessing the association between two *continuous* variables is known as *correlation*, while the technique for the second, prediction of one continuous variable from another is known as *regression*. Correlation and regression are often presented together and it is easy to get the impression that they are inseparable. In fact, they have distinct purposes and it is relatively rare that one is genuinely interested in performing both analyses on the same set of data. However, when preparing to analyse data using either technique it is always important to construct a scatter plot of the values of the two variables against each other. By drawing a scatter plot it is possible to see whether or not there is any visual evidence of a straight line or linear association between the two variables.

Correlation

As stated previously, as part of the leg ulcer trial HRQoL was measured at baseline, 3 months and 12 months follow-up. Plotting HRQoL at 3 months and 12 months indicates that there is a positive linear relationship between HRQoL at 3 months and 12 months (Figure 29.8).

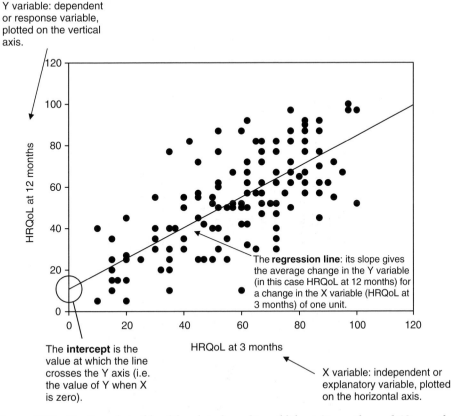

Figure 29.8   Scatter plot of health related quality of life at 3 months and 12 months.

Unsurprisingly, quality of life at 3 months is generally related to quality of life at 12 months i.e. low values at 3 months generally corresponded with low values at 12 months and high values at 3 months corresponded with high values at 12 months. In order to examine whether there is an association between the two variables, the *correlation coefficient* can be calculated. At this point, no assumptions are made about whether the relationship is causal i.e. whether one variable is influencing the value of the other variable. The standard method (often ascribed to Pearson) leads to a statistic called r. In essence r is a measure of the scatter of the points around an underlying *linear trend*: the greater the spread of points the lower the correlation. Pearson's correlation coefficient r must be between -1 and $+1$, with -1 representing a perfect negative correlation, $+1$ representing perfect positive correlation and 0 representing no linear trend.

The easiest way to check the validity of the hypothesis test is by examining a scatterplot of the data. This plot should be produced as a matter of routine when correlation coefficients are calculated, as it will give a good indication of whether the relationship between the two variables is roughly linear and thus whether it is appropriate to calculate a correlation coefficient. If the data do not have a normal distribution, a non-parametric correlation coefficient, Spearman's rho (r_s), can be calculated. The assumptions underlying the validity of the hypothesis test associated with the correlation coefficient are outlined in Box 29.7.

From Figure 29.9 it can be seen that the Pearson correlation coefficient between HRQoL at 3 months and 12 months is 0.718 and this is statistically significant.

Regression (including multiple regression)

Often it is of interest to quantify the relationship between two continuous variables, and given the value of one variable for an individual, to predict the value of the other variable. This is not possible from the correlation coefficient as it simply indicates the strength of the association as a single number; in order to describe the relationship between the values of the two variables, a technique called *regression* is used. Thus, using regression the value of HRQoL at 3 months could be used to predict the value at 12 months. HRQoL at 3 months is regarded as the X-variable; it is also called the independent, predictor or explanatory variable and it should be plotted on the horizontal axis of the scatter plot. HRQoL at

---

Box 29.7 The assumptions underlying the validity of the hypothesis test associated with the correlation coefficient.

- The two variables are observed on a random sample of individuals.
- The data for at least one of the variables should have a normal distribution in the population.
- For the calculation of a valid confidence interval for the correlation coefficient both variables should have a normal distribution.

Correlations

		Health related quality of life: 3 months	Health related quality of life: 12 months
Health related quality of life: 3 months	Pearson Correlation	1	.718**
	Sig. (2-tailed)	.	.000
	N	198	147
Health related quality of life: 12 months	Pearson Correlation	.718**	1
	Sig. (2-tailed)	.000	.
	N	147	155

**. Correlation is significant at the 0.01 level (2-tailed).

The Pearson correlation coefficient between HRQoL at 3 months and 12 months is 0.718. Its associated P value is given underneath it; in this case its value is 0.000 indicating that the result is statistically significant and there is sufficient evidence to reject the null hypothesis of no linear relationship between HRQoL at 3 months and at 12 months. It can be concluded that the two are correlated.

Correlations

			Health related quality of life: 3 months	Health related quality of life: 12 months
Spearman's rho	Health related quality of life: 3 months	Correlation Coefficient	1.000	.695**
		Sig. (2-tailed)	.	.000
		N	198	147
	Health related quality of life: 12 months	Correlation Coefficient	.695**	1.000
		Sig. (2-tailed)	.000	.
		N	147	155

**. Correlation is significant at the .01 level (2-tailed).

The Spearman correlation coefficient is 0.695 (P-value = 0.000). This is very similar to the results for the Pearson correlation coefficient, though this will not always be the case.

Figure 29.9 Output of correlation analysis in SPSS.

Box 29.8 Assumptions underlying regression analysis.

- The values of the response variable Y should have a normal distribution for each value of the explanatory variable X.
- The variance (or standard deviation) of Y should be the same at each value of X, i.e. there should be no evidence that as the value of Y changes, the spread of the X values changes.
- The relationship between the two variables should be linear.

---

12 months is regarded as the Y-variable; it is also known as the dependent or response variable and is plotted on the vertical axis of the scatter plot (Figure 29.8). Three important assumptions underlie regression analysis as outlined in Box 29.8.

Regression slopes can be used to predict the response of a new patient with a particular value of the predictor/explanatory/independent variable. However, it is important that the regression model is not used to predict outside the range of observations. In addition, it should not be assumed that just because an equation has been produced it means that X causes Y. The results of regressing HRQoL at 12 months on HRQoL at 3 months are displayed in Figure 29.10.

Looking at the table for the coefficients at the bottom of the figure it can be seen that the slope coefficient for HRQoL is 0.74 (p value = 0.000), indicating that HRQoL at 3 months has a significant effect on HRQoL at 12 months. The value of r^2 is often quoted in published articles and indicates the proportion (sometimes expressed as a percentage) of the total variability of the outcome variable that is explained by the regression model fitted. In this case 51.6% of the total variability in HRQoL at 12 months is explained by HRQoL at 3 months.

Regression as described above involves the investigation of the effect of a single explanatory variable on the outcome of interest. However, there is usually more than one possible explanatory variable influencing the values of the outcome variable and the method of regression can be extended to investigate the influence of more than one variable. In this case it is referred to as *multiple regression*, and the influence of several explanatory variables on the outcome of interest are investigated simultaneously. For example, in the leg ulcer trail, apart from HRQoL at 3 months, age and gender may have a role to play in HRQoL at 12 months and these may be fitted into the model to examine what their influence on HRQoL is, over and above that exerted by HRQoL at 3 months.

Regression or correlation?

Regression is more informative than correlation. Correlation simply quantifies the degree of linear association (or not) between two variables. However, it is often more useful to *describe* the relationship between the two variables, or even *predict* a value of one variable for a given value of the other and this is done using regression. If it is sensible to assume that one variable may be causing a response in the other then regression analysis should be used.

Conclusion

In summary this chapter has outlined the process of testing hypotheses and emphasised the usefulness of confidence intervals when drawing conclusions from the results of studies. In addition it has covered some of the basic statistical tests for the types of data outlined in the previous chapter. Armed with this information, for a given set of such data, it should be possible to decide upon the most appropriate analysis, carry out the chosen method and draw conclusions from the results.

Variables Entered/Removed[b]

Model	Variables Entered	Variables Removed	Method
1	HRQoL: 3 months[a]	.	Enter

a. All requested variables entered.

b. Dependent Variable: HRQoL: 12 months

Model Summary

Model	R	R Square	Adjusted R Square	Std. Error of the Estimate
1	.718[a]	.516	.512	16.27485

a. Predictors: (Constant), HRQoL: 3 months

R^2 is a number which gives the percentage of variability explained by the predictor variable, X, and gives an indication of how well the model explains the data.

ANOVA[b]

Model		Sum of Squares	df	Mean Square	F	Sig.
1	Regression	40910.179	1	40910.179	154.453	.000[a]
	Residual	38406.270	145	264.871		
	Total	79316.449	146			

a. Predictors: (Constant), HRQoL: 3 months

b. Dependent Variable: HRQoL: 12 months

Coefficients[a]

		Unstandardised Coefficients		Standardised Coefficients			95% Confidence Interval for B	
		B	Std. Error	Beta	t	Sig.	Lower Bound	Upper Bound
1	(Constant)	10.734	3.802		2.824	.005	3.220	18.248
	HRQoL: 3 months	.740	.060	.718	12.428	.000	.622	.858

a. Dependent Variable: HRQoL: 12 months

Regression coefficient for the value of the intercept. The value of 10.734 indicates that when HRQoL at 3 months is zero, HRQoL at 12 months is 10.734.

Regression coefficient for the slope of HRQoL at 3 months. The value of 0.74 indicates that for every unit change in HRQoL at 3 months there is a change in HRQoL at 12 months of 0.74 units.

The P value for the intercept is 0.005, which indicates that the value of the intercept (10.734) is unlikely when the null hypothesis (that its true value is zero) is true. Thus the result is said to be statistically significant. This is also the case for the slope coefficient.

Figure 29.10 SPSS output from regression analysis.

Further reading

Huff D (1991) *How to Lie With Statistics*. London, Penguin Books
Kinnear R, Gray CD (2004) *SPSS for Windows Made Simple*, Release 12. Hove, Psychology Press
See Chapter 28 for further references

Section 6
Putting Research into Practice

The final section of this book moves on from the practical process of doing research to consider how research can make a difference to nursing and health care. The book concludes with a glimpse into the future.

Chapter 30 deals with the very important stage of moving a research study on from an investigation into a piece of new knowledge, accessible to other members of the profession and the wider public. It is a practical guide to writing research reports, journal articles, presenting at conferences and other means of dissemination.

Chapters 31 and 32 take the next logical step of considering how health care practice integrates (or does not) the new knowledge generated by research into evidence-based practice. Chapter 31 looks at the theory underpinning evidence-based practice, and assesses different models of research utilisation relevant to nursing. Chapter 32 builds on this foundation to discuss change management in health care, and to give some practical examples of how research findings are being implemented in practice.

The book ends with a chapter that continues the discussion begun in Chapter 1 about the best way to build research capacity in nursing. Five policy imperatives are identified and appraised that are essential if nursing is to move forward to becoming a more 'research-based profession'. Since this phrase was first used in the Briggs Report in 1972 (Committee on Nursing 1972), nursing research has come a very long way. Even since the first edition of this text in 1984, the progress has been considerable. The chapter, and the book, therefore ends with three futuristic scenarios for the direction that might now be travelled. The reader is left to decide which, if any, of the scenarios should be pursued.

Reference

Committee on Nursing (1972) *Report of the Committee on Nursing (Briggs Report)* London, HMSO (Cmnd 5115)

30 Communicating and Disseminating Research

Kate Gerrish and Anne Lacey

Key points

- Research needs to be disseminated in various ways for different audiences.
- Journal articles and research reports are the main written forms of communication, and each needs to be written in an appropriate style.
- Presentations at conferences, verbally or in poster format, are effective ways of disseminating results and networking with other researchers.
- Websites, workshops and clinical guidelines can be used by researchers to tell others about their work.

Introduction

Although research may be an interesting and intellectually satisfying activity in its own right, there is little point in carrying out rigorous research unless it is disseminated in some way to those who can make use of the new knowledge generated. Public funding of research by bodies such as the Department of Health and Research Councils is done on the understanding that results will be made known to the public and, where appropriate, used to improve health care. Having said this, it is still true that many research reports never get very far beyond the desk of those carrying out the research and those funding it. Even publication in a journal does not guarantee that the appropriate community, professional or public, gets to hear about the research. So how do we ensure optimum communication from the research community to the professionals involved in health care, users of health care, and to the wider public?

Communicating with different audiences

The same piece of research may be disseminated in many different ways. First, a report is likely to be written as a permanent record of the research and to satisfy the needs of those commissioning, funding and supporting the study. If the research was undertaken as part of an educational programme, the report will take the form of a dissertation or thesis.

The research may also be reported as an article in a high status academic journal such as the *Journal of Advanced Nursing* or the *British Medical Journal*, where it is likely to be read by nurses and other health professionals in academic roles and by some students and advanced practitioners. Such journals have strict guidelines for the reporting of research, (see for example, *www.journalofadvancednursing.com*) or (*www.bmj.com*) that should be followed. The research findings may even be picked up from high-profile journals and reported in the media, if they are of public interest or controversial.

Research findings may also be written up, perhaps in a different form, in a popular professional journal such as *Nursing Standard*. Here they will be read by a wider range of practising nurses not necessarily engaged in academic study.

Increasingly, research is disseminated via a dedicated website, which may have links from other websites of a similar nature. Websites allow more visual and interactive communication, and so provide opportunities for creative presentation.

Finally, the research may be communicated verbally or as a poster at international, national, and local level in conferences, workshops and seminars, at journal clubs and research interest groups in the workplace.

Each of these ways of disseminating research findings requires a different style, different resources, and serves a different audience. We will address each of these means of dissemination in turn.

The research report

A research study is not complete until a report has been written and submitted to interested parties. The report serves as a complete record of what was done, how it was done, details of results and conclusions. Implications for practice may also be included where relevant. The report will be used to give an account of the research to those who commissioned and funded it, but can also become a means of dissemination to those who can make use of the findings. The length and style of the research report is highly variable. In research conducted for an educational degree, the report is the dissertation or thesis, written in academic language and, in the case of a doctoral thesis, running to 100,000 words or more. In contrast, a small project carried out in clinical practice may be reported in 20 pages or less. Whatever the length and style, however, the content is likely to be similar in format. It should be noted that universities usually produce guidelines on the presentation and content of a thesis and these should be adhered to.

The writing of a research report follows conventions that closely mirror the research process itself. These are outlined in Box 30.1. Sections of the report will vary according to the intended audience.

Box 30.1 Sections of a research report.

Abstract or executive summary
This should orientate the reader to the whole study. It is best written at the end after the detailed report is complete.

Introduction
This section describes the background to the study and the context in which it was undertaken.

Aims of the research
The aims, research questions and any hypotheses to be tested should be stated clearly.

Literature review
A comprehensive literature review will set out the available knowledge before the research commenced. The length and depth of this review will depend on the audience of the report. An academic dissertation requires a substantial section critically appraising the available evidence, whereas policymakers are likely to require a more concise summary.

Research design
A clear description of the conceptual framework used, the methodology adopted, and data collection methods selected is required to give the reader an understanding of the research design.

Access and ethical approval
All research conducted in a health care context should have obtained ethical and research governance approval, and a statement to this effect should be included. Other access negotiations and procedures for recruiting and gaining consent from research participants will be given. Copies of consent forms and information sheets may be included in an appendix.

Sampling
This section will provide details of how sampling was done, sample size calculations, and the composition and characteristics of the sample obtained.

Data collection
A full account of how data were collected, data collection tools and outcome measures used will be given here.

Data analysis
A description of how the data were analysed is necessary, as well as a full presentation of the results. For quantitative research, this will be in the form of tables and figures, with a narrative commentary. For qualitative research, the results will be presented in words, with verbatim quotations from interviews, fieldnotes, etc. as supporting evidence. Qualitative research reports often include discussion within the presentation of the results, rather than keeping the two sections separate as suggested below.

Discussion and conclusion
This section gives the researcher the opportunity to reflect upon the findings in the light of previous literature, and to draw conclusions. Implications for practice, suggested further research, and any limitations of the study are commonly included.

Writing an article for publication

Publishing research in an academic or professional journal provides a means of disseminating the findings to a wide, possibly international, audience. Authors also gain considerable personal satisfaction to see their work in print.

A published article on a research study will generally follow the same structure as a research report referred to in the previous section, albeit in a more condensed format. However, the content of the paper and style of writing will vary according to the target audience for the journal. An academic journal normally requires a detailed account of the research in which the author demonstrates rigour in carrying out the study as well as showing how the research contributes to advancing knowledge in the field. The style of writing tends to be formal. By contrast, the account of the research methodology in a professional journal is normally concise with more emphasis placed on the findings and implications for policy and practice. A journalistic approach that seeks to engage the reader's attention may be used.

Preparing a paper for submission

Selecting an appropriate target journal for publication requires some careful groundwork. The first step is to become familiar with the journal by reading some back issues. This will provide insight into the types of article the editor seeks to publish, the intended audience and the writing style. Most journals provide detailed guidance for contributors, which may be published in the journal itself or are available on the publisher's website. This guidance frequently provides information on the aims and scope of the journal to help authors decide whether their work is appropriate for a particular journal. A very useful website run by the Medical College of Ohio provides an index of all instructions for authors for health care journals at *http:mulford.mco.edu/instr/*

Once familiar with the type of articles published in different journals a decision can be made about which one to pursue. This decision should be informed by an objective appraisal of the match between the type of article published in the journal and the nature of the research to be published. If in doubt, advice should be sought from someone who is experienced at writing for publication, or from the journal editors themselves.

The guidelines for authors normally provide details of the expected content and format of the paper, and should be followed closely. Increasingly journals are moving towards electronic submission via a manuscript tracking system, which enables the publication process to be managed electronically and provides the opportunity for authors to check on progress with their paper.

Having decided on the journal and studied the guidance for authors, writing can begin. A novice will find it beneficial to co-author with someone with a track record of publication. Once a draft version of the paper has been written it is advisable to seek feedback from colleagues who can provide constructive advice on how it might be improved. A paper is likely to require several revisions before it reaches the stage where it is ready for submission. Before submitting the paper it is important to undertake a final proofread, check all references are correctly cited in the text and the reference list and ensure that it is presented in the required format.

The review process

All papers submitted to editors undergo some form of assessment in order to ascertain whether they are suitable for publication in a particular journal. Academic journals and an increasing number of professional journals seek an independent review (*peer review*) of the paper by one or more people who are judged to be experts in the field. Before a decision is made to send a paper for review the editor usually undertakes an initial assessment and it may be that the paper is considered unsuitable and rejected at this stage.

Usually a paper is reviewed 'blind', in other words the reviewer does not know the identity of the author and the feedback from the reviewer to the author is anonymised. However there are increasing calls for a more open review process and some editors are now considering making authors and reviewers aware of each other's identity (Smith 1997). Many journals provide guidance to reviewers on the areas they should consider when assessing a paper. Whereas journals differ in terms of their aims and readership, the criteria used to assess a paper are often similar. An example of general criteria used by reviewers is given in Box 30.2.

It will normally take several weeks for an author to receive feedback from the editor. The reviewers' comments are usually sent to authors together with an editorial decision. In exceptional circumstances the paper may be accepted as submitted. However, it is more common for authors to be asked to revise their paper on the basis of the feedback from reviewers. Where a paper is rejected outright the reviewers' feedback should provide an indication as to why it was considered unsuitable. Suggestions may also be made on how to develop the paper for publication elsewhere.

Box 30.2   General criteria used to review an article.

- relevance of topic to journal aims
- potential interest to readership
- originality and contribution to knowledge and/or practice
- scientific rigour
- clarity and coherence of the article
- style of writing, angle, level of presentation

When revising a paper the author should give serious consideration to the recommendations made by the reviewers. Where an author disagrees with a reviewer, the editor needs to be informed of the reasons why the author has not taken the recommendations on board. Indeed, many journals ask authors to submit a separate report providing details of how they have responded to the reviewers' comments. A revised paper may need to be sent out for further review so authors should anticipate a time delay.

The publication process

Once a paper has been accepted for publication the editor will notify the author and often provides an indication of the anticipated publication date. Before the paper is published authors will be asked to sign a copyright declaration form, which assigns the copyright of the paper to the publisher. Whereas assigning copyright imposes certain restrictions on the author's future use of the material it is designed to protect the interests of the author, for example should others plagiarise their work.

A few weeks before publication the author is sent the page proofs to check. These are presented in the format in which the paper will be printed in the journal and provide a clear indication of what the paper will look like in print. It is important that authors check the page proofs carefully for accuracy. However, only essential changes can be made at this stage, as more extensive editing is costly and will delay publication. Authors do need to be aware that some minor changes may have been made to their original manuscript. Usually this is to correct minor errors, but some editors of professional journals may make more significant changes. If an author is unhappy with any changes that have been made to the article it is essential that the editor is informed. At the end of the day, it is the author's work and he or she has the right to decide the ultimate content of the paper.

Many journals are now being published in electronic as well as written format, and some are only produced electronically. These 'e-journals' appear on the internet, and articles can be downloaded from them, but they never appear in print form. This is a new form of publication, and reduces the time taken for an article to be disseminated. Many of the journals have a stringent system of ensuring quality just as print journals do. Such journals commonly have no subscription system, however, authors may be asked to pay for publication of their article. The *International Electronic Journal of Health Education* is an early example of such a journal, running since 1998 (*www.aahperd.org/iejhe/*).

Political issues in the publication process

It may be necessary to seek permission to publish from the funding body that commissioned the research. This requirement is usually written into the research contract. The research funder may wish to see the paper before it is sent for publication and may require a disclaimer to be included which states that the views expressed in the paper are those of the authors and not the research funding body.

It is also good practice to acknowledge those who have made a contribution to the research but are not co-authors of the paper. This may include the funding body, individuals who have granted special permissions, for example agreeing to a questionnaire they have developed being used in the study, or who have provided particular support, such as a supervisor or project advisory panel members.

Where a research team rather than an individual has undertaken a study, it is generally appropriate for all members of the team to be co-authors of the article. This should be agreed in advance, as there can be difficulties if a member of the research team feels they were not given an opportunity to contribute to a paper. Disagreements about whose name will appear first are also likely if this is not made clear from the outset. Supervisors often co-author papers with their students, and normally the student's name appears as first author. Anyone who co-authors a paper should have made a significant contribution to the research study and/or to writing the paper. Increasingly editors require each author to sign a declaration confirming their contribution.

Researchers who are based in academic institutions in the UK may be required to submit their publications as part of the Research Assessment Exercise (RAE). This is a periodic assessment by national and international experts of the quality of research in a particular discipline, for example, nursing. The quality of published research is the main criterion used to judge the overall quality of research within a university. Numerical ratings of research quality ranging from 1 (most research at sub-national level) to 5* (most research of international standing) are linked to funding allocations and therefore universities take the RAE most seriously. High-status academic journals are regarded by many disciplines as the most appropriate avenue for research outputs to be included in the RAE. Whereas the RAE Nursing Panel has tended to be more eclectic, valuing a range of possible outputs, new researchers in university settings would do well to seek advice from more experienced colleagues on the most suitable journals in which to publish.

Presenting research at a conference

Presenting research at a conference helps to disseminate the findings more quickly than is possible by publication. Research findings can be presented in the form of an oral presentation or a poster at national or international conferences. Increasingly, health authorities and NHS trusts host conferences that provide the opportunity to disseminate research across the local health community and facilitate networking with colleagues who share similar interests. Such conferences are often quite small and provide an ideal opportunity for the novice presenter to hone their skills. Many national and international conferences focus on a particular area of nursing, for example clinical practice, management or education and presentations need to address the conference theme. However some conferences, such as the Royal College of Nursing Annual International Research Conference, focus specifically on research and invite presentations on a broad range of topics.

Whereas conference organisers may invite lead researchers to present their work, most researchers are required to submit an abstract for an oral or poster presentation for consideration by a selection panel. When deciding where to submit an abstract it is worth considering the material to be presented and the intended audience. For example, a study examining a new form of treatment for the management of leg ulcers by community nurses might form the basis of an abstract for a conference on community nursing, wound management or a research conference. If the intention is to disseminate the findings to a large number of clinical nurses then a conference related to a particular area of nursing may be most suitable. Research conferences, by contrast, provide the opportunity to discuss aspects of the research process as well as the findings with an audience who have a particular interest in research.

Writing a conference abstract

A major factor in having an abstract accepted for presentation is whether the author has followed the guidelines provided within the published 'call for abstracts'. This normally specifies:

- the conference themes
- the deadline date for submission
- the format and content of the abstract, including the maximum word length
- whether there is an option to present the work as either an oral presentation or a poster.
- the criteria by which the abstract will be judged

The abstract provides the only information that a selection panel has to make its decision about whether a proposed presentation is relevant and of suitable quality. It is essential to present information in a concise and informative way that grabs the interest of the reviewer, and ultimately the conference delegate. Box 30.3 gives an example of the criteria by which an abstract may be judged.

Abstracts which exceed the word length or which do not use the specified headings may be automatically rejected. Despite these constraints it is possible to convey a considerable amount of relevant information in relatively few words. For example 'A survey by self-completed questionnaire was undertaken with a random sample of ward-based nurses working in a large teaching hospital in England. Content validity and reliability of the questionnaire were established. Of a random sample of 700 nurses, 563 responded.' This covers the design, method, sample and setting in just 40 words. An example of an abstract is given in Box 30.4.

Deciding whether to present an oral paper or a poster is to some extent a matter of personal choice. Whereas novice presenters may feel more comfortable with a

Box 30.3 Abstract submission checklist.

ROYAL COLLEGE OF NURSING OF THE UNITED KINGDOM

ANNUAL INTERNATIONAL NURSING RESEARCH CONFERENCE

Abstract Submission Checklist (for concurrent session and poster presentation)

Abstracts submitted to the RCN's annual international nursing research conference are peer reviewed by an international panel. The criteria against which reviewers make their recommendations are detailed in the online abstract submission form. These criteria are listed here in the form of a checklist for you to use prior to submitting your abstract. You may also like to invite a 'critical friend' to review your abstract against these criteria before you submit it. If you have any ticks in the 'no' column you can then amend your abstract before you submit it and hence increase the potential for your abstract to be accepted and included in the conference programme.

		yes	no	n/a
1	The abstract about a research project or a research related issue (for example policy or a methodological issue).			
2	The abstract should specify how the paper will contribute to the development of knowledge and practice within health and health care.			
3	Material presented in abstracts must be concise and coherent, with the focus of the abstract stated clearly.			
4	The authors must make explicit what they intend to present.			
5	Abstracts of empirical studies must outline the research process and the focus of the analysis must be provided with an indication of the results.			
6	Sample size and sampling method used must be supplied where appropriate.			
7	Relevant contextual information must be given.			
8	The word limit must be adhered to. For concurrent and poster submissions the word limit is 300 and for symposia and workshops, 1000 words.			
9	Abstracts for poster and concurrent presentations should not contain any information about the author/s competence to deliver.			
10	Symposium and workshop abstracts must be accompanied by a CV demonstrating the principal author's competence to deliver.			

In addition, up to three references are normally cited and these must be provided using the Harvard referencing system
Reproduced with permission from RCN Research Society and RCN R&D Co-ordinating Centre.

Box 30.4   Example of a conference abstract.

Access to cardiac rehabilitation services
Some of the highest national coronary heart disease death rates are experienced in Barnsley, Rotherham and Doncaster, the areas that make up the South Yorkshire Coalfields (SYC). One intervention that aims to benefit patients with coronary heart disease and their relatives is cardiac rehabilitation. Questions exist regarding inequalities in access to cardiac rehabilitation and the contact and quality of services. The National Service Framework for coronary heart disease seeks to address these problems. A restructuring of cardiac rehabilitation services, with increased emphasis on primary care services is inevitable. Nurses play a key role in delivering the cardiac rehabilitation services of the future, which are equitable and accessible.

This paper outlines a qualitative research project that was funded by SYC Health Action Zone. Patients and staff participated in semi-structured interviews to explore barriers to accessing cardiac rehabilitation and their preferences for services for the future. A sample of 111 participated in group and individual interviews. The data were analysed using a Framework Analysis approach.

This presentation will focus on the role of health visitors in the delivery of cardiac rehabilitation services. A limited health visitor service was available in all three districts. The study revealed a number of organisational issues that prevented health visitors fully engaging in the service. The patients identified a range of service components they considered important. These included advice and reassurance, psychological support, consistent and personalised information, support for carers and support from the family doctor. The first two weeks post-discharge and six weeks post-discharge emerged as the most crucial in terms of need. The results will be discussed in relation to the future role of health visitors and public health nurses in cardiac rehabilitation.

(Oral presentation at the International Public Health Nursing Conference 2002 by A Tod and A Lacey)

relatively informal poster presentation, they should not underestimate the considerable effort and resources required to produce a high-quality poster as well as the time required during the conference itself to be available to discuss the poster. Although the idea of an oral presentation may appear daunting, with careful planning and the opportunity to practice by presenting the paper to colleagues beforehand, the novice researcher can get an enormous amount of personal satisfaction from delivering an oral presentation.

Oral presentations

The letter confirming acceptance of an oral presentation will normally include important information on the time allocated for the paper, where it appears on the conference programme and what audiovisual facilities will be available. However, presenters may not be notified in advance of the size and layout of the room in which they will present. There may be no indication of the likely size of the audience so they will need to plan for different eventualities.

Some presenters may feel that they need to read verbatim from a paper. Whereas this provides the opportunity to produce a coherent, well-constructed presentation, it can be difficult for the audience to concentrate on someone reading for any length of time. A presenter who uses notes or written prompt cards for guidance and who maintains eye contact with the audience is more likely to keep their attention.

The key to presenting a successful paper is to be realistic on how much information can be included within the time available. If planning to read a paper verbatim, a reasonable conversion rate is to consider 500 words as equivalent to five minutes' speaking time. If using PowerPoint slides, it is reasonable to prepare about one slide per two minutes of presentation. This means that only limited information on some aspects of a research study can be included.

Deciding what to include and what to leave out is probably the most difficult task. Delegates at a conference that attracts clinical nurses are likely to be interested in research findings and their implications for practice, whereas those attending a research conference are likely to be interested in the methodology used. Many conferences request that presenters allow time at the end of their paper for the audience to ask questions. Ensure that this is planned into the allotted time.

Including audiovisual aids enhances the presentation and helps maintain audience attention. It is essential to check in advance what facilities are available. Overhead projectors and slide projectors are increasingly being replaced by computer projection using PowerPoint. When planning to use PowerPoint presentations it is essential to check which version of the software is available. Animation features developed on the most recent version may not work with older versions. Advice should be sought from the conference organisers on how the computer file should be prepared, for example on floppy disc, CD or flash drive. Assistance on preparing audiovisual aids may be available locally in NHS trusts or universities, and can also be found on the internet.

Once the content has been decided upon and audiovisual aids prepared, it is essential to rehearse, preferably in front of a friendly colleague or friend. Keeping to time should be the most important priority. Conference programmes very often run to a tight schedule and it can be frustrating for delegates when a paper is cut short because the presenter has run out of time. It is also essential to practice using the audiovisual equipment to ensure a smooth transition in the presentation.

Once at the conference, check out the venue and the audiovisual facilities available as far in advance of the presentation as possible, seeking assistance from a technician if required. In terms of the actual delivery it is important to consider:

- posture, movement and hand actions – face the audience, stand rather than sit, avoid excessive movements and fiddling with paper clips, etc.
- eye contact and facial expression – look at the audience, adopt a relaxed facial expression and try to smile!
- voice – aim to achieve clarity and variety, speak clearly, slowly, and use appropriate intonation by raising, lowering and altering the tone of voice.

Poster presentations

Preparing a poster requires considerable time so it is essential to think about the presentation well in advance of the conference. Many NHS trusts and universities have departments that can assist with both design and production. The cost of producing a poster ranges from a few pounds to several hundred. Whereas a professionally presented poster produced with the assistance of a graphic designer is impressive, there is no reason why someone with a more modest budget cannot produce a very effective poster. Advice on designing posters is readily available via the internet. Computer software for wordprocessing, presentation and desktop publishing is increasingly available at the workplace and can be used to produce posters.

Details indicating the amount of space available will accompany the letter that confirms acceptance of the abstract. It is essential that the poster fits the parameters given. A poster should not be overcrowded with information as this will detract from its impact and delegates will quickly tire. The noise and bustle of a poster-viewing hall is rarely conducive to a serious read! Text should be sufficiently large to be read easily from a distance of at least one metre although the title should be larger to attract interest from a distance. There should be a balance between text and other visual stimuli such as graphs, figures or photographs. Material should be sequenced in a logical manner with the reader clearly guided through the content. Numbered headings or arrows can assist here.

There is a tendency when planning the content of a poster to be over-ambitious in terms of content. The key is to present information succinctly – short phrases rather than full sentences will often suffice. The title needs to be short and snappy to attract attention. The name and contact details of members of the research team should be included. It is usual to provide a brief introduction to the topic or project. Other areas to include depend on the poster topic. If the poster is about a research study, information needs to be included on the aims, sample, methods, findings and conclusions. Supporting materials that interested delegates can take away with them can also be produced. For example, a scaled-down version of the poster can be printed on A4 paper, or alternatively a more detailed written account of the research project prepared as a handout.

When designing a poster on a tight budget there may be a tendency to take the easy option of printing out a series of A4 PowerPoint slides and mounting these on the poster board. Whereas this kind of display can convey the essential information, its visual impact is not as great as a large poster. Many computer software packages allow for a larger format than A4 to be designed. Once the poster has been designed on the computer, it may be possible to have it printed within a local NHS trust or university. Alternatively a number of high street print companies will produce the poster from disc onto suitably sized paper and laminate it for a reasonable price. However, before the material is taken for printing it is essential to proofread carefully as errors cannot be rectified.

Consideration should be given to transporting the poster to the conference. It is recommended that it is taken as hand luggage in a waterproof container.

Although conference organisers may provide materials to mount the poster on the presentation board it is advisable to take an 'emergency kit', including for example, Velcro, double-sided tape, drawing pins and scissors.

Finally, it is important to remember that presenters are normally required to spend time beside the poster discussing it with interested parties. This is often during meal breaks and presenters need to think about how to manage their time. When it is necessary to leave a poster unattended during a specified conference viewing time, it is helpful to leave a note beside the poster indicating when the presenter will be available to answer questions.

Networking opportunities, research partnerships and collaborations

In addition to the more traditional means of dissemination through publications and conference presentations there are a number of other ways of disseminating research.

Websites

Large-scale, funded research projects often have a dedicated website which will include regular updates with progress of the study and may post interim findings before they are more widely available. University department or professional webpages in a NHS trust may provide the opportunity for a synopsis of ongoing or recently completed research to be posted.

Workshops and seminars

Both NHS and universities may have research interest groups who meet regularly to provide a forum for local researchers to present their work. A seminar, in which the audience is encouraged to discuss a paper in some detail, calls for a more participatory form of presentation than a traditional conference paper. Workshops may also be provided which enable participants to engage more actively in discussion and contribute their own ideas, often through working on specific tasks in small groups. This can be particularly useful for researchers who wish to work with potential 'users' of their research, such as patient groups, health care providers, educators and policy makers in order to consider the implementation of their findings.

Practice guidelines

Chapter 32 considers how research findings can be used to develop clinical guidelines and care pathways. Such guidance is normally based on a systematic review of several studies on a particular topic. However, the findings from an individual study may have important implications arising for practice. One way of making this information accessible to those who might apply it in their practice, is to produce practice guidelines. These are normally concise documents that identify how the research findings can be applied locally. For example, a study that has examined attitudes towards the use of information technology by nurses in a large hospital may identify particular education needs that can be incorporated into in-service training initiatives or used to inform curriculum development of nursing courses in a local university.

Conclusion

Dissemination of research, both while it is being undertaken and after its completion, is essential if the knowledge generated is going to be used by the nursing profession. Dissemination also gives an opportunity for researchers to learn from one another's experience, and to engage in networks with others working in a similar field. There are many forms of communication available to researchers, ranging from academic journal articles to informal local discussion groups. The mode of presentation needs to take account of these differing audiences.

References

Smith R (1997) Peer review: reform or revolution? Time to open up the black box of peer review (editorial). *British Medical Journal* 315: 759–760

Further reading

Burnard P (1996) *Writing for Health Professionals*, 2nd edition. London, Chapman & Hall
Gerrish K (2005) Getting published: practicalities, pitfalls and plagiarism. *Journal of Community Nursing* 19:8 13–15
Murray R (2004) *Writing for Academic Journals*. Buckingham, Open University Press

Websites

www.man.ac.uk/rcn/publish/index.htm – the RCN Research and Development Co-ordinating Centre contains tips and advice on getting published and information on different nursing and health journals, with links to their websites
mulford.mco.edu/instr/ – the Medical College of Ohio lists all instructions for authors for journals in the health and medical sciences
www2.warwick.ac.uk/services/cap/resources/eguides/classroom/ – Warwick University gives advice about all aspects of oral presentation

31 Evidence-Based Practice

Kate Gerrish

Key points

- Evidence-based practice involves integrating the best available research evidence with professional expertise while taking account of patient preferences.
- Evidence-based practice is a complex undertaking that involves identifying and appraising different sources of evidence, translating evidence into clear guidance for practice, implementing and finally evaluating the impact of change.
- Research findings may be applied directly to practice in the form of clinical protocols or practice guidelines, be used indirectly to inform nurses' understanding of practice or used persuasively to present a case for changes in policy or practice
- Barriers to achieving evidence-based practice relate to the nature of the evidence, the way in which the evidence is communicated, the knowledge and skills of the individual nurse or the characteristics of the organisation.

Introduction

During the past decade evidence-based practice has become a major concern of health care policy makers, providers and professional groups. Nurses, alongside other health care practitioners, recognise that high-quality care is dependent on being able to use robust evidence to support clinical interventions. Yet achieving evidence-based care is a complex undertaking. It requires considerable skill in identifying and appraising evidence in order to decide whether it is appropriate to use. The evidence then needs to be translated into guidance that can be understood and used by practitioners, before being introduced into everyday practice.

However, introducing change is far from straightforward. Commitment is needed from individual nurses together with support from colleagues within the multidisciplinary team and from managers. Finally, the impact of the change in practice needs to be evaluated. This activity needs to be supported by appropriate resources and take place in an environment where practitioners are comfortable with questioning practice and are willing to embrace change.

This chapter examines the concept of evidence-based practice in some detail. The debates about what constitutes 'good' evidence are explored and consideration given to different models of research utilisation and factors influencing evidence-based practice. This sets the scene for the following chapter, which examines the implementation of evidence-based practice through a number of different approaches.

The nature of 'evidence' in evidence-based practice

There is considerable debate within the nursing literature about whether the 'evidence' in evidence-based practice should relate solely to research evidence or if a broader definition is more appropriate, bearing in mind that there may be insufficient recent research evidence to support some nursing interventions. The potential contribution of different forms of evidence is identified in one of the most frequently used definitions of evidence-based practice: Sackett *et al.* (1996) define the concept of evidence-based medicine as:

> 'The conscientious, explicit and judicious use of current best evidence in making decisions about the care of individual patients. The practice of evidence-based medicine means integrating individual clinical expertise with the best available external evidence from systematic research.' (Sackett *et al.* 1996:72)

Whereas this definition focuses on the care required by individual patients, the concept of evidence-based practice can be extended to groups of patients, health care services and policy initiatives (Muir Gray 2004).

It is worth examining the above definition in more detail. The emphasis on *current best evidence* draws attention to the changing nature of evidence. As more research is undertaken on a particular topic, a body of knowledge is built up; however, this knowledge base is constantly evolving. Nurses should keep up-to-date with research findings in order to provide the best possible care. The reference to *external evidence from systematic research* implies that research evidence should be in the public domain and accessible. Furthermore, the process whereby the evidence was generated should be clearly stated and open to scrutiny. Sackett *et al.*'s definition also emphasises the part that *clinical expertise* should play in making decisions about the most appropriate care. This is particularly important in situations where research evidence is lacking or the findings are inconclusive or contradictory. Clinical expertise is the proficiency that practitioners gain through experience, and is reflected in effective assessment, and in thoughtful and compassionate use of individual patient's preferences in making decisions about their care (Sackett *et al.* 1996). Thus evidence-based practice should take account of the preferences of patients and their carers who will have their own views about the care they should receive.

Let us now consider the different components of evidence-based practice.

Research findings as evidence

As the previous chapters of this book have demonstrated, the systematic nature of research means that it should be possible to use research findings with a reasonable degree of confidence. However, all research has limitations. It is essential, therefore, that research reports are subject to critical scrutiny in order to decide whether or not the quality of the research is sufficient to support the conclusions drawn. Chapter 8 provides guidance on how to undertake a critical appraisal of published research. However, the skills of critical appraisal cannot be viewed in isolation from knowledge of the research process. In order to undertake a rigorous review of a research report it is essential to have a good understanding of different research designs, methods of data collection and analysis, as well as being aware of ethical considerations.

Evidence provided from a single research study is generally considered insufficient grounds to justify changing practice. Rather a body of research evidence on a particular topic needs to be established. Ideally, a systematic review of relevant research (as outlined in Chapter 21) should be undertaken in order to draw an overall conclusion about the cumulative evidence. This activity is time consuming and requires a sound understanding of research methodologies. It is therefore beyond the scope of many practising nurses unless undertaken as part of an education course. However, there are several organisations that publish systematic reviews of clinical interventions that can be accessed by nurses or which translate the information provided from systematic reviews into evidence-based guidelines (Box 31.1).

Even when a systematic review has been published it may still not provide conclusive evidence to guide practice. Gerrish *et al.* (1999) describe how their plans to work with managers and practitioners to implement long awaited guidance on the prevention and treatment of pressure sores (Effective Health Care 1995) were thwarted when the systematic review concluded that there was insufficient evidence to guide practice, and what evidence there was, proved contradictory. They then had to draw upon professional expertise to identify best practice to supplement tentative research findings.

Box 31.1   Organisations publishing information to support evidence-based practice.

Systematic reviews
Effective Health Care bulletins, published by the Centre for Reviews and Dissemination, University of York (*www.york.ac.uk/inst/crd/ehcb.htm*)
Bandolier (*www.jr2.ox.ac.uk/bandolier*)
The Cochrane Collaboration (*www.cochrane.org/index0.htm*)
The Joanna Briggs Institute (*www.joannabriggs.edu.au/pubs/systematic_reviews.php*)

Evidence-based guidelines
National Institute for Health and Clinical Excellence (NICE) (*www.nice.org.uk*)
Royal College of Nursing (*www.rcn.org.uk/resources/guidelines.php*)
Scottish Intercollegiate Guidelines Network (SIGN) (*www.sign.ac.uk*)

Professional expertise as evidence

There is debate within the nursing literature as to whether professional expertise should be considered 'evidence'. Closs (2003), for example, argues that although clinical expertise is essential to the delivery of high-quality care, it does not constitute evidence *per se*. From her perspective, evidence is derived from research findings that have been validated through the process of peer review and resulted in publication. She also cautions against assuming that experience will lead to excellence in practice. Although experienced nurses may be able to predict problems and needs that other nurses may not, they may hold personal opinions that have no factual basis and which do not form reliable evidence.

Other commentators take a much broader view of evidence derived from professional experience. Eraut (1994) describes this form of evidence as 'practical knowledge' and differentiates it from the 'technical' or 'propositional knowledge' derived from research. It is the knowledge that is embedded in practice and which is often tacit or intuitive. It is acquired by nurses working alongside role models or others considered experts. Recent research has highlighted the extent to which nurses draw upon the knowledge gained experientially in the workplace, for example from specialist nurses, members of the multidisciplinary team and professional networks (Thompson *et al.* 2001). Indeed, nurses draw upon these sources of knowledge more frequently than formal sources of knowledge such as published research reports (Gerrish & Clayton 2004).

Liaschenko and Fisher (1999) provide a useful way of conceptualising the knowledge that nurses use within the context of evidence-based practice. They identify three different forms of knowledge:

- *Scientific knowledge* is largely biomedical knowledge derived from research and includes, for example, nurses' knowledge of disease processes and treatment regimes.
- *Patient knowledge* includes knowledge about how an individual becomes identified as a patient, how the person responds to treatment, how to get things done for the patient and who else may be involved in providing services for the patient. Nurses use this practical 'know-how' knowledge gained through experience, alongside research-based knowledge to guide their practice.
- *Person knowledge* is gained through viewing a patient as an individual with a personal biography and who occupies a particular social space. Knowing a person means understanding something of what living with the disease or disability is like for the individual and seeing that individual as more than a patient in a health care system.

Liaschenko and Fisher indicate that experienced nurses draw upon these different forms of knowledge, especially when there may be conflict between an individual patient's preferences and the opinions of health care professionals or among the professionals themselves. For example, they use it to justify an alternative approach to disease management and to defend their actions to support an individual patient's choice, even when this may conflict with established biomedical or institutional practices.

The experiential forms of knowledge (patient and person) identified above can have a reciprocal, reinforcing relationship with scientific evidence. Ferlie *et al.* (1999) have shown that research evidence is more influential when it tallies with clinical experience; conversely, when research evidence and clinical experience do not match, its use in practice can be variable. They describe how the use of a drug was influenced by the beliefs of a group of orthopaedic surgeons, which were based on their experience. There was a disparity between the research evidence and clinical expertise and as a result the uptake of the new drug was 'patchy'.

Patient experience as evidence

The third source of evidence that contributes to clinical practice is that derived from the patient experience. Farrell and Gilbert (1996) draw a distinction between *individual* and *collective* involvement of patients and carers in health care, which provides a useful means of viewing patient experience as a form of evidence. *Individual* involvement concerns individual patients and their contact with particular practitioners during episodes of care whereas *collective* involvement entails the participation of groups or communities in health care planning or service delivery.

In order to involve *individual* patients and their carers effectively in decisions about their care it is important that their views and preferences are taken into account. Patients and carers will tend to draw upon their knowledge of their physical and psychological 'self', their social lives and their previous experiences of care. Integrating the experiential knowledge of patients with scientific knowledge requires considerable expertise. Closs (2003) proposes that nurses should share their knowledge of research findings underpinning clinical interventions with patients so that patients understand the appropriateness of the intervention and can exercise an informed choice when there are alternative courses of action available. Patients are also becoming more informed about health care. Access by the general public to health information has increased significantly in recent years, supported by a number of government initiatives and consumer organisations that provide information via the internet. Some of these initiatives, for example the Database of Patients' Experiences (DIPex) (*www.dipex.org*), links patients' experiences with research information. However, nurses may encounter a mismatch between the best research evidence and patient preferences. Rycroft-Malone *et al.* (2004) provide an example whereby robust research evidence that recommends the use of compression bandaging to treat venous leg ulcers may not tally with a patient's experience of discomfort caused by the bandaging. The individual practitioner's skills in identifying these issues and negotiating the most appropriate course of action would be essential to improving patient outcomes.

There are various means whereby a *collective* view of patient and carer perspectives can inform evidence-based practice initiatives. For example, at a national level, NICE ensures patient and carer representation on its committees and involvement in the development of national guidelines. At a more local level, clinical audit and patient satisfaction surveys undertaken by NHS organisations provide a means whereby a collective view of patient perspectives can be gleaned through patient feedback.

In summary, evidence-based practice requires a blending of the research-based and experiential knowledge of professionals with the individualised personal knowledge of patients and their carers. Such a stance recognises that no single person is the expert as of right but that everyone has expertise of a differing kind. Figure 31.1 illustrates how these three elements of evidence-based practice are inter-related in regard to the use of compression bandages to treat venous leg ulcers. Where there is a lack of congruence, for example between the research evidence, the practitioner's skills to apply the bandages correctly, or in the patient's willingness to try a new treatment, the outcomes for the individual patient are likely to be affected.

Research evidence
- Compression bandaging has improved healing rates compared to treatments using no compression.
- Compression therapy is more cost-effective because the faster healing rates saved nurses time.
- High compression achieves better healing rates than low compression.
- Multi-layer compression systems are more effective than single layer systems.

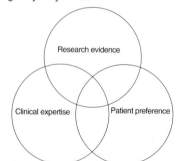

Clinical expertise
Practitioner is:
- knowledgeable of benefits of compression bandaging,
- trained in applying compression bandaging,
- skilled in patient education to promote patient understanding of leg ulcer management and concordance with treatment regime.

Patient preference
- Amenable to trying techniques offered.
- Willingness to comply with treatment regime.
- Experience of other treatment programmes.

Research evidence drawn from: Effective Health Care Bulletin (1997) Compression therapy for Venous Leg Ulcers, Centre for Reviews and Dissemination, University of York

Figure 31.1 An example of the relationship between the three components of evidence-based practice.

Hierarchies of evidence

If it is accepted that evidence-based practice involves drawing upon the different types of evidence outlined above, how then are decisions made about what constitutes the 'best' evidence? Muir Gray (1997) provides a classification that groups different sources of research evidence into five categories and ranks them in order of the strength of the evidence (*see* Box 31.2).

Box 31.2 Hierarchies of evidence.

I.   Systematic review multiple RCTs
II.   Randomised controlled trial
III. Non-randomised trails
IV.   Non-experimental studies
V.   Descriptive studies, expert committees

(*Muir Gray 1997*)

This form of classification, commonly known as a 'hierarchy of evidence' ranks different research designs in terms of the extent to which they prevent bias from influencing the findings of the research. The randomised controlled trial (RCT) in which the researcher seeks to minimise the effects of bias is judged to be the most robust form of evidence whereas expert opinion and descriptive studies are considered to be the weakest.

Hierarchies of evidence have played an important role in guiding the systematic reviews undertaken by the National Centre for Research and Dissemination and in informing the guidance produced by the National Institute for Health and Clinical Excellence (NICE). However, this approach has been criticised for devaluing the contribution of qualitative and participatory forms of research. Whereas some of this criticism may be justified, it is important to recognise that the hierarchy of evidence was developed to assist in judging the robustness of evidence examining the outcomes of different clinical interventions and treatments, and in this respect it can be a useful tool for deciding which sources of evidence are best able to link cause and effect. If a district nurse wants to know which type of dressing is most effective in healing venous leg ulcers, then an RCT that compares different types of dressing will clearly provide more robust evidence than the professional opinion of nurses who have experience of using different dressings.

However, where evidence is sought to provide guidance for practice on an aspect of care that is not focused on measurable outcomes, the hierarchy of evidence is inappropriate. For example, if a nurse wants to understand what the transition from independence to dependence is like for an older person in order to provide sensitive and appropriate care, then high-quality qualitative research is likely to provide appropriate evidence to inform practice. As the contribution of qualitative research becomes more valued, guidance is being developed on how to judge the robustness of evidence derived from this approach and use it to inform the development of clinical guidelines Chapters 8 and 21 provide more detail on critical appraisal of qualitative research.

What needs to be emphasised is the value of different research methodologies in providing guidance for practice and the need to acknowledge the contribution of different sources of knowledge where research evidence is lacking. In this

regard, Smith and Pell (2003) provide an amusing illustration of the inappropriate-
ness of placing too much emphasis on evidence derived from RCTs (Box 31.3).

Research utilisation

The different forms of evidence identified in the hierarchy of evidence lend themselves to different models of research utilisation. Much of the literature on
evidence-based practice focuses on the direct application of research findings to
practice often in the form of clinical protocols, practice guidelines or care pathways. Estabrooks (1998) refers to this as *instrumental* research utilisation.
Quantitative research, and in particular the RCT, is most suited to such direct
application. The hierarchy of evidence referred to earlier is generally used to
determine the robustness of evidence used in this model of research utilisation.
The difficulties of implementing research findings in practice have also been

---

Box 31.3   A cautionary note on RCTs.

Smith G, Pell J (2003) Parachute use to prevent death and major trauma related to gravitational challenge: systematic review of randomised controlled trials. *British Medial Journal*
327:1459–1461

Abstract
Objectives – To determine whether parachutes are effective in preventing major trauma
related to gravitational challenge.

Design – Systematic review of randomised controlled trials.

Data sources – Medline, Web of Science, Embase, and the Cochrane Library databases;
appropriate internet sites and citation lists.

Study selection – Studies showing the effects of using a parachute during free fall.

Main outcome – Death or major trauma, defined as an injury severity score measure >15.

Results – We were unable to identify any randomised controlled trials of parachute
intervention.

Conclusions – As with many interventions intended to prevent ill-health, the effectiveness
of parachutes has not been subjected to rigorous evaluation by using randomised controlled
trials. Advocates of evidence-based medicine have criticised the adoption of interventions
evaluated by using only observational data. We think that everyone might benefit if the most
radical protagonists of evidence-based medicine organised and participated in a double blind,
randomised, placebo controlled, crossover trial of the parachute.

demonstrated most clearly through this approach. Hunt's (1987) influential action research study, which sought to introduce research guidance on pre-operative fasting was unsuccessful, not because nurses and anaesthetists were not persuaded of the need to reduce the time that patients fasted pre-operatively on physiological grounds but because the complex health care organisation in which they worked was not able to accommodate an individualised approach to patient fasting. The context in which the research findings were being implemented was the influencing factor, not the research findings themselves or the attitudes of the practitioners concerned.

In recognising the importance of context, an alternative model of research utilisation is proposed by Weiss and Bucuvalas (1980). They suggest that research findings may be utilised but not necessarily always in a direct way that the instrumental model implies. Research findings may exert an influence through a process of subliminal diffusion, which informs a person's understanding. In this model of *indirect* research use, practitioners become aware of research findings, internalise them and use them to inform their practice in ways that are often not explicit (Estabrooks 1998). Qualitative research findings tend to be used more indirectly.

Research findings may also be used persuasively to argue for a change in policy or practice. Florence Nightingale's collation of epidemiological data during the Crimean War, which she then used to persuade government officials of the need for radical reform in the British military, is an example of the persuasive use of research at a macro-level. However, nurses use research as a means of persuasion in much more modest ways. For example, Gerrish *et al.* (1999) describe how a team of nurses in the operating theatres department in the hospital in which they worked used research examining the risk assessment of pressure damage to change surgeons' perceptions and gain support for the introduction of new theatre mattresses to minimise such risk.

The three models of research utilisation referred to above are helpful in thinking about different approaches to evidence-based practice. The instrumental model of research utilisation is reflected in the standard linear process of evidence-based practice outlined in Box 31.4, whereas the other two models identify how evidence can be used in more subtle ways to inform practice.

Box 31.4 The stages of evidence-based practice.

- Identify a problem or issue from practice.
- Formulate an answerable question.
- Identify the available evidence.
- Appraise the evidence.
- Develop guidance for practice.
- Plan strategy for introducing change.
- Implement change.
- Evaluate the impact of change.

The process of evidence-based practice

As Box 31.4 shows, there are a number of stages involved in evidence-based practice. Guidance on how to achieve the first four stages can be found in earlier chapters of this book (Chapters 6, 7, 8, and 21) whereas Chapter 32 deals with the implementation of evidence-based practice in more detail.

Although individuals or small groups of nurses may choose to take forward evidence-based initiatives, the implementation of evidence-based practice often forms part of a broader agenda in health care organisations to promote clinical effectiveness. The Department of Health has defined clinical effectiveness as:

'The extent to which specific clinical interventions when deployed in the field for a particular patient or population do what they are intended to do, i.e. maintain and improve health and secure the greatest possible health gain from the available resources.' (NHSE 1996:6)

Clinical effectiveness involves using sound evidence to improve care. However, this is a complex undertaking. Appleby *et al.* (1996) identify four steps involved.

- Evidence is generated by undertaking rigorous, large-scale clinical and economic evaluations of health care interventions.
- Evidence from multiple studies is systematically reviewed and brought together in a way that allows recommendations to be made for practice.
- The findings from systematic reviews are disseminated to those involved in the area in a format they can use.
- The evidence is used to change behaviour and influence decision-making by practitioners, managers and policy makers.

This approach to evidence-based practice is concerned primarily with process, that is ensuring that practitioners utilise the best available evidence to inform their practice, rather than with the outcome of that evidence for the patient. However, to use evidence to underpin practice and not to evaluate its effect on patients is short-sighted. Clinically effective practice can only occur when practitioners use the best available evidence to maximise patient outcomes. Evaluation is essential to monitoring outcomes of care.

Translating the aspirations of evidence-based practice into reality is far from straightforward and nurses need to be aware of what is entailed. There are barriers to achieving evidence-based practice that need to be overcome and certain conditions are necessary for the implementation of evidence-based practice. These will be considered in turn.

Barriers to achieving evidence-based practice

A number of research studies have sought to identify barriers to evidence-based practice by using an anglicised version of the Barriers to Research Utilisation scale developed by Funk *et al.* (1991) in the USA (Nolan *et al.* 1998; Parahoo 2000; Bryar *et al.* 2003). Other studies have developed specific instruments to examine different barriers to evidence-based practice (for example Gerrish & Clayton 2004; McKenna *et al.* 2004). The collective findings from these studies have identified barriers that can be grouped into four categories.

Barriers to do with the nature of the evidence

Although there has been a considerable increase over the past decade in the amount of research conducted by nurses and/or examining nursing practice, the lack of appropriate clinically relevant research in nursing is still seen to be problematic. Researchers have been accused of not asking questions that are relevant to clinical practice and there is a plethora of small-scale studies that focus on local need as opposed to large-scale definitive studies. The findings from such research may not be generalisable. Nursing research also varies considerably in terms of its quality and not all published research may have been carried out sufficiently rigorously.

Barriers to do with the way the evidence is communicated

Research is often published in academic journals rather than the more popular professional journals which clinical nurses are more likely to read. Evidence suggests that nurses tend not to read research journals (McCaughan *et al.* 2002), preferring instead to access research information via a third party, such as specialist nurses and medical staff, or through attending in-service training events and conferences. However, opportunities for practising nurses to attend conferences where up-to-date research is presented are limited. It can also be intimidating for practitioners who lack confidence in research to question researchers in a public forum.

The language of research can also act as a barrier. Research papers often use complex terminology and are written in a style that is not particularly accessible. Researchers may also fail to draw out the implications of their research for practice, leaving it to the reader to do the hard work. Nurses may encounter problems with interpreting and working with research products that are seen to be too complex. They perceive that research reports lack clinical credibility and fail to provide sufficient clinical direction (McCaughan *et al.* 2002).

Barriers to do with knowledge and skills of the individual nurse

Although nurses may be willing to use research they may lack the skills to do so. Studies examining barriers to research utilisation have consistently identified that nurses do not know how to access and appraise research information. In the past, the main concern has been whether nurses knew how to use library resources effectively. The increasing availability of evidence-based information on the internet means that nurses now need to be competent in using information technology

(IT) in the workplace. Yet, research has shown that nurses appear to lag behind other professional groups in their use of IT (Estabrooks *et al.* 2003).

One of the challenges of using the internet is coping with information overload. A seemingly straightforward search may result in a baffling array of research and other sources of evidence, some of which may be contradictory. Making sense of all this information is a daunting task even for the most determined practitioner.

Nurses have also been shown to lack skills in evaluating different sources of evidence and in drawing out the implications of research findings for practice. As Chapter 8 has shown, critical appraisal of research findings demands considerable knowledge about the research process and is time consuming. Whereas these skills now form part of both pre and post-registration nurse education, many nurses still do not consider themselves to be competent in this area (Gerrish & Clayton 2004).

Barriers to do with the organisation

Major obstacles that nurses encounter in implementing evidence-based practice relate to insufficient time to access and review research reports together with lack of authority and support to implement findings. Organisational factors have been identified as a major impediment to achieving evidence-based practice. In particular, lack of support from managers and doctors, problems with dissemination of information within the organisation, difficulties in the management of innovations including the time necessary to implement change and resource constraints are all seen to hinder the successful implementation of evidence-based practice (Closs & Cheater 1994; Newman *et al.* 1998). Additionally practitioners may experience restricted local access to information, for example library resources or the internet.

Implementing evidence-based practice

Whereas there is general consensus about what the barriers to evidence-based practice are, there is less agreement about how they might be overcome. Evidence-based practice requires complex actions on the part of organisations to facilitate its implementation, including high-level management commitment, putting in place systems for managing information and innovation and for individual skills development (Newman *et al.* 1998). Kitson *et al.* (1998) propose that the implementation of evidence-based practice depends on three factors. First, the nature of the evidence is important and this has been explored extensively earlier in this chapter. Second, structures and mechanisms are required to facilitate change. External and internal change agents can support the process of change, although consideration should be given to the personal characteristics of the facilitator, the style of facilitation and the role of the facilitator in terms of authority.

Finally, consideration of the context draws attention to the importance of the ward/team culture in terms of patient-centeredness; valuing team members and promoting a learning environment; the leadership styles of senior clinical nurses; and the audit and review procedures in place. Successful implementation of evidence-based practice is also dependent upon the resources available. These are many and varied and include the availability and access to library and IT resources, finances to support new treatments, an adequate number of nurses with appropriate skills, sufficient time for gathering and appraising research evidence and implementation activities and finally co-operation from peers, managers, and other professionals. Factors influencing the implementation of evidence-based practice are examined in more detail in the following chapter.

Conclusion

It is crucial that nurses use the best available evidence to inform their practice in order to provide high-quality patient care. Evidence derived from rigorous research is fundamental to the process of evidence-based practice but is not sufficient in its own right. Research evidence may be lacking or the findings may be inconclusive or contradictory. In recognising that knowledge derived from research is never absolute, nurses need to draw upon their own expertise and that of more experienced nurses to inform decisions about the most appropriate care for a particular patient. Clinical expertise should not been seen as a substitute for research evidence but rather as contributing to the decision-making process. It should be remembered that evidence-based practice is about providing care to patients and both patients and their carers will have their own views about the care they wish to receive. Therefore, nurses have a responsibility to share their knowledge of the best available evidence with patients in order to assist them to make informed choices.

Achieving evidence-based practice is a complex undertaking that involves identifying and appraising different sources of evidence, translating evidence into clear guidance for practice, implementing change and finally evaluating the impact of change. Earlier chapters of this book have examined the knowledge and skills nurses need to be able to critically appraise research findings in order to identify the best available evidence. The following chapter considers how the best available evidence can be implemented and the impact of change evaluated.

References

Appleby J, Walshe K, Ham C (1996) *Acting on the Evidence*. Birmingham, The NHS Confederation

Bryar R, Closs SJ, Baum G, Cooke J, Griffiths J, Hostick T, Kelly S, Knight S, Marshall K, Thompson D (2003) The Yorkshire BARRIERS project: diagnostic analysis of barriers to research utilisation. *International Journal of Nursing Studies* 40: 73–85

Closs SJ, Cheater F (1994) Utilisation of nursing research: culture, interest and support. *Journal of Advanced Nursing* 19: 762–773

Closs SJ (2003) Evidence and community-based nursing practice. In Bryer R, Griffiths J (eds) *Practice Development in Community Nursing*. London, Arnold, pp33–56

Effective Health Care (1995) The prevention and treatment of pressure sores. *Effective Health Care* 2:1

Eraut M (1994) *Developing Professional Knowledge and Competence*. London, Falmer Press

Estabrooks C (1998) Will evidence-based nursing practice make practice perfect? *Canadian Journal of Nursing Research* 30: 15–36

Estabrooks C, O'Leary K, Ricker K, Humphrey C (2003) The internet and access to evidence: how are nurses positioned? *Journal of Advanced Nursing* 42: 73–81

Farrell C, Gilbert H (1996) *Health Care Partnerships*. London, The King's Fund

Ferlie E, Wood M, Fitzgerald L (1999) Some limitations to evidence-based medicine: a case study from elective orthopaedics. *Quality in Health Care* 8:2 99–107

Funk S, Champagne M, Wiese R, Tornquist E (1991) BARRIERS: The Barriers to Research Utilization Scale. *Applied Nursing Research* 4: 39–45

Gerrish K, Clayton J, Nolan M, Parker K, Morgan L (1999) Promoting evidence-based practice: managing change in the assessment of pressure damage risk. *Journal of Nursing Management* 7: 355–362

Gerrish K, Clayton J (2004) Promoting evidence-based practice: an organisational approach. *Journal of Nursing Management* 12: 114–123

Hunt M (1987) The process of translating research findings into nursing practice. *Journal of Advanced Nursing* 12: 101–110.

Kitson A, Harvey G, McCormack B (1998) Enabling the implementation of evidence-based practice: a conceptual framework. *Quality in Health Care* 7: 149–158

Liaschenko J, Fisher A (1999) Theorising the knowledge that nurses use in the conduct of their work. *Scholarly Inquiry for Nursing Practice: An International Journal* 13: 29–40

McCaughan D, Thompson C, Cullum N, Sheldon T, Thompson D (2002) Acute care nurses' perceptions of barriers to using research information in clinical decision making. *Journal of Advanced Nursing* 39: 46–60

McKenna H, Ashton S, Keeney S (2004) Barriers to evidence-based practice in primary care. *Journal of Advanced Nursing* 45: 178–189

Muir Gray JA (1997) *Evidence-based Health Care*. Edinburgh, Churchill Livingstone

Muir Gray JA (2004) Evidence-based policy making (editorial). *British Medical Journal* 329: 988–989

National Health Service Executive (1996) *Promoting Clinical Effectiveness: a framework for action in and through the NHS*. London: NHS Executive.

Newman M, Papadopoulos I, Sigsworth J (1998) Barriers to evidence-based practice. *Clinical Effectiveness* 2: 11–20

Nolan M, Morgan L, Curran M, Clayton J, Gerrish K, Parker C (1998) Evidence-based care: can we overcome the barriers? *British Journal of Nursing* 7: 1273–1278

Parahoo K (2000) Barriers to, and facilitators of, research utilisation among nurses in Northern Ireland. *Journal of Advanced Nursing* 31: 89–98

Rycroft-Malone J, Seers K, Titchen A, Harvey G, Kitson A, McCormack B (2004) What counts as evidence in evidence-based practice? *Journal of Advanced Nursing* 47:1 81–90

Sackett DL, Rosenburg WM, Muir Gray JA, Haynes RB, Richardson WS (1996) Evidence-Based Medicine: what it is and what it isn't. *British Medical Journal* 312: 71–72

Smith G, Pell J (2003) Parachute use to prevent death and major trauma related to gravitational challenge: systematic review of randomised controlled trials. *British Medical Journal* 327: 1459–1461

Thompson C, McCaughan D, Cullum N, Sheldon T, Mullhall A, Thompson D (2001) The accessibility of research-based knowledge for nurses in United Kingdom acute care settings. *Journal of Advanced Nursing* 36: 11–22

Weiss C, Bucuvalas M (1980) *Social Science Research and Decision Making*. New York, Columbia University Press

Further reading

McSherry R, Simmons M, Abbott P (2002) *Evidence-informed nursing: a guide for clinical nurses*. London, Routledge

Evidence-Based Nursing, BMJ Publishing

World Views on Evidence-Based Nursing, Blackwell Publishing

Website

www.shef.ac.uk/scharr/ir/netting/ – *Netting the Evidence* is designed to facilitate evidence-based practice by providing access to organisations and learning resources, such as an evidence-based virtual library, software and journals

32 Implementing Evidence-Based Practice

Steve Campbell, Helen Hancock and Hilary Lloyd

Key points

- Different change management strategies, used individually or collectively, can be employed to facilitate the introduction of evidence-based practice.
- Change is more likely to be effective when there is local ownership of the need to change, and appropriate facilitation and educational support.
- Clinical practice guidelines are recommendations on the most appropriate treatment and care of people with specific conditions, based on the best available evidence.
- Published national guidelines that have been subject to rigorous review should be used and/or adapted for local use in preference to developing local guidelines.
- Evidence-based practice initiatives should be evaluated to ensure that the change has been effective and led to improvements in care.

Introduction

The extent to which evidence informs practice on a day-to-day basis is variable. The implementation of evidence-based practice is a complex process and requires knowledge, skill, planning and time. Definitions of evidence-based practice tend to imply that data speak for themselves, and in so doing ignore the human element of applying empirical evidence in practice. However, evidence-based practice does not just happen; someone has to make it happen. This chapter examines practical issues associated with the implementation of evidence-based practice, using examples that illustrate the process.

In nursing it is important to know not only 'how' to do something, but also to understand 'why' it is being done, in other words, to have knowledge of the evidence that underpins the practice. In this way it is linked with clinical effectiveness: doing the right thing in the right way and at the right time for the right patient (RCN 1996). By applying the principles of evidence-based practice, nurses can systematically examine what they do in order to ensure they are providing beneficial care. Factors affecting the implementation of evidence-based practice were considered in Chapter 31 and include a combination of available evidence, the development of skills, as well as wider factors such as working relationships, existing practices, attitudes and values.

Nurses are constantly being asked to find new ways of working in order to deliver health care that is both evidence-based and patient-centred. The NHS Plan (Department of Health 2000a) called for improvement in service provision, better use of research and the delivery of evidence-based health care. In order that evidence-based practice is promoted, it is essential to understand the change strategies that facilitate the effective introduction and application of research findings. There is no ideal method or approach; the choice will be determined by the requirements of the change to be implemented and the particular situation in which change is to take place.

Change

The first step in the process of implementing evidence-based practice is the identification of new, accepted, evidence that informs practice. Chapters 7, 8 and 21 consider how research findings can be identified, critically appraised and synthesised into a systematic review of the evidence for a particular topic area. The recommendations arising from a systematic review can then be used to review current practice. Whereas new evidence may confirm that current practice equates to practice based on the best available evidence, in many instances the evidence identifies a need to change policy and/or practice. There are a number of different levels of change required in clinical practice in order that evidence-based practice is implemented:

- a significant change that needs to be addressed immediately, such as a new treatment algorithm for resuscitation following cardiac arrest
- a change so slight and obvious it can be immediately implemented, such as turning off unnecessary lights at night to improve patients' sleep and maintain normal night and day sleep-wake patterns
- a change that needs to be addressed by the local team such as a new practice protocol to be developed from the latest evidence
- a change that needs addressing by the organisation as a whole, such as care delivery throughout the patient journey in the organisation, using national standards or guidelines. For example, the NICE guidance for Epilepsies (2004) recommends that all epilepsy patients have a structured annual review.

Change theory

There are a great many change theories and strategies offered by change theorists, knowledge of which is important in order to understand change and to articulate it to others. It is useful at this point to summarise the key theories as they offer valuable guidance in the complex process of initiating, managing and sustaining change. It is important to remember that in clinical practice a combination of several strategies can be applied.

Many change theories have their roots in the work of Lewin (1951), who described the process of successful change in three stages:

- *Unfreezing* – where the need for change is recognised. At this early stage professionals should be encouraged, supported and motivated in the direction of the desired change through an introduction to the (new) evidence and their involvement in the process of change.
- *Movement* – where the change process gets underway. Familiarisation with the (new) evidence results in an alteration in beliefs and behaviour so that desired change(s) begin to occur.
- *Refreezing* – where there is an acceptance and integration of the change. The new behaviour(s) and belief(s) become owned by the professionals. At this stage encouragement through positive feedback and support is important in order that change is achieved and maintained.

Change strategy

Selection of the most appropriate strategy, which is dependent upon the desired change, provides the underpinnings of an action plan and is vital to the success of any change. Haffer (1986) describes three strategies that are commonly used to effect change:

- *The power coercive approach* is based on the belief that those in authority have legitimate power to introduce change. People involved comply due to pressure, coercion and sanctions. This is a 'top-down' approach and is instigated in a hierarchical manner. It is advantageous in that it can bring about rapid change, but is often met with resistance, making permanent and effective change problematic.
- *The empirical rational approach* is based on the belief that people are largely guided by reason and that if given information, will choose the appropriate course of action. This is another 'top-down' approach and is subject to the pitfalls of the power coercive approach. It capitalises on the fact that the majority of individuals are rational beings and will therefore comply but does not take irrational individuals into account.
- *The normative re-educative approach* is based on the belief that those most likely to be affected by change should be involved in the change and that giving them ownership of the project makes it more likely to succeed. This is a 'bottom-up' participative approach and is the most democratic approach. Any changes are likely to be long-lasting, but it is very time-consuming and may be difficult for individuals who are used to taking orders.

Cleghorn and Headrick (1996) refer to the Plan–Do–Study–Act (PDSA) cycle of change that is often used in health care. The first phase: 'Planning' sets objectives and asks questions in an attempt to predict the kinds of change that is necessary. The 'Do' phase is about carrying out the plan, documenting problems and unexpected observations and starting to analyse the evidence. 'Studying' completes this analysis, compares the evidence to expected outcomes and makes a summary of the resultant learning. 'Act' makes the changes and prepares for starting the cycle again.

Much of the literature on change theory gives the impression that change is or can be a rational, controlled and orderly process. In practice, however, change is often chaotic, involving shifting goals and disjointed activities. Change is a complex process: however, there are several strategies that can be used to ensure, as far as is possible, that change within the context of the implementation of evidence-based practice is effective. There is no single method that could be reliably expected to change practice in all circumstances and settings. It is worth considering that a combination of these approaches can help to compensate for the limitations of each. Box 32.1 presents a practical example of how this combined approach can be applied to the implementation of change relating to the management of post-operative pain.

Given the complexity of change, there are guiding principles that can be adapted to the implementation of evidence-based practice in a variety of situations. The NHS Centre for Reviews and Dissemination's (1999) findings about helpful approaches to implementing change and evidence-based practice are summarised in Box 32.2.

Change strategies are only useful if they can be applied to clinical practice. The following section provides examples of how these strategies have been used to implement evidence-based practice in the authors' work setting.

An individual-led approach to implementing evidence-based practice

The following is an example of the process of change required to effect the introduction of a hospital-wide early warning scoring system (EWSS) by a nurse consultant in critical care outreach.

The evidence

The policy document *Comprehensive Critical Care* (Department of Health 2000b) gave a 'high priority' recommendation that critical care outreach services and EWSS should be introduced in order to address some of the shortfalls in patient care and outcomes. An EWSS is a simple physiological scoring system with an identifiable trigger threshold enabling the identification of patients at risk of critical illness. EWSS are based upon the allocation of 'points' to physiological observations, the calculation of a total 'score' and the designation of an agreed calling 'trigger' level (Morgan *et al.* 1997; Stenhouse *et al.* 2000; Subbe *et al.* 2001). More recently, EWSS have been referred to as 'Track and Trigger Warning Tools' (National

Box 32.1 Using a combination of strategies in the planning and implementation of change.

Hancock H (1996) Implementing change in the management of post-operative pain. *Intensive and Critical Care Nursing* 12: 359–362

Despite overwhelming evidence about effective post-operative pain management, existing practice did not achieve this. Therefore, it was necessary to implement change so that clinical practice was based on up-to-date evidence. The process of change was supported by a combination of strategies to ensure that the change was successful, timely and sustained. The following strategies were used during the change process.

Membership of the project management group
Membership of the project management group included representatives from all professional groups affected by the proposed change, i.e. management, medicine, nursing, allied health professions and research. Involving staff at both senior and junior levels within the organisation was vital to ensure ownership and effective implementation and evaluation of the change. This inclusive normative re-educative approach is in contrast to the power coercive approach where change is autocratically imposed from above.

Education and training
The development of an interactive, targeted education programme to underpin the change in practice was co-ordinated by the management group, and delivered by junior group members. Education may be effective in developing practitioners' knowledge, skills and attitudes in relation to the proposed change and implementation of evidence-based practice. Its delivery by junior group members was in accordance with the normative re-educative approach to change, which promotes a participative, non-threatening, bottom-up approach. In order that change occurs quickly, some power coercive strategies such as the monitoring of clinical practice and patient outcomes were used in combination with this approach.

Link members for each unit or ward area
Nominated by their ward or department manager, link members attended the education programme and were then given responsibility for disseminating the information and monitoring practice within their own area. They received ongoing support from the project management group and were given the opportunity to voice concerns, clarify any questions and provide feedback regarding the implementation of the evidence into practice. Using both an empirical-rational and a normative-re-educative approach enabled participation in and ownership of the desired change. Individuals were given the opportunity to oversee the implementation of evidence-based practice and this contributed to the success of the change in practice.

The combination of the three change strategies in this example promoted an effective change process and resulted in the implementation of evidence-based practice. There was evidence of reduced pain scores for patients following the change. The solution to addressing the inadequacies of previous practice required an effective change management strategy to ensure the implementation of evidence-based methods of pain management.

> **Box 32.2** Approaches to implementing change.
>
> - Be clear about the proposed change, why it is necessary, what is to be achieved, what the anticipated outcomes will be, and what evidence supports it.
> - Assess how prepared practitioners are to implement the proposed change and consider how the proposal for change will be presented to them.
> - Identify and, where possible, include representatives from all groups and individuals involved in, affected by or influencing the proposed change(s) in practice; a wide range of people may be involved, including health professionals, patients, managers, policy makers, researchers, and the public.
> - Ensure that this group feeds information and plans back to their colleagues so that those not directly involved are provided with the opportunity to discuss and influence the change.
> - Identify any potential barriers to the change and consider how these might be addressed.
> - Identify any factors that may support the change, including individuals and resources.
> - Most change strategies are effective under some circumstances; none are effective under all circumstances.
>
> (*NHS Centre for Reviews and Dissemination 1999*)

Outreach Forum 2003). Existing evidence about the reliability and benefit of EWSS is based on a consensus of professional opinion.

Plan

A needs analysis was undertaken in order to identify the most appropriate EWSS for the local patient population. This included an assessment of patient acuity, case mix, vital observations and resources.

The process of implementation

From the evidence collected, an aggregate EWSS was selected by the nurse consultant. The rationale for the particular choice was presented to senior clinicians. After some discussion, it was agreed that the chosen EWSS (*see* Box 32.3) would be piloted on a number of wards for adults. Following successful piloting the EWSS has been accepted and introduced hospital-wide.

This example demonstrates how evidence can be implemented into practice through the leadership of an individual. A recent evaluation has shown improvements in the quality and completeness of patients' observations and in referral to, and a more efficient use of, critical care.

Box 32.3   The Adult Early Warning Scoring System.

Measure	Score			
	0	1	2	3
Heart rate	51–100	41–50 101–110	<40 111–130	>130
Systolic blood pressure	101–160	81–100 161–200	71–80 >200	<70
Respiratory rate	9–14	15–20	<8 21–29	>30
Temperature	36.1–37.5	35.1–36.0 >37.5	<35	
CNS	alert	to voice	to pain	unconscious

Seek senior help immediately if the patient scores 3/5 or more on EWSS.

A co-ordinated approach to implementing evidence-based practice

The benefits of good teamwork in achieving change should not be underestimated. Teams are often more powerful in changing practice than individuals, with key members of the team influencing others to drive change forward.

The patient journey is a feature of the NHS Modernisation Agency's aim of understanding and redesigning patient processes. It entails mapping who does what to the patient throughout their episode of health care in order to identify how care can be improved. Through the application of evidence, patient involvement and leadership, it can be used to identify problems with, and steer improvements to, core patient processes or clinical management pathways. Improvement Leaders' Guides (*www.modern.nhs.uk/improvementguides*) provide helpful guidance on process mapping, analysis and redesign techniques. The following is an example of the application of this approach in relation to stroke patients.

The evidence

Stroke is a complex condition that requires a multifaceted approach to care. There is strong evidence that a comprehensive, coordinated, specialist multiprofessional service for stroke patients positively affects outcomes (*see* Box 32.4). In particular, care on a stoke unit reduces mortality and improves functional outcome in comparison to care on a general medical ward (Stroke Unit Trialists' Collaboration 2003).

Box 32.4   Evidence supporting stroke care.

Department of Health (2001) *The National Service Framework for Older People: Standard 5: Stroke.* London, Department of Health

Effective Stroke Care *www.effectivestrokecare.org*

Indredavik B. Bakke F. Slordahl SA. Rokseth R. Haheim LL. (1999) Stroke unit treatment. 10-year follow-up. *Stroke.* 30: 1524–1527

Kwan J, Sandercock P (2004) In-hospital care pathways for stroke. *The Cochrane Database of Systematic Reviews* 2004, Issue 4. Chichester, John Wiley

Royal College of Physicians (2004) *National Clinical Guidelines For Stroke,* 2nd edition. Intercollegiate Stroke Working Party. London, Royal College of Physicians

Royal College of Physicians (2005) *National Sentinel Stroke Audit Report 2004.* Intercollegiate Stroke Working Party. London, Royal College of Physicians

Stroke Unit Trialists' Collaboration (2003) Organised inpatient (stroke unit) care for stroke. The *Cochrane Database of Systematic Reviews* Issue 4. Sulter G, Elting JW, Langedijk M, *et al.* (2003) Admitting acute ischemic stroke patients to a stroke care monitoring unit versus a conventional stroke unit: a randomized pilot study. *Stroke* 34: 101–104

Box 32.5   Key roles for facilitating change in the patient journey.

Clinical champion	Brings leadership and vision to the group and ensures that rigorous evidence is sought and followed on the journey
Patient journey facilitator	Brings user involvement to the group by conducting interviews with patients and carers. This person is an outsider to the service and facilitates the whole process
Patient journey chair	Manages the development of the patient journey within the group and ensures the smooth progress, dealing with any blockages or issues as they arise.
Local facilitator	Brings the picture of the current service to the group. This person represents service needs and has an in-depth knowledge of the organisation.

The plan

Harvey *et al.* (2002) claim that the implementation of evidence-based practice is most successful when evidence is scientifically robust and when there is appropriate facilitation of change using the skill of external and internal facilitators. In recognition of the need to implement the evidence in a co-ordinated way, a multidisciplinary project team was set up to map, analyse and redesign care delivery. In addition, key roles were established, to drive the patient journey process (*see* Box 32.5).

The process of implementation

The existing journey for stroke patients was mapped and patient interviews undertaken (Campbell *et al.* 2004). This information was used together with published evidence to inform the development of a new patient journey. A project plan for its delivery was drawn up, discussed and agreed. This work led to the development of a comprehensive, coordinated, multiprofessional service for stroke patients, which meets the needs of the patients and their carers. The continued improvement of care and achievement of action plans is monitored through the group, which has now become the Stroke Services Implementation Group. In particular, the number of patients now being cared for in the stroke unit has increased considerably.

This example demonstrates how integrating published evidence with that obtained from patients has led to the delivery of evidence-based patient-centred care. By involving all members of the clinical team, ownership of the change is secured and this increases not only the success of the initiative but also its sustainability.

Clinical practice guidelines

Clinical practice guidelines are recommendations on the most appropriate treatment and care of people with specific diseases and conditions, based on the best available evidence. Designed to help health care professionals assimilate, evaluate and implement current best practice, clinical guidelines are a method of bridging the gap between research and everyday practice (SIGN 1999). There are two main sources of clinical guidelines: national and local guidelines.

National clinical guidelines are published by various professional and health care bodies. Box 32.6 provides examples of the main organisations that produce national guidelines.

Two examples of guidelines produced by national bodies are:

- The British Hypertension Society (Williams *et al.* 2004) recommends that systolic blood pressure for non-diabetic patients should be maintained below 140 mmHg.
- The National Service Framework for Coronary Heart Disease (Department of Health 2000c) states that 80% of patients who have a myocardial infarction should be prescribed aspirin, beta blockade and statin therapy.

Local clinical guidelines are normally produced to address specific health care issues not covered by national guidelines. Developing valid guidelines requires considerable expertise and resources that are often beyond the scope of health care practitioners. Wherever possible, it is recommended that existing guidelines that have included a systematic and rigorous review of the available evidence are adapted for local use. If no such guideline exists and it is considered necessary to

Box 32.6   Information on national clinical guidelines.

National Institute for Health and Clinical Excellence (NICE)

NICE (*www.nice.org.uk/*) is an independent organisation responsible for providing national guidance on the promotion of good health and the prevention and treatment of ill health. It produces three types of guidance:

- clinical guidelines on the appropriate treatment and care of people with specific diseases and conditions within the National Health Service (NHS) in England and Wales
- technology appraisals, which provide guidance on the use of new and existing medicines and treatments within the NHS in England and Wales
- interventional procedures, which provide guidance on whether interventional procedures used for diagnosis or treatment are safe enough and work well enough for routine use in England, Wales and Scotland. They also provide some information on the implementation of guidelines

Department of Health

The Department of Health (*www.dh.gov.uk/Home/fs/en*) sets standards and guidelines and National Service Frameworks (NSFs) for care across the NHS, social care and public health. NSFs are long term strategies for improving specific areas of care. They set national standards and identify key interventions for a defined service or care group and set measurable goals to be achieved within an agreed time scale. The Department of Health also provides guidance on the implementation of these standards, guidelines and NSFs.

Royal College of Nursing (RCN)

As part of its clinical effectiveness work, the RCN develops national nurse-led guidelines. The College is also involved in informing the development of other guidelines, providing a nursing perspective through membership of steering groups. The RCN website (*www.rcn.org.uk/*) provides links to these partner organisations.

Royal College of Physicians (RCP)

The Royal College of Physicians works to improve standards by influencing clinical practice through the generation of guidelines and audits. The website (*www.rcplondon.ac.uk/*) includes all UK guidelines produced in the previous five years (older guidelines may be included if new evidence does not exist) that are considered relevant to the RCP and non-UK guidelines that are relevant to UK practice.

National Electronic Library for Health (NeLH)

The NeLH (*www.nelh.nhs.uk/*) provides health care professionals with information to support the delivery of evidence-based health care. It has links to a number of relevant organisations as well as to specialist and health libraries and to a guidelines finder, which provides an index to over 1200 UK guidelines with links to downloadable versions.

develop one, then it is important that as rigorous a method as possible is used within the resources available. The increasing availability of high-quality, published, systematic reviews make the task somewhat easier, however the number of systematic reviews on specific nursing topics is limited. In developing a local guideline it is important to acknowledge any potential limitations that arise from the nature of the evidence upon which the guideline is based, or the methods used in developing the guideline (Fedder *et al.* 1999). Chapter 21 considers the process of undertaking a systematic review of research evidence in preparation for developing practice guidelines.

Once a relevant guideline has been identified, it should be appraised in order to assess its validity. National guidelines published by organisations such as National Institute for Health and Clinical Excellence (NICE) or Scottish Intercollegiate Guideline Network (SIGN) have gone through a rigorous process of development and validation. However, adopting recommendations from guidelines of questionable validity may lead to ineffective use of resources, inappropriate care or even harm to patients (Fedder *et al.* 1999).

Implementing clinical practice guidelines

Even though national clinical guidelines exist, it does not necessarily mean that they are used by practitioners. A systematic review of strategies for changing professional behaviour identified that passive methods of disseminating and implementing guidelines, for example publication in journals or mail shots to targeted health care professionals, rarely led to the desired changes in behaviour (Freemantle *et al.* 1996). As Chapter 31 identified, factors that facilitate or hinder the implementation of evidence-based practice may relate to the organisation or the individual practitioner and the influence of their peer group. A coherent dissemination and implementation strategy is therefore necessary in order to increase the likelihood of clinical guidelines being used. Such strategies need to capitalise on known positive factors and address any obstacles to implementation (Fedder *et al.* 1999).

Like other aspects of evidence-based practice, clinical guideline implementation presents a major challenge and the principles of change management outlined earlier in this chapter should be applied. It is important to remember that guidelines that are relevant, introduced to address a specific problem, and which have local ownership are more likely to be implemented successfully. Guideline implementers also need to pay attention to organisational factors to ensure that implementation plans fit in with the organisation's strategy and resource commitments. Key recommendations for implementing clinical practice guidelines are presented in Box 32.7.

An example of implementing a clinical guideline in the hospital in which the authors work is given below.

Box 32.7   Recommendations for implementing clinical practice guidelines.

- The ways in which guidelines are developed, implemented and monitored influence the likelihood of adherence.
- Guidelines are more likely to be effective if they take into account local circumstances, are disseminated by an active educational intervention, and implemented by specific reminders relating directly to professional activity.
- Guidelines should be based firmly on reliable evidence of clinical and cost effectiveness.
- Recommendations should be explicitly linked to the evidence. Few national or local guidelines are sufficiently based on evidence.
- National initiatives are needed to help provide the evidence base that can be incorporated into national and local guidelines.
- Priority should be given to the development and introduction of local guidelines where nationally produced rigorous guidelines exist or where the evidence base is readily available. Priority should be given to areas where current practice diverges from best practice providing the potential for significant gains in health.
- A coherent programme of research is needed to ensure that guidelines are used to their full potential.

Effective Health Care Bulletin (1995) Implementing clinical practice guidelines: University of York

Implementing a clinical guideline

The evidence

The evidence in relation to confirming the position of a paediatric enteral feeding tube indicated that blue litmus paper may not distinguish between the acidic pH of gastric contents and other fluids (Rollins 1997; Colagiovanni 1999). As a result, a malpositioned enteral feeding tube had the potential to go undetected if blue litmus paper was used to test the aspirate to confirm placement of the tube in the stomach. The limited published evidence together with expert opinion resulted in a guideline specifying that pH paper, *not* blue litmus paper should be used for this purpose (NHS Quality Improvement Scotland 2003; Northern Ireland Clinical Resource Efficiency Support Team (CREST) 2004; National Patient Safety Agency 2005).

The plan

A comprehensive plan was developed to facilitate the implementation of the guideline within the hospital. This process involved a team of paediatric nurses, physicians, managers and parents. The team discussed the new guidance in view of the potential for harm with existing practice, and developed the following standard: 100% of children who require a fine bore nasogastric or enteral feeding tube will have a tube passed and correct placement confirmed by pH paper or X-ray prior to its use.

The standard statement was important in order to establish and convey the requirements of care, but also to enable outcomes to be measured, care monitored and further action taken if necessary.

The process of implementation

The implementation of the guideline was supported by a number of initiatives. An education and training package was introduced for all staff together with a competency-based assessment programme. An information leaflet was produced for parents who were included as a central part of ensuring safety and achieving the standard. An ongoing audit process was introduced in order to monitor adherence to the standard. Finally, a continuing programme of support was established to provide identified link members with the opportunity to voice concerns, clarify any questions and provide feedback regarding patient care standards.

Evaluation

It is essential that any change in clinical practice, whether based on clinical guidelines, published research or on the consensus of professional opinion is evaluated. This is to ensure that the change has been effective and that it has resulted in an improvement in care delivery, policy or the service at which it was aimed. It is important to evaluate both the process used to implement change and the outcome of the change itself.

By evaluating the process, lessons can be learnt about 'what was effective' (i.e. did it result in a behaviour change of those involved) as well as about 'how things might be done better next time'. This entails looking at the strategies used to introduce change.

Evaluating whether the proposed change has taken place and is effective in terms of achieving the desired outcomes is often more difficult than evaluating the change process. The success of the change can be relatively easy to evaluate if there is, as in the example of the stroke patient journey presented earlier, a clearly measurable outcome. In many cases, however, the situation is more complex, such as in the implementation of the EWSS, where there may not be a single measurable outcome. Similarly, it may be that more detailed, and ongoing information is required about the change. Chapter 19 introduces some of the principles of evaluation that might be applied to evaluate the implementation of evidence-based practice.

Audit procedures may also be used to evaluate the implementation of evidence-based practice. This entails setting evidence-based standards against which practice can be monitored. Existing practice is then assessed against these standards and reassessed at a suitable time following the introduction of change. Audit is particularly useful for assessing compliance with clinical guidelines.

Evaluation is a complex process. When planning to introduce a change to current practice it is advisable to involve someone with particular skills in evaluation methods, for example a representative from the research or audit department, in the project management group.

Conclusion

The publication of research findings does not ensure that practitioners will use them to inform care delivery. Achieving evidence-based practice is a complex undertaking. Nurses need to develop a critical and questioning approach to their work in order to be receptive to changing practice on the basis of new evidence. Such evidence should be evaluated to determine its quality and relevance to patient care and research findings translated into key recommendations for practice, for example in the form of clinical practice guidelines. Different change management strategies, used individually or collectively, should be drawn upon to facilitate the introduction of evidence-based practice in order to ensure ownership of the initiative and behavioural change. Finally, it is essential that any change in clinical practice is evaluated to ensure that the change has been effective and led to improvements in care.

Acknowledgements

We would like to acknowledge the Nurse Consultant in Critical Care, the Stroke Patient Journey Team and the Paediatric Nutrition Team at City Hospitals Sunderland NHS Foundation Trust for their contribution to the examples of the implementation of evidence-based practice included in this chapter.

References

Campbell SJ, Gibson AF, Watson W, Husband G, Bremner K (2004) Comprehensive service and practice development: City Hospitals Sunderland's experience of patient journeys. *Practice Development in Health Care* 3: 115–126

Cleghorn GD, Headrick LA (1996) The PDSA cycle at the core of learning in health professions education. *Joint Commission Journal of Quality Improvement.* 22: 206–212

Colagiovanni L (1999) Taking the tube. *Nursing Times Supplement* 95: 921 63–66

Department of Health (2000a) *The NHS Plan: a plan for investment, a plan for reform.* London, Stationery Office

Department of Health (2000b) *Comprehensive Critical Care: a review of adult critical care services.* London, Department of Health

Department of Health (2000c) *The National Service Framework for Coronary Heart Disease.* London, Department of Health

Effective Health Care Bulletin (1995) *Implementing Clinical Practice Guidelines.* University of Leeds

Fedder G, Eccles M, Grol R, Griffiths C, Grimshaw J (1999) Using clinical guidelines. *British Medical Journal* 318: 728–730

Freemantle N, Harvey E, Grimshaw J, Wolf F, Bero L, Grili R (1996) The effectiveness of printed materials in changing behaviour of health care professionals. *The Cochrane Library* Issue 3. Oxford, Update Software

Haffer A (1986) Facilitating change: choosing the appropriate strategy. *Journal of Nursing Administration* 16: 4 18–22

Hancock H (1996) Implementing change in the management of post-operative pain. *Intensive and Critical Care Nursing* 12: 359–362

Harvey G, Loftus-Hills A, Rycroft-Malone J (2002) Getting evidence into practice: the role and function of facilitation. *Journal of Advanced Nursing* 37: 577–586

Lewin K (1951) *Field Theory and Social Sciences.* New York, Harper and Row

Morgan R, Williams F, Wright M (1997) An early warning scoring system for detecting developing critical illness. *Clinical Intensive Care* 8: 100

National Outreach Forum (2003) *Critical Care Outreach 2003: Progress in Developing Services.* NHS Modernisation Agency

National Patient Safety Agency (2005) *How to confirm the correct position of nasogastric feeding tubes in infants, children and adults. www.npsa.nhs.uk/site/media/documents/857_Insert-finalWeb.pdf*

NHS Quality Improvement Scotland (2003). *Nasogastric and gastrostomy feeding for children being cared for in the community. www.nhshealthquality.org/nhsqis/files/GastrostomyNMPDU. doc*

NHS Centre for Reviews and Dissemination (1999) *Effective Health Care: Getting Evidence into Practice* 9: (1) 1–16. NHS CRD, University of York

NICE (2004) *The epilepsies: the diagnosis and management of the epilepsies in adults and children in primary and secondary care. NICE guideline: www.nice.org.uk/pdf/CG020NICEguideline. pdf*

Northern Ireland Clinical Resource Efficiency Support Team (2004) *Guideline for the management of enteral feeding in adults. www.crestni.org.uk/publications/tube_feeding_guidelines.pdf*

Rollins H (1997) A nose for trouble. *Nursing Times* 93:49 66–67

Royal College of Nursing (1996) *Clinical Effectiveness: a Royal College of Nursing guide.* London, RCN

SIGN (1999) *SIGN Guidelines: an introduction to SIGN methodology for the development of evidence-based clinical guidelines.* Edinburgh, SIGN Publication No. 39

Stenhouse C, Coates S, Tivey M, Allsop P, Parker T (2000) Prospective evaluation of a modified early warning score to aid earlier detection of patients developing critical illness on a general surgical ward. *British Journal of Anaesthesia* 84:5 663

Subbe CP, Kruger M, Rutherford P, Gemmel L (2001) Validation of a modified early warning score in medical admissions. *QJM: An International Journal of Medicine* 94:10 521–526

Stroke Unit Trialists' Collaboration (2003) Organised inpatient (stroke unit) care for stroke. *The Cochrane Database of Systematic Reviews.* Issue 4 Chichester, John Wiley

Williams B, Poulter NR, Brown MJ, Davies M, McInnes GT, Potter JP, Sever PS, Thom S (2004) The BHS Guidelines Working Party Guidelines for Management of Hypertension: report of the fourth working party of the British Hypertension Society, BHS IV. *Journal of Human Hypertension* 18: 139–185

33 The Future of Nursing Research

Ann McMahon and Anne Lacey

Key points

- Five inter-related policy imperatives are discussed which are essential if nursing research is to thrive in the future.
- The future of nursing as a clinical academic discipline depends upon improvement in performance in university research ratings, and resolution of the inherent conflicts between priorities of research and teaching.
- There are many possible ways in which nursing research may develop – three possible scenarios are presented, and the reader encouraged to consider which, if any, is preferable for the future.

Introduction

The aim of this book has been to introduce the reader to research or, to put it differently, to the processes through which knowledge is generated, to inform nursing practice. The purpose of this final chapter is to look forward, and the chapter ends with a provocative series of possible scenarios for the future of nursing research.

In Chapter 1 it was argued that there were key, inter-related policy imperatives within nursing that had a degree of strategic alignment with national corporate Research and Development (R&D) policy initiatives. In nursing it was also recognised as fundamentally important to strengthen the professional voice within all strategic R&D decision-making arenas, particularly where this impacted directly on priorities for R&D, and research funding streams.

Five policy imperatives

Figure 33.1 shows the imperatives as five interlocking circles. Each of these will now be discussed in turn, after which we will engage in a critical discussion of nursing as a research-based clinical academic discipline.

Capacity building

The four countries of the UK are committed to developing research capacity. Capacity building refers to the process of individual and institutional develop-

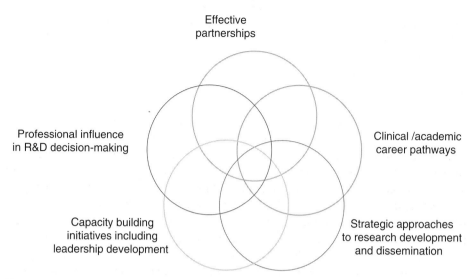

Figure 33.1   UK nursing R&D policy imperatives.

ment resulting in higher levels of skills and greater ability to undertake research (Trostle 1992). The rationale for developing research capacity, according to the Department of Health R&D website, is to maintain and improve health within a knowledge-based, patient-centred health service (*www.dh.gov.uk*). Since the nursing professions make up 80% of the health care workforce they are clearly fundamental to this endeavour. Chapter 4 outlined some of the programmes offering funding, training and fellowships to nurses in the UK. Details of all these initiatives can be found on the Royal College of Nursing (RCN) Research and Development Coordinating Centre website (*www.man.ac.uk/rcn*), which aims to make the infrastructure to support R&D in nursing more visible, and hence more accessible.

Capacity building is not a unidisciplinary concern, however. Various professional groups including GPs, dentists, professions allied to medicine and those working in social care are all conscious of a need to 'catch up' with the research capacity exhibited by certain disciplines within the medical profession (Butterworth 2004). Nurses need to engage with this wider, multidisciplinary agenda, which aims to develop health services research as an applied discipline, able to address the needs of modern health and social care practice (Department of Health 2000).

A national network of Research and Development Support Units (RDSUs) has now been established within England (*www.national-rdsu.org.uk*), and similar developments have occurred in Northern Ireland, Scotland and Wales. RDSUs offer research training, advice and support and mentorship to NHS staff in their geographical area, and in many cases also offer the opportunity to develop links with a multidisciplinary university department for health services research. Some RDSUs also operate primary care and other research networks, and incorporate

Clinical Trials Support Units. By maximising the use of such resources, nurse researchers can minimise the risk of marginalising nursing research from wider academic debates.

Career pathways

Capacity building initiatives alone are not enough. Those who develop their research capability must be afforded the opportunity to do so within the context of a clearly defined career pathway. Traditional stereotypical views of research careers are based on the assumption that research activity is carried out by academics based in universities or by clinical research nurses working in research teams that are usually led by medical doctors. The former are seen to have a recognised academic career pathway within higher education and the latter to have minimal career development opportunity. Kenkre and Foxcroft (2001a; b; c; d; e), however, have mapped out five research career pathways in nursing which include clinical practice, clinical research, academic, management and pharmaceutical (*www.man.ac.uk/rcn/rs/career.htm*). In publishing these pathways, Kenkre and Foxcroft sought to illustrate the potential transferability of skills from one context to another and encourage nurses working in research to move across the different pathways. There are currently however many practical barriers to transferability including terms and conditions of employment (Butterworth 2004).

While Kenkre and Foxcroft seek to ease transferability across academic career pathways there is a more radical move towards the greater integration in research career pathways. Indeed the Scottish Executive has stated that clinical/academic career pathways are

'the key platform for the future development of nursing and midwifery research in Scotland' (Scottish Executive Health Department 2002:23)

There is a strong argument that without the development of flexible and integrated career pathways the NHS will continue to have a sense that it 'loses' those it has nurtured to doctoral level if they transfer, for example, into the higher education sector and vice versa.

While some health care provider organisations and universities have established joint research appointments (Royal College of Nursing Working Party 2004) these posts are relatively new, and have not been formally evaluated. However there is a risk that joint appointments may not always be sustainable because universities and health care organisations serve different purposes and often appear to embark on the creation of joint appointments in research to serve their individual institutional needs. There are few examples where integrated appointments are made to champion agendas which integrate research with practice development or 'modernisation' processes to enable practice-based research and research-based practice to flourish (Royal College of Nursing Working Party 2004).

Increasingly Government funding for R&D is dependent upon demonstrable benefits to the economy and to society, and the university sector is becoming more responsive to these demands. For example, the establishment of a 'third line' funding stream within the higher education sector with parity of esteem for careers in 'knowledge transfer' with the more traditional teaching or research academic careers arguably has the potential to open many doors for nursing. 'Knowledge transfer' can be regarded as a very similar concept to 'practice development' (McCormack and Garbett 2003).

Recent concerns regarding the current state of medical and dentistry academic careers have been addressed under the auspices of the UK Clinical Research Collaboration (UKCRC) 'Walport Report' (Academic Careers Subcommittee of the MMC and UKCRC 2005). This initiative has paved the way for a comprehensive examination of the issues that will need to be addressed and the resources deployed to establish sustainable clinical academic careers in nursing. Until, however, experienced clinical nurses are afforded the opportunity to gain clinically credible research expertise and experience, the divide between clinical and academic careers in nursing will remain. Similarly, academic departments will be unable to recruit experienced nurses into research posts while academic salaries do not equate to those available in senior clinical roles such as nurse consultants. There are grounds for hope, however; recent statements from the national governments in the UK have indicated that a similar process to that established by the 'Walport Report' (Academic Careers Subcommittee of Modernising Medical Careers (MMC) and UKCRC 2005) for doctors and dentists might be funded for nurses. Current examples of nurse innovators managing an integrated clinical academic career portfolio are cited in the RCN Position Statement 'Promoting Excellence in Care through Research and Development' (Royal College of Nursing Working Party 2004). Pioneers such as these are able to demonstrate their capacity to develop clinically-based research projects and programmes of research that are making a difference to patients' experiences and their health outcomes.

Strategic approaches to R&D

A strategic approach to the development of career pathways in research needs to be matched by a more strategic approach to R&D. Traditionally nurses who have undertaken research have done so because they have had a concern that they wanted to address. More often than not they have undertaken their research in full or part fulfilment of a qualification and they have covered the costs of their research from their personal resources (Higher Education Funding Council for England 2001). This model of research activity is no longer sustainable. Coupled with the diminishing funding potential for research in nursing (The Policy Research Department (PRISM) 1998), it is recognised that nursing, alongside other disciplines, is now required to be much more strategic in its research endeavours. Increasingly, nurses who wish to pursue a research career will be required to either carry out research that has already been identified as a priority, or seek out a research team who are already carrying out research within their area of concern.

This will facilitate the growth of a body of knowledge within a specific field and will significantly increase the nurses' potential to secure resources to carry out research.

Increasingly, NHS organisations are developing clear research themes, in order to satisfy the demands of the Department of Health R&D funding levy. These themes need to show evidence of collaboration with university departments and other NHS organisations as appropriate. Nurses working in clinical practice need to be linked to such themes, working with researchers and clinicians from other disciplines where appropriate, in order to gain support for their research activity and find academic collaborators.

Professional influence in strategic R&D decision-making

The large amount of nursing research that has been undertaken as 'own account' (HEFCE 2001) might be a result of the relative paucity of professional influence in strategic R&D decision-making arenas. For example, the UKCRC was established to bring together the major stakeholders that influence clinical research in the UK; there is, however, at the time of writing, no nursing voice on the UKCRC board. Equally, there is no dedicated research council for nursing, despite calls for such a development over many years (Proctor 1997, Rafferty *et al.* 2000, Rafferty *et al.* 2002).

There is a cyclical argument that to become more strategic and focused in their research endeavours nurse researchers need to attract significant funding. This requires nurses to have a strong voice within strategic R&D decision-making arenas and in order to achieve this, nurses must become more strategic and focused in their research endeavours. To address this, the first step for nursing is to examine where it needs to exert greater influence. It was acknowledged in Chapter 1 that a rise in UK R&D investment in basic research was beginning to impact negatively on investment in clinical research, the funding base from which nursing draws its limited resources (The Policy Research Department (PRISM) 1998). The Welcome Trust, which produced this analysis, based on citations of funding sources in research publications, identified three main sectors for UK biomedical (basic and clinical) research, namely UK Government, UK private-non-profit, and industry. Table 33.1, which draws on data from the PRISM report, provides examples within each of these three main sectors and illustrates the trends in biomedical research funding.

The Welcome Trust reports that within the UK Government category, the research councils are the major research funders. The ability of nursing to secure Medical Research Council funding to date has, however, been marginal (RAE 2001). Equally, as illustrated in Table 33.1, while the percentage of investment reported in research outputs from this sector has remained stable, there are significant increases in the percentage of investment reported in both the private-non-profit sector and the global industry sector.

To break out of the vicious circle described above, nursing must undertake an analysis of the effectiveness of its influence within each of these sectors and

Table 33.1 UK R&D funding sectors.

Investment sector	Examples	% UK investment cited in biomedical research outputs	
		1988	1995
UK Government	government health departments higher education funding councils research councils	33.9	33.8
Private-non-profit	charities foundations hospital trustees	24.4	31.8
Industry	pharmaceutical biotechnology World Bank	13.9	17.4

develop tailored strategic lobbying strategies based on these results. The shape of these strategies will depend to a large extent on the direction the profession elects to take in this regard. Capacity building resources are increasingly being offered on an interdisciplinary competitive basis. Without a collective concerted effort to change the culture in nursing, where there is a reported shortfall in the number of applications for R&D resources in a multidisciplinary competitive context (Mead *et al.* 1997) there is a danger that this may lead to a fall in the number of applicants.

There are essentially two schools of thought regarding how nursing might secure a greater slice of the R&D resource cake. The first is that nursing should swim with the tide, embrace the brave new world, and ensure that nursing has a strong voice within this multidisciplinary research arena. The potential benefits of pursuing such a position is that when successful, nursing may be recognised as an equal player alongside other professional and academic groups. The danger is that nurses themselves might lose sight of their distinctly nursing values and purpose (Royal College of Nursing 2003). In the worst case scenario, there may be a nurse at the top table but with no way of identifying who she is, as she has become indistinguishable from her medical colleagues.

The counter argument is that the only way that nursing's distinctive contribution to the R&D table can be fully appreciated is through the establishment of a Nursing Research Council with the resources to commission nursing research to inform nursing policy and practice. The benefits of this scenario would lie in the ring fencing of funding for nursing research and in the capacity to strengthen the distinct voice of nursing research. The danger would lie in the potential to further marginalise the voice of nursing from the interdisciplinary research arena.

If nursing elects to swim with the tide it will need to put balances and checks in place to ensure that when at the top table it does offer a truly distinct perspective. If the profession chooses to swim against the tide, evidence suggests that these balances and checks will need to be in place regardless. Commentators on the equivalent of a UK nursing research council in the United States have suggested that nurses in the US may have lost sight of their distinctiveness (Rafferty & Traynor 1997).

Effective partnerships

There is growing evidence that the voice of nursing research is slowly but surely exerting more of an influence among policy makers. One of the most effective ways of doing this is through collaboration. To this end the UK nursing professional organisations (e.g. Royal College of Nursing, Royal College of Midwives and Community Practitioners and Health Visitors Association) have joined forces to create a strategic research alliance (CHIVE, RCN, RCM Research Collaborative). Collectively they identify and address shared concerns, and develop a lobbying strategy to exert more influence.

Effective partnerships such as this are recognised as key to success on a number of levels. Resources to develop nursing research capacity have been secured through a mixed portfolio of funding, from the Higher Education Funding Councils, the UK health departments, and the private-non-profit sector, with the Health Foundation providing the major share. These resources have not only been secured through partnerships, they have also been allocated through partnerships. The individual nurse who applies for a national or local research fellowship must do so in partnership with a recognised Higher Education Institution.

A partnership between academia, and nurses in clinical practice is also required if nursing research is to prosper. A study published in 1991 illustrated how an academic (Tierney) worked with a clinician (Taylor) and her colleagues on a ward that cared for women receiving chemotherapy for breast cancer. Through working in partnership a decision was reached to focus on conducting a literature review to examine the management of alopecia, a distressing side effect of chemotherapy (Tierney and Taylor 1991). This clinically relevant research activity both informed nursing practice (Tierney 1987; 1990) and future research thus leading to further academic publications (Tierney 1991; 1992).

There are many other examples of academic/clinician partnership working, with their endeavours frequently presented jointly at conferences. While such partnerships clearly have the capacity to lead to better-informed patient care, the time and energy required to develop and sustain effective partnerships for research should not be underestimated.

Another model that endeavours to ensure that nursing research is relevant and has the potential to inform nursing practice is through the establishment of nursing research leadership positions within health care settings. There are a number of nurse consultant posts in R&D and clinically-based professorial positions throughout the UK. Such postholders often hold a formal joint appointment between an academic institution and a health care organisation or they are employed by one organisation and have an honorary contract with the other. It is recommended that these leadership positions are underpinned by a robust clinical academic career structure (Royal College of Nursing Working Party 2004) and the firm commitment and support of nurses in executive positions and academic deans is a prerequisite. Such posts also require a jointly developed role profile coupled with a realistic measure of performance and copious amounts of support and encouragement!

There are at least three facets to R&D leadership roles in health care organisations. First they seek to establish nursing research projects and programmes of research in their respective organisations. Second, they aim to influence the wider R&D agenda to both secure more resources for nursing research and ensure that a nursing perspective is incorporated into collaborative research activities when they are led by other disciplines. And thirdly such posts often have a strong focus on the development of nursing practice where the aim is to enable research to inform practice and practice to inform research.

The future of nursing as a clinical academic discipline – a higher education perspective

Since the first nursing degrees in the late 1960s, nursing has had a place in the UK universities as an academic discipline. The debate continues, however, at an international level, about whether nursing should be a graduate profession (Greenwood 2000), with much nurse education worldwide still taking place outside universities. In the UK the move of all nurse education into the university sector during the 1990s did not result in an immediate acceptance of nursing as a research-based academic discipline. Nursing's relatively poor performance in the Research Assessment Exercise (RAE, *see* Chapter 30 for a fuller discussion) since then has not helped this cause (Tierney 1994, Traynor and Rafferty 1999, Watson and Robinson 2001). Many nursing departments are located in the 'new' universities where research activity has not traditionally been strong, and where funding for research activity in teaching departments is poor.

Academic nursing departments, apart from a handful of dedicated nursing research units, carry a burden of teaching that surpasses that in most other disciplines, and their dependence upon funding from NHS contracts for professional training ensures that this will remain a high priority. Given this commitment, it is understandable that research activities are not prioritised except by a small minority of academic staff, despite a reported desire of nursing academics to be recognised as research active (Deans *et al.* 2003). There are two possible solutions to this problem.

One is for nursing departments to draw in more external research funding from charities, research councils, government departments and even private industry. This funding could then be used to free up nursing academic staff to become involved in research without incurring conflicting priorities with teaching commitments. This presupposes, however, that casual staff can be found to backfill and cover teaching sessions while academics are engaged on research projects. This may not be easy to achieve. Nevertheless nursing departments could then make progress from their existing low base of external research funding, increasing nursing research capacity, contributing to a national and local research agenda, and also improving the department's rating in the RAE. This route is a viable one if nurse academics can be successful in winning competitive research funding grants while engaged in traditional teaching commitments.

The second solution is more radical, probably less desirable, but may be more realistic. Two streams of academic nursing departments could be established, some universities focusing on excellence in teaching and promoting evidence-based practice. These departments would not enter the RAE or encourage their staff to engage in empirical research, but would receive the bulk of funding for pre-registration nurse training. Other departments would take the research active route, teaching only at postgraduate level and relying for a major part of their income on external research funding. Academics working in these departments would be expected to achieve research outputs of publications, research grants and scholarly activities, rather than carrying a heavy teaching load. There are signs at the time of writing that it is already beginning to happen, and only time will tell whether it will be fruitful in terms of improving the quality of nursing research.

Many would not agree that this is the way academic nursing should go. However such critics need to face the relatively poor performance of nursing departments in research activity over the last decade, and consider whether heavy teaching commitments can be successfully combined with proactive research activity. It is possible that the two streams of nursing academic departments outlined above could be combined within a single department, enabling cross-fertilisation between teaching and research – this would perhaps be the optimal situation.

Finally, nursing as an academic discipline needs to address the issue of research careers as outlined earlier in the chapter. Compared with other academic disciplines, nursing lacks the tradition of keeping its brightest undergraduate students within academia to undertake higher degrees and engage in research from an early stage in their careers. The case against this has always been that nursing is a practical discipline and new graduates need to gain clinical experience. While this is true, ways can surely be envisaged of allowing young PhD students to engage in clinical practice on a part-time basis, or during vacation periods, while maintaining the momentum of their academic careers. The contribution and added value of a PhD training to clinical practice must be made explicit, and doctorally-prepared nurses must become requisite members of the NHS workforce if the anti-academic culture, still evident in some health care settings, is to be overcome. The current route into academia for clinical nurses is too long and too uncertain to sustain a dynamic body of new researchers within the discipline. It is also not cost effective to wait until a clinical nurse is in a senior position before negotiating her transfer back into academia.

Three scenarios for the future of nursing research

We end this chapter, and the book, with a deliberately provocative look at three scenarios for the future development of nursing research. The scenarios are caricatures, designed to throw into sharp perspective the possibilities, challenges and pitfalls that could lie ahead for nursing research. We leave the reader to decide which of the scenarios they wish to see, or whether they can create a better alternative scenario, and how the preferred scenario may be brought into reality.

The status quo

Nurses remain small players in the research field. They have developed a certain expertise in many different approaches to research, and the profession has a small elite with higher degrees who meet together regularly and collaborate on nursing research. They have developed some international links with nurses in North America, Australasia and Europe. However, nursing departments in universities perform poorly in research compared with other disciplines, and research taking place within them is largely funded through educational sources and small grants. Some research takes place in clinical practice, but the majority is self-funded and conducted by lone enthusiasts. Medical research largely ignores nursing research and nurses make little contribution to the wider health services research agenda.

The purist approach

Nursing research has decided to go it alone. A Nursing Research Council (NRC) has been successfully established, and more funding is flowing from national sources into nursing academic departments. The NRC works with only a fraction of the funds that its big brother the MRC enjoys, but successful lobbying by the profession has begun to improve this situation. University nursing departments have pared themselves down so that most nurse educators are not research active, but specialise in teaching and promoting evidence-based practice. Research-active nursing departments, however, enjoy considerable success internationally and in university research ratings, and are acknowledged by colleagues in other disciplines as producing rigorous and erudite research outputs. There is also increasing evidence of more effective nursing research leadership within health care organisations and a fully-funded clinical academic career structure has been established.

Nursing research journals have proliferated to accommodate the volume of material being submitted. However, the highest-rated research that takes place in academic nursing departments is rarely read by clinical nurses, as the language is impenetrable and the subject matter seems to have little relevance to the everyday pressures of caring for patients. The direct influence of this nursing research on practice is limited, but there are some centres of excellence in the UK that are spearheading the development of clinically relevant research at a local level. This is influencing nursing as a whole, and other health professions see nursing as a good example of a profession that has developed skills in knowledge transfer.

The brave new world

Nursing research has grasped the nettle of engagement in mainstream health services research. Nurses are involved at every level of national R&D strategy, and are doing battle to ensure that topics of relevance to clinical nurses are high on the agenda for funding bodies. High quality, multidisciplinary research that addresses real problems in health care is increasingly led by nurses working self-confidently with teams that include statisticians, health economists, social scientists, medical and allied health professionals. A career structure has been established whereby nurses can engage in research immediately after training or at any stage thereafter without losing parity of pay or clinical credibility. Nurse consultants aim to combine participation in externally funded research with clinical and policy roles, though it is acknowledged that this sometimes results in severe job strain. Implementation of evidence-based practice is moving on apace, however, as clinical nurses see research findings which are relevant and accessible.

Academic nursing departments have developed research-based teaching methods that allow full-time researchers to contribute to teaching alongside specialists in educational delivery. Successful university departments have had to become strongly linked to local NHS organisations in primary and secondary care, ensuring they are firmly grounded in the needs of everyday clinical practice, and enabling research collaborations to be developed. This has resulted, however, in the closure of some nursing academic departments that were unable to develop this 'real-world research' perspective and have consequently lost their funding. Similarly, nurses who wish to engage in curiosity-led, unfounded research are having difficulty in finding any support for their work and some argue this has led to the stifling of innovation in health care.

None of the three scenarios above is perfect, and all three are drawn as caricatures. It is our hope that the reader will allow them to stimulate thought and debate, so that nurse researchers of the future can self-confidently move forward to promote their preferred model in dialogue with policy makers, colleagues in other disciplines, and international research partners.

References

Academic Careers Sub-Committee of the MMC & UKCRC (2005) *Medically and dentally qualified academic staff: recommendations for training the researchers and educators of the future.* UK Clinical Research Collaboration and Modernising Medical Careers London (Walport Report)

Butterworth T (2004) *Developing and sustaining a world-class workforce of educators and researchers in health and social care*, StLaR HR Plan Project Phase II Strategic Report, London

Deans C, Congdon G, Sellers ET (2003) Nurse education in English universities in a period of change: expectations of nurse academics for the year 2008. *Nurse Education Today* 23 146–154

Department of Health (2000) *Towards a Strategy for Nursing Research And Development: proposal for action*. London, Department of Health

Greenwood J (2000) Critique of the graduate nurse: an international perspective. *Nurse Education Today* 20, 17–23

Higher Education Funding Council for England (2001) Promoting research in nursing and the allied health professions. *www.hefce.ac.uk/Pubs/hefce/2001/01_64.htm* Research report 01/64. Higher Education Funding Council for England

Kenkre J, Foxcroft DR (2001a) Career pathways in research: clinical practice. *Nursing Standard* 16:4 40–43

Kenkre J, Foxcroft DR (2001b) Career pathways in research: clinical research. *Nursing Standard* 16:5 41–44

Kenkre J, Foxcroft DR (2001c) Career pathways in research: academic. *Nursing Standard*, 16:7 40–44

Kenkre J, Foxcroft DR (2001d) Career pathways in research: support and management. *Nursing Standard* 16:6 33–35

Kenkre J, Foxcroft DR (2001e) Career pathways in research: pharmaceutical. *Nursing Standard*, 16:8 36–39

Mead D, Moseley L, Cook R (1997) The performance of nursing in the research stakes: Lessons from the field. *NT Research* 2: 5 335–344

McCormack B, Garbett, R (2003) The characteristics, qualities and skills of practice developers. *Journal of Clinical Nursing* 12: 315–323

Policy Research in Science and Medicine (PRISM) (1998) *Mapping the Landscape: national biomedical research outputs 1988–1995*. London, The Wellcome Trust

Proctor S (1997) Developing research capacity in nursing. *Journal of Nursing Management* 5: 321–323

Rafferty AM, Traynor M (1997) On the state of play in nursing research. *Journal of Interprofessional Care* 11: 43–48

Rafferty AM, Bond S, Traynor M (2000) Does nursing, midwifery and health visiting need a research council? *Nursing Times Research* 5: 325–335

Rafferty AM, Newell R, Traynor M (2002) Nursing and midwifery research in England: working towards establishing a dedicated fund. *Nursing Times Research* 7: 243–254

Royal College of Nursing (2003) *Defining Nursing*. London, Royal College of Nursing

Royal College of Nursing Working Party (2004) Promoting Excellence in Care Through Research and Development. a RCN position statement. London, Royal College of Nursing

Scottish Executive Health Department (2002) *Choices and Challenges: the strategy for research and development in nursing and midwifery in Scotland*. Edinburgh, SEHD

Tierney AJ (1987) Preventing chemotherapy-induced alopecia in cancer patients: is scalp cooling worthwhile? *Journal of Advanced Nursing* 12: 303–310

Tierney AJ (1990) Chemotherapy support. *Nursing Times* 86: 54–55

Tierney AJ (1991) Side effects expected and experienced by women receiving chemotherapy for breast cancer. *British Medical Journal* 302: 272

Tierney AJ (1992) Knowledge, expectations and experiences of patients receiving chemotherapy for breast cancer. *Scandinavian Journal of Caring Sciences* 6: 75–80

Tierney AJ (1994) An analysis of nursing's performance in the 1992 assessment of research in British universities. *Journal of Advanced Nursing* 19: 593–602

Tierney AJ, Taylor J (1991) Research in practice: an 'experiment' in researcher-practitioner collaboration. *Journal of Advanced Nursing* 16: 506–510

Traynor M, Rafferty AM (1999) Nursing and the research assessment exercise. *Journal of Advanced Nursing* 30: 186–192

Trostle J (1992) Research capacity building and international health: Definitions, evaluations and strategies for success. *Social Science and Medicine* 35: 1321–1324

Watson R, Robinson J (2001) The United Kingdom research assessment exercise 2001. *Journal of Advanced Nursing* 35: 635–637

Websites

www.nccrcd.nhs.uk – the National Co-ordinating Centre for Research Capacity Building website lists all the nationally-funded and sponsored initiatives to develop research capacity in health and social care. RDSUs are listed under 'infrastructure'

www.man.ac.uk/rcn/ – RCN Research and Development Co-ordinating Centre website contains a comprehensive listing of R&D structures and support agencies in the four countries of the UK. Readers can also sign up to a regular e-mail circulation that provides weekly updates of research policy, funding, training, conferences and jobs

www.scotland.gov.uk/Resource/Doc/46932/0013926.pdf – *Choices and Challenges*, the strategy for research and development in nursing and midwifery in Scotland published in 2001

www.nes.scot.nhs.uk/nmapresearch/documents/booklet.pdf – *Making Choices, Facing Challenges* booklet published in 2005 complements Choices and Challenges and aims to enable nurses, midwives and allied health professionals in Scotland to develop their research careers

www.national-rdsu.org.uk/ – network of research and development support units (RDSUs) in England

Glossary

Abstract A concise summary of a research study, journal article or conference presentation, often limited to 200 words. It is usually found at the beginning of a research article or report, and may be used alone in indexes and conference proceedings.

Action research Research that is characterised by the active participation of the researcher in the study. It may be carried out as part of a change process. It has a strong emphasis on context, and the participation of non-researchers. Research methods are often **qualitative**, but can also include **quantitative** data.

Audit A rigorous procedure for measuring and improving the quality of care or clinical outcomes against an agreed standard at local or national level.

Bias The systematic influence of factors other than those being investigated. Bias should be eliminated or minimised, as it reduces the **validity** of the study.

Blinding The process, used in **experimental design**, whereby participants are unaware whether they are allocated to the experimental or control group. It may necessitate the use of a **placebo**. Data collectors and professional staff may also be blinded to the experimental group – this is known as **double blinding**, and is used to reduce bias.

Case study The use of a single person, event or context in a research study in order to study a phenomenon in depth. Case study research may use multiple 'cases' to explore a subject area.

Cohort study A form of research within the epidemiological tradition, where a group of research participants is recruited and followed up over time. Common examples are birth cohorts (all children born in a particular time period) and disease cohorts (all patients diagnosed in a particular year).

Conceptual framework An abstract set of concepts and theories that are related to one another and may be used to organise ideas and guide analysis within a study. A conceptual framework may be derived from a particular philosophical position.

Confidence interval A range within which the true value of a parameter (e.g. mean or proportion) is estimated to lie.

Control group A group of research participants recruited to be compared with an experimental or intervention group. The control group are not given the experimental treatment or condition, but may be given a placebo treatment or condition.

Correlation The extent to which variation in one variable is related to variation in another.

Covert observation A form of participant observation in which those being observed are not aware of the researcher's activity or intentions. Often involves some degree of deception and may therefore be considered unethical.

Cross tabulation A comparison, expressed in a table, of two or more categorical variables to show how they are related to one another e.g. age group, gender and smoking

Data cleaning A process of examining data, once collected, to remove error and omissions. Usually applied to quantitative data once it has been entered into computer software for analysis.

Deduction The process of testing theories by the collection of data and analysis. Underlies much **quantitative research**, especially **experimental design**, and is opposed to **induction**.

Delphi technique A research method where a panel of experts are asked to rank statements or concepts in order of priority in a series of rounds to reach a consensus.

Dependent variable The variable which forms the outcome of a study. Experimental studies are designed to explain changes in the dependent variable, possibly caused by an **independent variable**. In studies of nurse related cross infection, wound sepsis might be the dependent variable, where handwashing technique is the independent variable.

Dissemination The process of informing others about the results of a particular research study. This may be by verbal, written, audiovisual or electronic means.

Emic The view from within a culture or research setting, recognised only by those who participate in that culture – opposed to **etic**.

Empirical That which can be observed, experienced and measured through the human senses, as opposed to theoretical, which is concerned with thought processes.

Epidemiology The science of measuring the prevalence and incidence of disease and other phenomena in large populations.

Epistemology The philosophical theory of knowledge. Research approaches are based upon differing bodies of knowledge, known as their underlying epistemology.

Ethnography An approach to qualitative research which focuses on culture and sub-cultures within a society. Ethnographers study behaviour, interaction, customs, rituals, values and institutions and attempt to interpret them in a narrative account.

Etic The view from outside a research setting or culture, whereby a researcher seeks to interpret the culture to a wider audience – opposed to **emic**

Evaluation An attempt to assess the worth or value of something.

Evaluation research A type of research which has the purpose of assessing the worth or value of something (e.g. of practice, intervention, innovation, or service).

Evidence based practice Integrating the best available research evidence with professional expertise, taking into account patient or user preferences.

Experimental design A research design characterised by testing a **hypothesis** under controlled conditions. The method is **quantitative**, and favoured in pure scientific and medical research.

Experimental group A group of research participants who are exposed to an experimental treatment or condition. Often called an **intervention** group. May be compared to a **control** group.

External validity The extent to which a research study can be **generalised** to other populations and contexts. Often called **generalisability**.

Fieldwork Data collection that takes place in the everyday context of the research participants. Commonly used in **qualitative** research using interviews and **participant observation**.

Focus group A group of individuals assembled to take part in a group interview, with the purpose of collecting data and observing the effect of group interaction. Often used in **qualitative** and market research.

Gatekeeper A term used for a person occupying a role that enables the researcher access to a setting or to research participants. May be a head teacher for access to schoolchildren, or a practice manager for access to primary healthcare facilities.

Generalisability The extent to which the findings from a research study can be applied to other populations and contexts.

Grounded theory A specific **inductive** methodology in **qualitative** research. Data collection and analysis take place simultaneously, with the ultimate goal of development of new theory.

Hawthorne effect A phenomenon observed in research, whereby the research participants change their behaviour purely as a result of taking part in an experiment. This effect is a threat to the **validity** of the study.

Health services research A broad term used to describe research into health care systems, evaluation of health care, and clinical effectiveness of interventions. Health services research uses a wide range of methodologies and is multidisciplinary in nature, but excludes laboratory and biomedical research.

Hypothesis A statement about the relationship between two or more variables, which can be tested **empirically**.

Independent variable The variable that is thought to cause, or explain in some way, another variable, called the **dependent** variable. In studies of nurse-related cross infection, wound sepsis might be the dependent variable, where handwashing is the independent variable.

In-depth interview An interview technique used in **qualitative** research in which the interviewer imposes minimal structure on the conversation in order to explore the perceptions or experience of the participant. Commonly used in **phenomenology** and **grounded theory** where little is known about the subject of interest.

Induction The process of drawing conclusions and building theory from data that has been collected and analysed. Often used in **qualitative research** and opposed to **deduction**.

Inferential statistics Statistical techniques whereby hypotheses are tested and inference made from a sample to a wider population.

Informed consent The process of ensuring that research participants are fully aware of what the study involves, and freely agree to take part. This usually requires a formal signature after verbal and written information has been given.

Internal validity The extent to which effects observed in a research study are truly caused by the variables under study, and not due to any **bias**, **unreliability**, or other sources of error.

Interpretivism The belief that human beings continuously interpret and make sense of their environment, and so research into their behaviour and social processes must take the meaning of events into account. This approach underlies **qualitative** research methods, and may be opposed to **positivism**.

Intervention group See **experimental group**.

Likert scale A scale, usually used in **questionnaires**, where the respondent is asked to agree or disagree with a series of statements in order to measure an attitude or other variable.

Mean The statistical measure obtained by adding all scores for a variable together and dividing the sum by the number of items. Often known as a mathematical average.

Median The statistical measure that is the middle value when a range of scores is arranged in ascending or descending order.

Meta-analysis The statistical re-analysis of data from a number of studies, to reach an interpretation of their combined data. Often found in **systematic reviews**. May also be attempted in a non-statistical form for **qualitative** studies.

Mode The numerical value from a **frequency distribution** that occurs most often. This may have no relation to the middle value.

Objectivity Observation or measurement that relies upon physical reality not amenable to individual interpretation. Examples would include temperature measurement, wound size. Can be argued that even such observations may be open to **subjectivity**.

Overt observation A form of observation where the researcher's intentions and actions are fully open to those being observed.

Paradigm A way of viewing reality, informed by a particular theoretical perspective, belief, or set of assumptions.

Participant observation Used in **qualitative research**, the researcher takes part in the research context and may assume a role e.g. researcher becomes a nursing assistant in an A&E department in order to observe the interaction of patients and staff. May be **overt** (open) or **covert** (hidden).

Peer review A system of assessing the quality of research proposals, conference presentations and journal articles, where respected researchers and other peers of the author are asked to comment critically upon the work. Used in the university **Research Assessment Exercise**.

Phenomenon An occurrence, circumstance, experience or fact that is perceptible to the senses.

Phenomenology An inductive approach to **qualitative** research that focuses on understanding the human experience from 'the inside'. Phenomenologists interpret the meaning of the 'lived experience' of study participants through their description.

Pilot study A preliminary study carried out before the full research, to test out data collection instruments and other procedures.

Placebo A non-active substance or form of intervention used for the control group in experimental designs to avoid bias. Trial participants may be **blinded** to whether they are taking the active treatment or the placebo.

Population All possible participants or items that could be included in a sample. Might be all qualified nurses in an NHS trust, or all patient records in a primary care practice. A **sample** is usually then selected from the population for study.

Positivism A theoretical position derived from eighteenth century philosophy, believing that scientific truth can only be derived from that which is observable by the human senses. Positivists would apply the methods of traditional scientific enquiry to the study of human behaviour. **Quantitative** research methods rely on this tradition, rather than **interpretivism**.

Power calculation A statistical calculation that is carried out to determine sample size in a quantitative study, to ensure enough participants or items are included to increase the probability of observing any real effects and reduce the probability of errors.

Qualitative research The broad term used to denote research designs and methods that yield non-numerical data, and are based upon an **interpretative** philosophy. Analysis is usually based on narrative and thematic methods.

Quantitative research The broad term used to denote research designs and methods that yield numerical data, and are based upon a **positivist** philosophy. Analysis is usually based on statistical methods.

Quasi-experimental design A form of experiment where it is not possible or ethical to randomise participants to comparison groups.

Questionnaire A data collection tool, paper or web based, where respondents are asked to complete a series of structured questions or items. Answers are often in 'tick box' format.

Randomised controlled trial (RCT) An experimental design where participants are randomly allocated to comparison groups, sometimes using a **placebo**. Often referred to as the 'gold standard' for evaluating treatment and to form the basis for evidence based practice. Most clinical trials of treatments use this design.

Random sampling A form of sampling where units are chosen from a population in a systematic but random way, to ensure each unit has an equal (and non-zero) chance of being selected.

Reflexivity The process, used in **qualitative research**, whereby the researcher reflects continuously on how their own actions, values and perceptions impact upon the research setting and affect the data collection and analysis.

Regression Prediction of one continuous variable from another, using a particular statistical technique

Reliability A measure of the consistency and accuracy of data collection. A data collection instrument may be said to be unreliable if it generates different readings on repeated measurements at the same time of the same person. Low reliability can cause a research study to lack **validity**, but high **reliability** does not necessarily ensure **validity**.

Representative sample A sample that contains a similar proportion of important variables (e.g. age, gender, medical condition) as the population from which it is drawn.

Research assessment exercise (RAE) The system used by the funding council for higher education (HEFCE) in the UK to assess the quality of research undertaken in universities. The assessment is related to subject discipline and strength of research output, as measured by publications, external funding grants won, and peer esteem.

Research governance A system of regulation of research activity in health and social care organisations introduced in England and Wales in 2001.

Rigour The strength of a research design in terms of adherence to procedures, accuracy, and consistency.

Sample A sub-set of a **population** drawn for the purpose of research. A sample may be made up of individuals, clinical material such as blood samples, organisations, or events.

Sampling The process of selecting a sample. The sampling technique used will affect **validity** of the research.

Sampling frame The list of units, individuals, or organisations in a population, from which a sample is drawn. Common sampling frames are (for individuals) electoral rolls, GP registration lists, school registers and (for organisations) yearbooks of NHS organisations, mailing lists of schools of nursing in UK.

Secondary analysis Re-analysis of data collected for another purpose, or for a previous research study.

Semi-structured interview An interview technique whereby the interviewer uses pre-determined topics and questions, but retains the flexibility to follow up ideas raised by the participant. Commonly used in **qualitative** research where there is a policy agenda, as in **health services research**.

Stakeholder Someone in an organisation or other focus of a study who has an interest (stake) in the evaluation, or other research, and its outcomes. Includes participants, clients, workers and management.

Standard deviation A statistical measure of the spread of data in a sample. It measures dispersion from the **mean**.

Stratification The process of dividing a population into known strata by important variables (e.g. gender) before taking a **sample**.

Structured abstract A form of **abstract** where the information is given under prescribed headings (e.g. aim, method, results, conclusion). Some academic journals and conferences insist on presentation in this style.

Structured interview A form of interview where questions are pre-set both in topic and sequence. Commonly used in **quantitative** research.

Structured observation A form of observation used in **quantitative** research where events or actions being observed are recorded in pre-determined categories, often using checklists or handheld computers as data collection tools.

Subjectivity Observation or measurement that is seen to be influenced by the perception of the individual. Examples would include the experience of pain or gender discrimination. Opposed to **objectivity**.

Survey A research design that collects information from a **sample** or **population**, to obtain descriptive and **correlational** data. A whole **population** survey is called a census.

Systematic review A rigorous and systematic literature search, using a well-defined question, and strict criteria for study inclusion and evaluation. It may also involve amalgamating statistical data from different studies in **meta-analysis**.

Thick description Detailed account of cultural behaviours and practices, described in context. Used in **ethnography**.

Triangulation The use of two or more data sources, theoretical perspectives or methods in a research study to compare findings and hence achieve greater **validity**.

Validity The extent to which data, and its interpretation, reflects the phenomenon under investigation without **bias**. Studies and instruments used to collect data are unlikely to be **valid** unless they are also **reliable**. Some qualitative researchers prefer to use terms such as credibility and trustworthiness to describe this concept.

Vignettes Brief scenarios that can be given verbally or in writing to research participants to stimulate a response.

Index